Pelican Books
Awakenings

Dr Oliver W. Sacks was born in London,
and educated at St Paul's School, Queen's
College, Oxford, and the Middlesex
Hospital, prior to further work and
training in the United States.
Following a period of research in
neurophysiology and neurochemistry,
he returned to clinical work,
interesting himself especially in
migraine, tics, behavioural development
and disorder in children, and the care of
post-encephalitic patients. Professor
A. R. Luria has said of his book
Awakenings, 'The ability to *describe*
which was so common to the great
neurologists and psychiatrists of the
nineteenth century . . . is almost lost
now. This excellent book shows that
the important tradition of clinical
case-studies can be revived, and with
great success . . . It is truly a great
book.' Dr Sacks is Instructor in
Neurology at the Albert Einstein
College of Medicine and Consultant
Neurologist to several New York
hospitals.

OLIVER SACKS

AWAKENINGS

. . . and now, a preternatural
birth in returning to life
from this sickness

DONNE

PENGUIN BOOKS

Penguin Books Ltd,
Harmondsworth, Middlesex, England
Penguin Books Australia Ltd,
Ringwood, Victoria, Australia
Penguin Books (N.Z.) Ltd,
182–190 Wairau Road, Auckland 10, New Zealand

First published by Gerald Duckworth & Co. 1973
Revised edition published in Pelican Books 1976

Made and printed in Great Britain by
C. Nicholls & Company Ltd
Set in Linotype Juliana

To the memory of
Wystan Hugh Auden

'Healing',

Papa would tell me,
'is not a science,
but the intuitive art
of wooing Nature.'

W.H.A. (from *The Art of Healing*)

Thanks are due to the following for permission to reproduce material included in the inset: plates on pages 1, 2 *top*, and 3, to the *Daily Mail*; 4, 6 *top*, 6 *bottom*, 7 *bottom*, and 8 *top left*, to Yorkshire Television. Plates on pages 5, 7 *top*, 7 *middle*, 8 *top right*, 8 *bottom left*, and 8 *bottom right*, were contributed by the author.

CONTENTS

ACKNOWLEDGEMENTS

My first debt is to the staff, and – above all – the patients at Mount Carmel Hospital, without whom this book could never have been written.

I am deeply grateful to Miss Marjorie Kohl, M.A., who has been my constant helpmate in the care of our patients; to friends and relatives, for their encouragement and insights; and to my publisher, Mr Colin Haycraft, who by his delicate and profound *maieuticê technê* has finally delivered me of this overdue work. I must express special thanks to the *Listener*, who have allowed me to quote freely from a recent article of mine ('The Great Awakening', 26 October 1972), and the ensuing correspondence which appeared in their columns. I am grateful to the following for quotations from copyright material: from Ernest Jones, *The Life and Work of Sigmund Freud*, to Mrs Katherine Jones, The Hogarth Press Ltd and Basic Books Inc.; from *The Complete Poems* of D. H. *Lawrence*, to Laurence Pollinger Ltd and the Estate of the late Mrs Frieda Lawrence, William Heinemann Ltd and The Viking Press Inc.; from Ludwig Wittgenstein, *Philosophical Investigations*, to the literary executors of Ludwig Wittgenstein, Basil Blackwell & Mott Ltd and The Macmillan Company, New York; from John Maynard Keynes, *Collected Writings*, to the Royal Economic Society, Macmillan, London and Basingstoke, Ltd and St Martin's Press Inc.; from T. S. Elliot, *Collected Poems 1909–1962*, to Faber & Faber Ltd and Harcourt Brace Jovanovich Inc.

February 1973

O. W. S.

A. R. Luria, almost alone among contemporary physicians, has preserved or revived the almost-forgotten art of clinical biography. His great case-histories combine an extraordinary accuracy and wealth of detail with the ease and sensibility and style of a novel. They have been instrumental, despite the differences in theme and approach, in moving me towards the feeling and format of *Awakenings* – and it was my consciousness of this which led me to bring out an essay on Luria ('The Mind of A. R. Luria', *Listener*, 28 June) on the same day as *Awakenings* was published. Professor Luria at once wrote me two letters, one defining his own position, the other generously praising *Awakenings*. I have found my reading of Luria, over many years, and my correspondence with him, during the past few weeks, a source of especial inspiration and pleasure.

September 1973

O. W. S.

By a painful irony, it may require an act of separation, and even the abruption of death, to show one what has been most important in one's life. The sudden and tragic death of W. H. Auden has given me an intense sense of my debt to him, and the extent of his influence on my life and thought. He was the first man to see the manuscript of my book *Migraine*; he discussed it at length with me, encouraged me to complete it, and reviewed it with great generosity on its final publication. Similarly he was the only man – apart from my publisher – to see the first proofs of *Awakenings*; he was intrigued by its themes; he helped me to harmonize its peculiar problems of content and form; he spoke very warmly of it, in his last letters to me and other friends; and he had intended to review it on its publication in America. Auden's interest in medicine was deep and lifelong; it was his patrimony – for he was the son of a distinguished medical practitioner; abhorring specialists and 'medical engineers', he felt an instinctive affinity and affection for certain medical friends who, like himself, preserved the spaciousness and sympathies of a former age (no fewer than four poems, in his last book, are dedicated to such friends); he himself had an extraordinary clinical flair and 'feeling', and had he not been a very great poet, I think he would have been a very great physician. I always found Auden the kindest of friends and the wisest of mentors, a man who conveyed a profound scepticism but a still profounder faith. Auden, above all contemporaries, was an 'awakener' to me; and so in gratitude and love I dedicate *Awakenings* to his memory.

October 1973

O. W. S.

PREFACE

The theme of this book is the lives and reactions of certain patients in a unique situation – and the implications which these hold out for medicine and science. These patients are among the few survivors of the great sleeping-sickness epidemic (*encephalitis lethargica*) of fifty years ago, and their reactions are those brought about by a remarkable new 'awakening' drug (laevodihydroxyphenylalanine, or L-DOPA). The lives and responses of these patients, which have no real precedent in the entire history of medicine, are presented in the form of extended case-histories or biographies: these form the major part of the book. Preceding these case-histories are introductory remarks on the nature of their illnesses, the sort of lives they have led since first being taken ill, and something about the drug which has transformed their lives. Such a subject might seem to be of very special or limited interest, but this, I believe, is by no means the case. In the latter part of the book, I have tried to indicate some of the far-reaching implications which arise from the subject – implications which extend to the most general questions of health, disease, suffering, care, and the human condition in general.

In a book such as this – about living people – a difficult, perhaps insuperable, problem arises: that of conveying detailed information without betraying professional and personal confidence. I have had to change the names of my patients, the name and location of the hospital where they live, and certain other circumstantial details. I have, however, tried to preserve what is important and essential – the real and full *presence* of the patients themselves, the 'feeling' of their lives, their characters, their illnesses, their responses – the essential qualities of their strange situation.

The general style of this book – with its alternation of narrative and reflection, its proliferation of images and metaphors, its remarks, repetitions, asides and footnotes – is one which I have been impelled towards by the very nature of the subject-matter. My aim is not to make a system, or to see patients as systems, but to picture a world, a variety of worlds – the landscapes of being in which these patients reside. And the picturing of worlds requires not a static and systematic formulation, but an active exploration of images and views, a continual jumping-about and imaginative *movement*. The stylistic (and epistemological) problems encountered have been precisely those described by Wittgenstein in the Preface to *Philosophical Investigations* when he spoke of the necessity of depicting landscapes (thoughtscapes) by images and 'remarks':

> ... This was, of course, connected with the very nature of the investigation. For this compels us to travel over a wide field of thought criss-cross in every direction. The ... remarks in this book are, as it were, a number of sketches of landscapes which were made in the course of these long and involved journeyings. The same or almost the same points were always being approached from different directions, and new sketches made ... Thus this book is really only an album.

Running throughout the book is a metaphysical theme – the notion that it is insufficient to consider disease in purely mechanical or chemical terms; that it must be considered equally in biological or metaphysical terms, i.e. in terms of organization and design. In my first book (*Migraine : Evolution of a Common Disorder*, 1970) I suggested the necessity of such a *double* approach, and in the present work I develop this theme in much greater detail. Such a notion is far from new – it was understood very clearly in classical medicine. In present-day medicine, by contrast, there is an almost exclusively technical or mechanical emphasis, which has led to immense advances, but also to intellectual regression, and a lack of proper attention to the full needs and feelings of patients. This book represents an attempt to regain and restore this metaphysical attention.

I have found the writing unexpectedly difficult, although its ideas and intentions are simple and straightforward. But one cannot go straight forward unless the way is clear, and the way is *allowed*. One struggles to gain the right perspective, focus, and tone – and then, one loses it, all unawares. One must continually fight to regain it, to hold accurate awareness. I cannot better express the problems which have challenged me, and which my readers must challenge, than in the splendid words of Maynard Keynes in the Preface to his *General Theory* :

The composition of this book has been for the author a long struggle of escape, and so must the reading of it be for most readers if the author's assault upon them is to be successful – a struggle of escape from habitual modes of thought and expression. The ideas which are here expressed so laboriously are extremely simple and should be obvious. The difficulty lies, not in the new ideas, but in escaping from the old ones, which ramify, for those brought up as most of us have been, into every corner of our minds.

Force of habit, and resistance to change – so great in all realms of thought – reaches its maximum in medicine, in the study of our most complex sufferings and disorders of being; for we are here compelled to scrutinize the deepest, darkest and most fearful parts of ourselves, the parts we all strive to deny or not-see. The thoughts which are most difficult to grasp or express are those which touch on this forbidden region and re-awaken in us our strongest denials and our most profound intuitions.

New York
February 1973   O. W. S.

PREFACE AND ACKNOWLEDGEMENTS
FOR THE PENGUIN EDITION

I have made no alterations of substance to this new edition of *Awakenings*, but I have *added* a good deal of further material, both in the way of further clinical observations, and wide-ranging reflections arising from these. In order not to disturb the general format of the book, I have put all this additional matter in the form of *footnotes*: these 'footnotes' sometimes have the form and length of miniature essays, and in aggregate now constitute about one third of the book's length. I have been moved to add these further observations and reflections, for the most part, in response to the many penetrating and interesting queries raised by readers and reviewers of the original edition. I should stress, however, that the footnotes *are* footnotes, and that the narrative centre of the book is still in its *tales* – the twenty short histories or biographies which picture the life stories of my patients, and their complex, infinitely variable responses to the strangest of illnesses and the most dramatic of drugs. Most of these patients, whose stories I described up to the summer of 1972, are still alive and reasonably well – a few, indeed, are notably better than they were two years ago; but a few have also deteriorated or died, for complex and sometimes disquieting reasons (I exemplify this in the tragic follow-up of Rolando P.). Further, in order to bring home that I am speaking of real people, who are the survivors of a vast but strangely forgotten epidemic, I have added a pictorial supplement, showing some of my patients at different times in a variety of different moods and situations – a *collage* of old photographs and newspaper cuttings, which will bring to life, as no retrospect can, what the epidemic was *really like*, fifty years ago. I have also added a number of photographs of patients from Mount Carmel, some of whose stories are told in the book. It is my hope that these additions will enhance the range, the clarity, and the vividness of this book.

Many of these illustrations have been taken from the television film which was made about *Awakenings*, and from original documents and photographs unearthed during the preparation of this film: I am deeply indebted to Mr Duncan Dallas, of Yorkshire Television, for permission to use this material. I am also most grateful to Miss Julia Vellacott, of Penguin Books, for her advice and assistance in collating all additions with the original text to produce this new and enlarged edition.

London
October 1974

O. W. S.

INTRODUCTION

PARKINSON'S DISEASE AND PARKINSONISM

In 1817, Dr James Parkinson – a London physician – published his famous *Essay on the Shaking Palsy*, in which he portrayed, with a vividness and insight that have never been surpassed, the common, important and singular condition we now know as Parkinson's disease.

Isolated symptoms and features of Parkinson's disease – the characteristic shaking or tremor, and the characteristic hurrying or festination of gait and speech – had been described by physicians back to the time of Galen. Detailed descriptions had also appeared in the non-medical literature – as in Aubrey's description of Hobbes's 'Shaking Palsy'. But it was Parkinson who first saw every feature and aspect of the illness as a whole, and who presented it as a distinctive human condition or *form of behaviour*.[1]

1. It is true, in a sense, that Parkinson had many 'predecessors' (Gaubius, Sauvages, de la Noë, and others) who had observed and classified various 'signs' of Parkinsonism. But there was a radical difference between Parkinson and these men – perhaps more radical than Parkinson himself allowed or admitted. Observers of Parkinsonism, before Parkinson himself, had been content to 'spot' various characteristics (in much the same way as one 'spots' trains or planes), and then to arrange these characteristics in classificatory schemes (somewhat as a butterfly-spotter, or would-be entomologist, might arrange his specimens according to colour and shape). Thus Parkinson's predecessors were entirely concerned with 'diagnosis' and 'nosology' – an arbitrary, pre-scientific diagnosis and nosology, based entirely on superficial characteristics and relationships: the Zodiacal charts of Sauvages and others represent a sort of pseudo-astronomy, first attempts to come to grips with the unknown. Parkinson's own initial observations were also made 'from the outside', so to speak,

Between 1860 and 1890, working amid the large population of chronically ill patients at the Salpêtrière in Paris,
Charcot filled in the outline which Parkinson had drawn. In
addition to his rich and detailed characterizations of the ill-

---

from seeing Parkinsonians in the streets of London, inspecting their
peculiarities of motion from a distance. But his observations were
deeper than those of his predecessors, deeper-rooted and more deeply
related. Parkinson resembles a *genuine* astronomer, and London the
field of his astronomical observations, and at this stage, through
his eyes, we see Parkinsonians as bodies-in-transit, moving like
comets or stars. Soon, moreover, he came to recognize that certain
stars form a *constellation*, that many seemingly unrelated phenomena
form a definite and constant 'assemblage of symptoms'. He was the
first to recognize this 'assemblage' as such, this constellation or
syndrome we now call 'Parkinsonism'.

This was a clinical achievement of the first magnitude, and
Parkinsonism was one of the first neurological syndromes to be recognized and defined. But Parkinson was not merely talented – he was
a man of genius. He perceived that the curious 'assemblage' he had
noted was something more than a diagnostic syndrome – that it
seemed to have a coherent inner logic and order of its own, that the
constellation was a sort of *cosmos* ... Sensing this, he now realized
that inspection-at-a-distance, however acute, was insufficient if he
wished to understand its nature; he realized it was necessary to
meet actual patients, to engage them in clinical and dialogic encounter. With this he adopted an entirely different stance and concurrently with this a quite different language. He ceased to see
Parkinsonians as remote objects in orbit, and saw them as patients
and fellow human beings; he ceased to use diagnostic jargon, and
used words indicative of *intention* and *action*; he ceased to see
Parkinsonism as 'an assemblage of symptoms' and now thought
of being-Parkinsonian as a strange form of *behaviour*, a peculiar and
characteristic mode of *Being-in-the-World*. Thus Parkinson, compared
to his 'predecessors', was a radical, a revolutionary, in two different
ways: first in establishing a genuine empiricism – a science of 'facts'
and their inter-relations; second, in making a still more radical
move in intellectual mid-course, by moving from an empirical to an
existential position. We cannot but be reminded of Hume's evolution in the preceding century – of how he first tried to understand
Human Nature as 'a bundle of perceptions', but finding this synthetic

ness, Charcot perceived the important relations and affinities which existed between the symptoms of Parkinson's disease and those of depression, catatonia and hysteria: indeed, it was partly in view of these striking relationships that Charcot called Parkinsonism 'a neurosis'.

In the nineteenth century, Parkinsonism was almost never seen before the age of fifty, and was usually considered to be a reflection of a degenerative process or defect of nutrition in certain 'weak' or vulnerable cells; since this degeneration could not actually be demonstrated at the time, and since its cause was unknown, Parkinson's disease was termed an idio-syncrasy or 'idiopathy'. In the first quarter of this century, with the advent of the great sleeping-sickness epidemic (*encephalitis lethargica*), a 'new' sort of Parkinsonism appeared, which had a clear and specific cause: this encephalitic or post-encephalitic Parkinsonism,[2] unlike the idiopathic illness, could affect people of any age, and could assume a form and a severity much graver and more dramatic than ever occurred in the idiopathic illness. A third great cause of Parkinsonism has been seen only in the last twenty years, and is an unintended (and usually transient) consequence or 'side-effect' of the use of phenothiazide and butyrophenone drugs – the so-called 'major tranquillizers'. It is said that

view incoherent and inadequate, was forced to see 'Personal Identity' as an unanalysable whole, to accept as elemental the con-cept of *existence* (*which cannot be arrived at, but can only be started from . . .*). By a curious (and, one feels, symptomatic) irony Hume is always cited as the great exemplar of empiricism, 'for-getting' that he renounced empiricism and moved to existentialism; similarly, Parkinson is always praised as a great empirical physician, and one who always stuck to 'facts' and 'syndromes'; whereas, in reality, he moved from his empirical position to become one of our first and greatest existential physicians.

2. The term 'post-encephalitic' is used to denote symptoms which have come on *following* an attack of *encephalitis lethargica*, and as a direct or indirect consequence of this. The onset of such symptoms may be delayed until many years after the original attack.

in the United States alone there are two million people with Parkinsonism: a million with idiopathic Parkinsonism or Parkinson's disease; a million with drug-induced Parkinsonism; and a few hundred or thousand patients with post-encephalitic Parkinsonism – the last survivors of the great epidemic. Other causes of Parkinsonism – coal-gas poisoning, manganese poisoning, syphilis, tumours, etc. – are excessively rare, and are scarcely likely to be seen in a lifetime of practice by the ordinary physician.

Parkinson's disease has been called the 'shaking palsy' (or its Latin equivalent – *paralysis agitans*) for some centuries. It is necessary to say at the outset that the shaking or tremor is by no means a constant symptom in Parkinsonism, is never an isolated symptom, and is often the least problem which faces the Parkinsonian patient. If tremor is present, it tends to occur at rest and to disappear with movement or the intention to move;[3] sometimes it is confined to the hand, and has a characteristic 'pill-rolling' quality or (in Gowers's words) a quality 'similar to that by which Orientals beat their small drums'; in other, and especially in post-encephalitic patients, tremor may be extremely violent, may affect any or every part of the body, and tends to be increased by effort, nervousness or fatigue. The second commonly mentioned symptom of Parkinsonism, besides tremor, is stiffness or rigidity; this has a curious plastic quality – often compared to the bending of a lead pipe – and may be of intense severity.[4] It must be stressed, however, that neither

3. There are many actors, surgeons, mechanics and skilled manual workers who show severe Parkinsonian tremor at rest, but not a trace of this when they concentrate on their work or move into action.

4. It was observed by Charcot, and is observed by many Parkinsonian patients themselves, that rigidity can be loosened to a remarkable degree if the patient is suspended in water or swimming (see below the cases of Hester Y., Rolando P., Cecil M., etc.). The same is also true, to some extent, of other forms of stiffness and 'clench' – spasticity, athetosis, torticollis, etc.

tremor nor rigidity is an essential feature of Parkinsonism; they may both be completely absent, especially in the post-encephalitic forms of disease with which we shall especially be concerned in this book. The essential features of Parkinsonism, which occur in every patient, and which reach their extremest intensity in post-encephalitic forms of disease, relate to disorders of movement and 'push'.

The first qualities of Parkinsonism which were ever described were those of *festination* (hurry) and *pulsion* (push). Festination consists of an acceleration (and with this, an abbreviation) of steps, movements, words or even thoughts – it conveys a sense of impatience, impetuosity and alacrity, as if the patient were very pressed for time; and in some patients it goes along with a *feeling* of urgency and impatience, although others, as it were, find themselves hurried against their will.[5] The character of movements associated with festination or pulsion are those of quickness, abruptness and brevity. These symptoms, and the peculiar 'motor impatience' (akathisia) which often goes along with them, were given full weight by the older authors: thus Charcot speaks of the 'cruel restlessness' suffered by many of his patients, and Gowers of the 'extreme restlessness ... which necessitates ... every few minutes some slight change of posture'. I stress these aspects – the alacrity and pressure and precipitation of movement – because they represent, so to speak, the less familiar 'other side' of Parkinsonism, Parkinsonism-on-the-boil, Parkinsonism in its expansile and explosive aspect, and as such have peculiar relevance to many of the 'side-effects' of L-DOPA which patients exhibit.

The opposite of these effects – a peculiar slowing and diffi-

---

5. Thus festination ('*scelotyrbe festinans*') is portrayed by Gaubius in the eighteenth century: 'Cases occur in which the muscles, duly excited by the impulses of the will, do then, with an unbidden agility, and with an impetus not to be repressed, run before the unwilling mind.'

culty of movement – are more commonly stressed, and go by the general and rather uninformative name of 'akinesia'. There are many different forms of akinesia, but the form which is exactly antithetical to hurry or pulsion is one of active *retardation* or *resistance* which impedes movement, speech and even thought, and may arrest it completely. Patients so affected find that as soon as they 'will' or intend or attempt a movement, a 'counter-will' or 'resistance' rises up to meet them. They find themselves embattled, and even immobilized, in a form of physiological conflict – force against counter-force, will against counter-will, command against countermand. For such embattled patients, Charcot writes: 'There is no truce' – and Charcot sees the tremor, rigidity and akinesia of such patients as the final, futile outcome of such states of inner struggle, and the tension and tiredness of which Parkinsonian patients so often complain as due to the pre-emption of their energies in such senseless inner battles. It is these states of push and constraint which one patient of mine (Leonard L.) would always call 'the goad and halter'.[6] The appearance of passivity or inertia is deceiving: an obstructive akinesia of this sort is in no sense an idle or restful state, but (to paraphrase de Quincey) '... no product of inertia, but ... resulting from mighty and equal antagonisms, infinite activities, infinite repose'.[7]

6. Analogous concepts are used by William James, in his discussion of 'perversions' of will (*Principles*, 2, xxvi, esp. pp. 537-49). The two basic perversions delineated by James are the 'obstructive' will and the 'explosive' will; when the former holds sway, the performance of normal actions is rendered difficult or impossible; if the latter is dominant, abnormal actions are irrepressible. Although James uses these terms with reference to neurotic perversions of the will, they are equally applicable to what we must term Parkinsonian perversions of the will: Parkinsonism, like neurosis, is a *conative* disorder, and exhibits a formal analogy of conative structure.

7. At this point we must introduce a fundamental theme which will re-appear and re-echo, in various guises, throughout this book. We have taken a first, amazed look at the phenomena of Parkinson-

In some patients, there is a different form of akinesia, which is not associated with a feeling of effort and struggle, but with one of continual repetition or perseveration: thus Gowers records the case of one patient whose limbs '... when raised remained so for several minutes, and then slowly fell'

---

ism – its sudden starts and stops, its odd speedings and slowings. Our approach, our concepts, our terms have so far been of a purely mechanical or empirical type: we have seen Parkinsonians as bodies, but not yet as *beings* ... if we are to achieve any understanding of *what it is like to be Parkinsonian*, of the actual nature of *Parkinsonian existence* (as opposed to the parameters of Parkinsonian motion), we must adopt a different and complementary approach and language.

We must come down from our position as 'objective observers', and meet our patients face-to-face; we must meet them in a sympathetic and imaginative encounter: for it is only in the context of such a collaboration, a participation, a relation, that we can hope to learn anything about *how they are*. They can tell us, and show us, what it is like being Parkinsonian – they can tell us, but nobody else can.

Indeed we must go further, for if – as we have reason to suspect – our patients may be subject to experiences as strange as the motions they show, they may need much help, a delicate and patient and imaginative collaboration, in order to formulate the almost-unformulable, in order to communicate the almost-incommunicable. We must be co-explorers in the uncanny realm of being-Parkinsonian, this land beyond the boundaries of common experience; but our quarry in this strange country will not be 'specimens', data or 'facts', but images, similitudes, analogies, metaphors – whatever may assist to make the strange familiar, and to bring into the thinkable the previously unthinkable. What we are told, what we discover, will be couched in the mode of 'likeness' or 'as if', for we are asking the patient to make *comparisons* – to compare being-Parkinsonian with that mode-of-being which we agree to call 'normal'. All experience is hypothetical or conjectural, but its intensity and form vary a great deal: thus patients able to achieve some detachment, or patients only partially or intermittently affected, will describe their experiences in metaphorical terms; whereas patients who are continually and completely engulfed by their experience will tend to describe it in hallucinatory terms ...

– a form of akinesia which he correctly compares to catalepsy; this is generally far more common and far more severe
in patients with post-encephalitic forms of Parkinsonism.

These characteristics – of impulsion, of resistance, and of
perseveration – represent the active or positive characteristics of Parkinsonism. We will later have occasion to see that
they are to some extent interchangeable, and thus that they
represent different phases or forms or transformations of
Parkinsonism. Parkinsonian patients also have 'negative'
characteristics – if this is not a contradiction in terms. Thus
some of them, Charcot particularly noted, would sit for hours
not only motionless, but apparently without any impulse to
move: they were, seemingly, content to do nothing, and they
lacked the 'will' to enter upon or continue any course of
activity, although they might move quite well if the stimulus or command or request to move came from another person – *from the outside*. Such patients were said to have an
absence of the will – or 'aboulia'.

Other aspects of such 'negative' disorder or deficiency in
Parkinsonian patients relate to feelings of tiredness and lack
of energy, and of certain 'dullness' – an impoverishment
of feeling, libido, motive and attention. To a greater or less
degree, all Parkinsonian patients show alteration of 'go',
impetus, initiative, vitality, etc., closely akin to what may be
experienced by patients in the throes of depression.[8]

Thus Parkinsonian patients suffer simultaneously (though
in varying proportions) from a pathological absence and a
pathological presence. The former cuts them off from the
fluent and appropriate flow of normal movement (and – in
severe cases – the flow of normal perception and thought),
and is experienced as a 'weakness', a tiredness, a deprivation,
a destitution; the latter constitutes a preoccupation, an abnor-

8. A special form of negative disorder, not described in the classical
literature, is depicted on p. 141.

mal activity, a pathological organization, which, so to speak, distends or inflates their behaviour in a senseless, distressing and disabling fashion. Patients can be thought of as *engorged* with Parkinsonism – with pathological excitement ('erethism') – as one may be engorged with pain or pleasure or rage or neurosis. The notion of Parkinsonism as exerting a pressure on the patient seems to be supported, above all, by the phenomenon of 'kinesia paradoxa' which consists of a sudden and total (though transient) disappearance or deflation of Parkinsonism – a phenomenon seen most frequently and most dramatically in the most intensely Parkinsonian patients.[9]

It is scarcely imaginable that a profound deficiency can suddenly be made good, but it is easy to conceive that an intense pressure might suddenly be relieved, or an intense charge discharged. Such conceptions are always implicit, and sometimes explicit, in the thinking of Charcot, who goes on, indeed, to stress the close analogies which could exist between the different forms or 'phases' of Parkinsonism and those of neurosis: in particular Charcot clearly saw the formal similarity or analogy between the three clearly distinct yet interchangeable phases of Parkinsonism – the compliant-

9. Thus one may see such patients, rigid, motionless, seemingly lifeless as statues, abruptly called into normal life and action by some sudden exigency which catches their attention (in one famous case, a drowning man was saved by a Parkinsonian patient who leapt from his wheelchair into the breakers). The return of Parkinsonism, in circumstances like these, is often as sudden and dramatic as its vanishing: the suddenly 'normal' and awakened patient, once the call-to-action is past, may fall back like a dummy into the arms of his attendants. Less abrupt and complete, but of more therapeutic relevance, is the *partial* lifting of Parkinsonism, for long periods of time, in response to interesting and activating situations, which *invite* participation in a non-Parkinsonian mode. Different forms of such therapeutic activation are exemplified throughout the biographies in this book, and explicitly discussed in two long footnotes towards the end (see pp. 319 and 323).

perseverative, the obstructive-resistive, and the explosive-precipitate phases – with the plastic, rigid and frenzied forms of catatonia and hysteria. These insights were reinforced during the 1920s, by observation of the extraordinary amalgamations of Parkinsonism with other disorders seen in the encephalitis epidemic. They were then completely 'forgotten', or thrust out of the neurological consciousness. The effects of L-DOPA – as we shall see – compel us to reinstate and elaborate the forgotten analyses and analogies of Charcot and his contemporaries.

THE SLEEPING-SICKNESS[10]
(ENCEPHALITIS LETHARGICA)

In the winter of 1916–17, in Vienna and other cities, a 'new' illness suddenly appeared, and rapidly spread, over the next three years, to become world-wide in its distribution. Its manifestations were so varied that no two patients ever presented exactly the same picture, and so strange as to call forth from physicians such diagnoses as epidemic delirium, epidemic schizophrenia, epidemic Parkinsonism, epidemic disseminated sclerosis, a typical rabies, a typical poliomyelitis, etc., etc. It seemed, at first, that a thousand new diseases had suddenly broken loose, and it was only through the profound clinical acumen of Constantin von Economo, allied with his pathological studies on the brains of patients who had died, and his demonstration that these, besides showing a unique pattern of damage, contained a sub-microscopic, filter-passing agent (virus) which could transmit the disease

10. The term 'sleeping-sickness' is used in America to designate both the African, parasite-borne, endemic disease (*trypanosomiasis*) and the epidemic, virus-borne, *encephalitis lethargica*; in England, however, the latter is often called 'sleepy-sickness'.

to monkeys, that the identity of this protean disease was established. *Encephalitis lethargica* – as von Economo was to name it – was a Hydra with a thousand heads.

Although there had been innumerable smaller epidemics in the past, including the London sleeping-sickness of 1672–3[11], there had never been a world-wide pandemic on the scale of that which started in 1916–17.[12] In the ten years that

11. It is of historical (and perhaps epistemological) interest that Leibniz (whose ideas I shall often quote in this book) was himself in London at the time of the London sleeping-sickness, and there met Sydenham (who had described it under the name of 'febris comatosa'), and the aged and then deeply-Parkinsonian Hobbes. The vast majority of Leibniz's 40,000-odd letters are still unsorted and unpublished; perhaps, one day, we will discover descriptions of Parkinsonism, and *encephalitis lethargica*, written by the hand of Leibniz himself.

12. I have elsewhere (*British Medical Journal*, 9 October 1971) detailed the 2,000-year-long history of these epidemics: the following extract is taken from my B.M.J. letter:

The older literature is full of vivid accounts of feverish somnolent illnesses followed, within months or years, by the development of characteristic slowness, poverty and difficulty of movement, masking, rigidity, tremors, and, on occasion, torticollis, dystonias, oculogyria, strabismus, blepharoclonus, myoclonus, catatonus, somnolence, etc., etc. The unique symptomology of such cases, so circumstantially described in the older literature, is scarcely compatible with any other illness but encephalitis lethargica with Parkinsonian and other typical sequelae. Many such accounts are collected and scrutinized in the encyclopaedic works of von Economo and Jelliffe. Von Economo, while allowing that such retrospective diagnosis can only be tentative, concludes: 'We may assume with some degree of certainty that encephalitis lethargica had already appeared *repeatedly* before the Great War, both sporadically in the shape of isolated cases and in epidemics which again and again attracted notice for a short period on account of the ... singular combinations of symptoms displayed ...'

A few of these former cases and epidemics may be recalled. In 1580, Europe was swept by a serious febrile and lethargic illness ('Morbus epidemicus per totam fere Europam *Schlafkrankheit* dictus ...'), which led to Parkinsonian and other neurological sequelae.

it raged, this pandemic took or ravaged the lives of nearly
five million people before it disappeared, as mysteriously and

---

A similar serious epidemic occurred in London between 1673 and
1675, and is described by Sydenham as 'febris comatosa'; hiccough
was a prominent symptom in this epidemic (as in the Vienna encephalitis of 1919). Albrecht of Hildesheim, in 1695, provided an
elaborate account of oculogyric crises, Parkinsonian symptoms, diplopia, strabismus, etc. following an attack of somnolent brain-fever
in a 20-year-old girl ('De febre lethargica in strabismo utriusque
oculi desinente'). A severe epidemic of *Schlafkrankheit* occurred in
Tübingen in 1712 and 1713, and was followed in many cases by persistent slowness of movement and lack of initiative ('aboulia').
Minor epidemics of 'coma somnolentum' with Parkinsonian features occurred in France and Germany during the latter half of the
eighteenth century, alternating with hyperkinetic epidemics of hiccough, myoclonus, chorea, and tics. Many isolated cases of *juvenile*
Parkinsonism, variously associated with diplopia, oculogyria, tachypnoea, retropulsion, tics, and obsessional disorders were described by
Charcot, and were almost certainly post-encephalitic in origin. In
Italy, following the great influenza epidemic of 1889-90, the notorious
'*nona*' appeared – a devastatingly severe somnolent illness which
was followed by the development of Parkinsonian and other sequelae
in almost all of the few survivors.

A knowledge of such historical accounts, and of the peculiar
comings and goings of encephalitis lethargica in previous centuries,
is of more than academic importance. A graphic description of the
'*nona*', given by his mother to the young von Economo, enabled
him to recognize and characterize this illness when it re-appeared in
its catastrophic form in 1917; this is movingly described in the preface of his book. Jelliffe, in his many writings at the time of the great
encephalitis epidemic, asks again and again how it could happen
that a disease which had obviously existed since the days of Hip-
pocrates could be 'discovered' only *now*, and how it was possible
for an illness which had been described unmistakably innumerable
times to be 'forgotten' anew by each generation. Such forgettings
are as dangerous as they are mysterious, for they give us an un-
warranted sense of security. In 1927, with the virtual cessation of
new cases of encephalitis lethargica, the medical profession heaved
a huge sigh of relief, and did its best to forget the horrors of the
previous decade. Von Economo warned against this, saying that the
causative virus was not extinct, but only in a dormant or non-virulent

suddenly as it had arrived, in 1927.[13] A third of those affected died in the acute stages of the sleeping-sickness, in states of coma so deep as to preclude arousal, or in states of sleeplessness so intense as to preclude sedation. Patients who suffered but survived an extremely severe somnolent / insomniac attack of this kind often failed to recover their original aliveness. They would be conscious and aware – yet not fully awake; they would sit motionless and speechless all day in

---

phase, from which it would inevitably re-emerge as it had done innumerable times since the dawn of recorded history.

*

The best descriptions of the epidemic and its sequelae have been provided by von Economo and by Jelliffe in the following works:

Von Economo, C., *Encephalitis Lethargica: Its Sequelae and Treatment*, Oxford University Press 1931.

Jelliffe, S. E., *Post-encephalitic Respiratory Disorders*, Nervous and Mental Disease Publishing Co., Washington, 1927.

Jelliffe, S. E., *Psychopathology of Forced Movements and the Oculogyric Crises of Lethargic Encephalitis*, Nervous and Mental Disease Publishing Co., Washington, 1932.

13. There was some coincidence and overlap of the great encephalitis pandemic with the world-wide 'flu' pandemic – as thirty years earlier the Italian '*nona*' was preceded by a virulent if local influenza epidemic. It is probable, but not certain, that the influenza and the encephalitis reflected the effects of two different viruses, but it seems possible, and even probable, that the influenza epidemic in some way paved the way for the encephalitis epidemic, and that the influenza virus potentiated the effects of the encephalitis virus, or lowered resistance to it in a catastrophic way. Thus, between October 1918 and January 1919, when half the world's population was affected by the influenza or its consequences, and more than twenty-one million people died, the encephalitis assumed its most virulent form. If the sleeping-sickness was mysteriously 'forgotten', the same is true of the great influenza (which had been the most murderous epidemic since the Black Death of the Middle Ages). In the words of H. L. Mencken, written in 1956: 'The epidemic is seldom mentioned, and most Americans have apparently forgotten it. This is not surprising. The human mind always tries to expunge the intolerable from memory, just as it tries to conceal it while current.'

their chairs, totally lacking energy, impetus, initiative, motive, appetite, affect or desire; they registered what went on about them without active attention, and with profound indifference.[14] They neither conveyed nor felt the feeling of life; they were as insubstantial as ghosts, and as passive as zombies: von Economo compared them to extinct volcanoes. Such patients, in neurological parlance, showed 'negative' disorders of behaviour, i.e. no behaviour at all. They were ontologically dead, or suspended, or 'asleep' – awaiting an awakening which came (for the tiny fraction who survived) fifty years later.

If these 'negative' states or *absences* were more varied and severe than those seen in common Parkinson's disease, this was even truer of the innumerable 'positive' disorders or pathological *presences* introduced by the sleeping-sickness: indeed, von Economo, in his great monograph, enumerated more than five hundred distinct forms or varieties of these.

Parkinsonian disorders, of one sort or another, were perhaps the commonest of these disorders, although their appearance was often delayed until many years after the acute epidemic. Post-encephalitic Parkinsonism, as opposed to ordinary or idiopathic Parkinsonism, tended to show less in the way of tremor and rigidity – indeed, these were sometimes completely absent – but much severer states of 'explosive' and 'obstructive' disorders, of akinesia and akathisia, push and resistance, hurry and impediment, etc., and also much severer states of the complaint-perseverative type of akinesia which Gowers had compared to catalepsy. Many patients, indeed, were swallowed up in states of Parkinsonian akinesia so profound as to turn them into living statues – totally motionless for hours, days, weeks, or years on end. The very

14.   his heart transfixed,
              Comatose in her cave, cares little
              What the senses say ...
                                        W. H. AUDEN

much greater severity of these encephalitic and post-encephalitic states revealed that *all* aspects of being and behaviour – perceptions, thoughts, appetites, and feelings, no less than movements – could also be brought to a virtual standstill by an active, constraining Parkinsonian process.

Almost as common as these Parkinsonian disorders, and frequently co-existing with them, were *catatonic* disorders of every sort. It was the occurrence of these which originally gave rise to the notion of an 'epidemic schizophrenia', for catatonia – until its appearance in the encephalitis epidemic – was thought to be part-and-parcel of the schizophrenic syndrome. The majority of patients who were rendered catatonic by the sleeping-sickness were *not* schizophrenic, and showed that catatonia might, so to speak, be approached by a direct physiological path, and was not always a defensive manoeuvre undertaken by schizophrenic patients at periods of unendurable stress and desperation.[15]

The general forms or 'phrases' of encephalitic catatonia were closely analogous to those of Parkinsonism, but were at a higher and more complex level, and were usually experienced as subjective states which had exactly the same form as the observable behavioural states. Thus some of these patients showed automatic compliance or 'obedience', maintaining (indefinitely, and apparently without effort) any posture in which they were put or found themselves, or 'echoing' words, phrases, thoughts, perceptions or actions in an unvarying circular way, once these had been suggested to them (palilalia, echolalia, echopraxia, etc.). Other patients

15. Post-encephalitic patients, when they can speak – which in the severest cases was not rendered possible until half a century later, when they were given L-DOPA – are thus able to provide us with uniquely detailed and accurate descriptions of states of catatonic 'entrancement', 'fascination', 'block', 'negativism', etc., which schizophrenic patients, usually, are unable or unwilling to do, or which they will only describe in distorted, magical, 'schizophrenic' terms.

showed disorders of a precisely antithetical kind ('command negativism', 'block', etc.) immediately preventing or countermanding any suggested or intended action, speech or thought: in the severest cases, 'block' of this type could cause a virtual obliteration of all behaviour and also of all mental processes (see the case of Rose R., for example). Such constrained catatonic patients – like constrained Parkinsonians – could suddenly burst out of their immobilized states into violent movements or frenzies: a great many of the tics seen at the time of the epidemic, and subsequently, showed themselves to be interchangeable with 'tics of immobility' (or catatonia).

An immense variety of involuntary and compulsive movements were seen during the acute phase of the encephalitis, and for a few years thereafter: myoclonic jerks and spasms; states of mobile spasm (athetosis), dystonias and dystonic contortions (e.g. torticollis), with somewhat similar functional organizations to that of Parkinsonian rigidity; desultory, forceless movements dancing from one part of the body to another (chorea); and a wide spectrum of tics and compulsive movements at every functional level – yawning, coughing, sniffing, gasping, panting, breath-holding, staring, glancing, bellowing, yelling, cursing etc. – which were enactions of sudden *urges*.[16]

16. In Thom Gunn's poem 'The Sense of Movement', there occurs the following, pivotal line:
   'One is always nearer by not being still.'
This poem deals with the basic *urge to move*, as it may take possession of motorcycle riders, driving them to strenuous, ceaseless movement, to driving which is seemingly without end or aim, which seems to be a mere *akathisia* – but which in reality is always *towards*, towards somewhere or something or some state-of-mind, something which continually beckons and calls, but which is unconscious, and too deep to be formulable ... This is not so for the Parkinsonian: the Parkinsonian is *no* nearer for not being still. His urges are truly aimless and senseless – 'beneath intention' and 'beneath comprehension'. He is no nearer to anything by virtue of his motion; and,

At the 'highest' level the *encephalitis lethargica* presented itself as neurotic and psychotic disorders of every kind, and a great many patients affected in this way were originally considered to have 'functional' obsessional and hysterical neurosis, until the development of other symptoms indicated the encephalitic aetiology of their complaints. It is of interest, in this connection, that 'oculogyric crises' were considered to be purely 'functional' and hysterical for several years after their first appearance.

Clearly differentiated forms of affective compulsion were common in the immediate aftermath of the sleeping-sickness, especially erotomanias, erethisms and libidinal excitement, on the one hand, and tantrums, rages and destructive outbursts on the other. These forms of behaviour were most clearly and undisguisedly manifest in children, who sometimes showed abrupt changes of character, and suddenly became impulsive, provocative, destructive, audacious, salacious and lewd, sometimes to a quite uncontrollable degree: such children were often labelled 'juvenile psychopaths' or 'moral aments'.[17] Sexual and destructive outbursts were rarely

---

in this sense, his motion is not genuine movement, as his lack of motion is not genuine rest. The road to Parkinsonism is a road which leads nowhere; the land of Parkinsonism is paradox and dead-end.

17. Among the many eminent physicians who were deeply concerned with the changes in character which might be wrought by the sleepy-sickness was Dr G. A. Auden (father of the poet W. H. Auden). Such changes, Dr Auden stressed, could not always be regarded as purely deleterious or destructive in nature. Less zealous to 'pathologize' than many of his colleagues, Dr Auden noted that some of those affected, especially children, finding themselves subject to complex stimulations or 'de-repressions' of affect, might be 'awakened' from a pre-existing emotional dullness into a genuine (if morbid) brilliance, into unexpected and unprecedented heights and depths. This notion of a disease with a 'Dionysiac' potential was often discussed in the Auden household, and formed an enduring theme in W. H. Auden's thought and writing. Many other artists at this time, perhaps most notably Thomas Mann, were struck by the

outspoken in adults, being 'converted' (presumably) to other, more 'allowable', reactions and expressions. Jelliffe,[18] in particular, who undertook lengthy analysis of some highly intelligent post-encephalitic patients, showed unequivocally how accesses of erotic and hostile feeling could be and were 'converted', not only into neurotic and psychotic behaviour, but into tics, 'crises', catatonia and even Parkinsonism. Adult post-encephalitic patients thus showed an extraordinary ability to 'absorb' intense feeling, and to express it in indirect physiological terms. They were gifted – or cursed – with a pathologically extravagant expressive facility or (in Freud's term) 'somatic compliance'.

Nearly half the survivors became liable to extraordinary crises, in which they might experience, for example, the simultaneous and virtually instantaneous onset of Parkinsonism, catatonia, tics, obsessions, hallucinations, 'block', increased suggestibility or negativism, and thirty or forty

world-wide spectacle of a disease which could – however temporarily, however ambiguously – raise cerebral activity to a more awakened and creative pitch: in *Doctor Faustus* the Dionysiac fever is attributable to neurosyphilitic infection; but a similar allegory of extraordinary excitement, followed (and *paid for*) by attrition and exhaustion, could as well apply to post-encephalitic infection (see p. 41 on the 'up' and 'down' phases of this). Thus the twofold effects of the original illness – Stimulation–Destruction: Elevation–Depression: Awakening–Tribulation: Hubris–Nemesis – themselves foreshadowed the later effects of L-DOPA.

18. Smith Ely Jelliffe, a man equally eminent as neurologist and psychoanalyst, was perhaps the closest observer of the sleeping-sickness and its sequelae. This was his summing-up, looking back on the epidemic: 'In the monumental strides made by neuropsychiatry during the past ten years no single advance has approached in importance that made through the study of epidemic encephalitis. No individual group of disease-reactions has been ... so far-reaching in modifying the entire foundations of neuropsychiatry in general ... *An entirely new orientation has been made imperative.*' (Jelliffe, 1927, op. cit.)

other problems; such crises would last a few minutes or hours, and then disappear as suddenly as they had come. They were highly individual, no two patients ever having exactly the same sort of crises, and they expressed, in various ways, fundamental aspects of the character, personality, history, perception and fantasies of each patient.[19] These crises could be greatly influenced, for better or worse, by suggestion, emotional problems or current circumstances. Crises of all sorts became rare after 1930, but I stress them and their characteristics because they show remarkable affinities to certain states induced by L-DOPA, not merely in post-encephalitic patients, but in the normally much stabler patients with common Parkinson's disease.

One thing, and one alone, was (usually) spared amid the ravages of this otherwise engulfing disease: the 'higher faculties' – intelligence, imagination, judgement, and humour. These were exempted – for better or worse. Thus these patients, some of whom had been thrust into the remotest or

19. Not infrequently a single, sensational *moment-of-being* is 'caught' by a crisis, and preserved thereafter. Thus Jelliffe (1932) alludes to a man whose first oculogyric crisis came on during a game of cricket, when he had suddenly to fling one hand up to catch a high ball (he had to be carried off the field still entranced, with his right arm still outstretched and clutching the ball). Subsequently, whenever he had an oculogyric crisis, these would be ushered in by a *total replay* of this original, grotesque and comic moment: he would suddenly feel it was 1919 once again, an unusually hot July afternoon, that the Saturday match was in progress again, that Trevelyan had just hit a probable 'six', that the ball was approaching him, and that he had to catch it – RIGHT NOW! Similar, dramatic moments-of-being may also be incorporated into epileptic seizures, especially those of psychomotor type; Penfield and Perot, who have provided the most detailed accounts of this, suggest that 'fossilized memories' may be preserved in the cortex-memories which are normally dormant and forgotten, but which can suddenly come to life and be re-activated under special conditions. Such phenomena endorse the notion that our memories, or beings, are 'a collection of moments' (see footnote to pp. 305–6).

strangest extremities of human possibility, experienced their states with unsparing perspicacity, and retained the power to remember, to compare, to dissect, and to testify. Their fate, so to speak, was to become unique witnesses to a unique catastrophe.

THE AFTERMATH OF THE SLEEPING-SICKNESS (1927–67)

Although many patients seemed to make a complete recovery from the sleeping-sickness, and were able to return to their former lives, the majority of them subsequently developed neurological or psychiatric disorders, and, most commonly, Parkinsonism. Why they should have developed such 'post-encephalitic syndromes' – after years or decades of seemingly perfect health – is a mystery, and has never been satisfactorily explained.

These post-encephalitic syndromes were very variable in course: sometimes they proceeded rapidly, leading to profound disability or death; sometimes very slowly; sometimes they progressed to a certain point and then stayed at this point for years or decades; and sometimes, following their initial onslaught, they remitted and disappeared. This great variation of pattern is also a mystery, and seems to admit of no single or simple explanation.

Certainly it could not be explained in terms of microscopically visible disease-processes, as was considered at one time. Nor was it true to say that post-encephalitic patients were suffering from a 'chronic encephalitis', for they showed no signs of active infection or inflammatory reaction. There was, moreover, a rather poor correlation between the severity of the clinical picture and that of the pathological picture, insofar as the latter could be judged by microscopic or chemical

means: one saw profoundly disabled patients with remarkably few signs of disease in the brain, and one saw evidences
of widespread tissue-destruction in patients who were scarcely
disabled at all. What *was* clear, from these discrepancies,
was that there were many other determinants of clinical
state and behaviour besides localized changes in the brain; it
was clear that the susceptibility or propensity to Parkinsonism, for example, was not a fixed expression of lesions in the
'Parkinsonism-centre' of the brain, but dependent on innumerable other 'factors' in addition.

It seemed, as Jelliffe[20] and a few others repeatedly stressed,
as if the '*quality*' of the individual – his 'strengths' and
'weaknesses', resistances and pliancies, motives and experiences, etc. – played a large part in determining the severity,
course and form of his illness. Thus, in the 1930s, at a time
of almost exclusive emphasis on specific mechanisms in
physiology and pathology, the strange evolutions of illness
in these post-encephalitic patients recalled Claude Bernard's
concepts of the *terrain* and the *milieu interne*, and the im-
memorial ideas of 'constitution', 'diathesis', 'idiosyncrasy',
'predisposition', etc., which had become so unfashionable in
the twentieth century. Equally clear, and beautifully analysed by Jelliffe, were the effects of the external environment, the circumstances and vicissitudes of each patient's
life. Thus, post-encephalitic illness could by no means be considered a simple disease, but needed to be seen as an individual creation of the greatest complexity, determined not
simply by a primary disease-process, but by a vast host of
personal traits and social circumstances: an illness, in short,
like neurosis or psychosis, a coming-to-terms of the sensitized
individual with his total environment.[21] Such considerations,
of course, are of crucial importance in understanding the
total reactions of such patients to L-DOPA.

20. See p. 267 n.
21. See notes on pp. 44 and 45.

There remain today a few survivors of the encephalitis who, despite Parkinsonism, tics, or other problems, still lead active and independent lives (see for instance the case of Cecil M.). These are the fortunate minority, who for one reason or another have managed to keep afloat, and have not been engulfed by illness, disability, dependence, demoralization, etc. – Parkinson's 'train of harassing evils'.

But for the majority of post-encephalitic patients – in consequence of the basic severity of their illness, their 'weaknesses', their propensities, or their misfortunes – a much darker future was in store. We have already stressed the inseparability of a patient's illness, his self, and his world, and how any or all of these, in their manifold interactions, through an infinity of vicious circles, can bring him to his nadir of being. How much is contributed by this, and that, and that, and that, can perhaps be unravelled by the most prolonged, intimate contact with individual patients, but cannot be put in any general, universally applicable form. One can only say that most of the survivors went down and down, through circle after circle of deepening illness, hopelessness and unimaginable solitude, their solitude, perhaps, the least bearable of all.

As *Sicknes* is the greatest misery, so the greatest misery of sicknes, is *solitude* ... *Solitude* is a torment which is not threatened in *hell* itselfe.

DONNE

The character of their illness changed. The early days of the epidemic had been a time of ebullition or ebullience, pathologically speaking, full of movements and tics, impulsions and impetuosities, manias and crises, ardencies and appetencies. By the late twenties, the acute phase was over, and the encephalitic syndrome started to cool or congeal. States of immobility and arrest had been distinctly uncommon in the early 1920s, but from 1930 onwards started to roll in a great sluggish, torpid tide over many of the survivors.

enveloping them in metaphorical (if not physiological) equivalents of sleep or death. Parkinsonism, catatonia, melancholia, trance, passivity, immobility, frigidity, apathy: this was the quality of the decades-long 'sleep' which closed over their heads in the 1930s and thereafter. Some patients, indeed, passed into a timeless state, an eventless stasis, which deprived them of all sense of history and happening. Isolated circumstances – fire alarms, dinner-gongs, the unexpected arrival of friends or news – might set them suddenly and startlingly alive for a minute, wonderfully active and agog with excitement. But these were rare flashes in the depths of their darkness. For the most part, they lay motionless and speechless, and in some cases almost will-less and thoughtless, or with their thoughts and feelings unchangingly fixed at the point where the long 'sleep' had closed in upon them. Their minds remained perfectly clear and unclouded, but their whole beings, so to speak, were encysted or cocooned.

Unable to work or to see to their needs, difficult to look after, helpless, hopeless, so bound up in their illnesses that they could neither react nor relate, frequently abandoned by their friends and their families, without specific treatment of any use to them – these patients were put away in chronic hospitals, nursing homes, lunatic asylums, or special colonies; and there, for the most part, they were totally forgotten – the lepers of the present century; there they died in their hundreds of thousands.

And yet some lived on, in diminishing numbers, getting older and frailer (though usually looking younger than their age), inmates of institutions, profoundly isolated, deprived of experience, half-forgetting, half-dreaming of the world they once lived in.

LIFE AT MOUNT CARMEL[22]

Mount Carmel was opened, shortly after the First World War, for war-veterans with injuries of the nervous system, and for the expected victims of the sleeping-sickness. It was a cottage hospital, in these early days, with no more than forty beds, large grounds, and a pleasant prospect of surrounding countryside. It lay close to the village of Bexley-on-Hudson, and there was a free and friendly exchange between the hospital and the village: patients often went to the village for shopping or meals, or silent movies, and the villagers, in turn, frequently visited the hospital; there were dates, and dances, and occasional marriages; and there were friendly rivalries in bowls and football, in which the measured deliberation of the villagers would be met by the abnormal suddenness and speed of movement characteristic of so many encephalitic patients, fifty years ago.

All this has changed, with the passage of years. Bexley-on Hudson is no longer a village, but a crowded and squalid

22. W. H. Auden once visited Mount Carmel, and may have had it in mind when he wrote 'Old People's Home'; certainly the poem (written in 1970) vividly conveys the 'feeling' of Mount Carmel c. 1970:

> ... The élite can dress and decent themselves,
> are ambulant with a single stick, adroit
> to read a book all through, or play the slow movements of
> easy sonatas ... Then come those on wheels, the average
> majority, who endure TV, and, led by
> lenient therapists, do community-singing, then
> the loners, muttering in limbo ...
> ... their generation
> is the first to fade like this, not at home but assigned
> to a numbered frequent ward, stowed out of conscience
> as unpopular luggage.

suburb of New York; the leisurely life of the village has
gone, to be replaced by the hectic and harried anti-life of
New York; Bexleyites no longer have any time, and rarely
spare a thought for the hospital among them; and Mount
Carmel itself has grown sick from hypertrophy, for it is now
a 1,000-bed Institution which has swallowed its grounds; its
windows no longer open on pleasant gardens or country, but
on ant-nest suburbia, or nothing at all.

Still sadder, and more serious, has been the change in its
character, the insidious deterioration in 'atmosphere' and
care. In its earlier days – indeed, before 1960 – the hospital
was both easy-going and secure; there were devoted nurses
and others who had been there for years, and most of the
medical positions were honorary and voluntary, calling forth
the best side, the kindness, of visiting doctors; and though
its patients had grown older and frailer, they could look forward to excursions, day-trips, and summer-camps. In the past
ten years, and especially the last three years, almost all this
has changed. The hospital has assumed somewhat the aspect
of a fortress or prison, in its physical appearance and the
way it is run. A strict Administration has come into being,
rigidly committed to 'efficiency' and rules; 'familiarity'
with patients is strongly discouraged. Law and order have
been ousting fellow-feeling and kinship; hierarchy separates
the inmates from staff; and patients tend to feel they are
'inside', unreachably distant from the real world outside.
There are, of course, gaps in this totalitarian structure, where
real care and affection still maintain a foothold; many of the
'lower' staff – nurses, aides, orderlies, physiotherapists,
occupational therapists, speech therapists, etc. – give themselves unstintingly, and with love, to the patients; volun-
teers from the neighbourhood provide non-professional care;
and, of course, *some* patients are visited by relatives and
friends. The hospital, in short, is a singular mixture, where
freedom and bondage, warmth and coldness, human and

mechanical, life and death, are locked together in perpetual combat.[23]

In 1966, when I first went to Mount Carmel, there were still some eighty post-encephalitic patients there, the larg-

23. We have seen that Parkinsonism and neurosis are innately coercive, and share a similar *coercive structure*. Rigorous institutions are also coercive, being, in effect, *external neuroses*. The coercions of institutions call forth and aggravate the coercions of their inmates: thus one may observe, with exemplary clarity, how the coerciveness of Mount Carmel aggravated neurotic and Parkinsonian tendencies in post-encephalitic patients; one may also observe, with equal clarity, how the 'good' aspects of Mount Carmel – its sympathy and humanity – reduced neurotic and Parkinsonian symptoms.

If we put the matter in political terms (with reference to Locke's *Two Treatises of Government* and Hobbes's *Leviathan*), we might say that Mount Carmel in its 'good' aspects formed a democratic and Lockean federation, while in its 'bad' aspects is formed a despotic and Hobbesian Leviathan. Auden, in one of his last poems, singles out Hobbes as one of the 'clever nasties' who have plagued humanity, and assuredly Leviathan depends upon an atrocious view of human nature – that Man will destroy himself in universal anarchy or war unless forcibly constrained by absolute and unconditional authority. It is upon such a political philosophy that all totalitarian states and total institutions are founded – it is the philosophy of 1984. It is significant and sinister that such a view has also been entertained by many schools of physiology and psychology: thus Hughlings Jackson's theory of *Hierarchy* in the nervous system is a vision of irresponsible and anarchic 'lower centres' which will destroy the organism unless held in check by the monarchic 'higher centres' of the cerebral cortex. (Jackson's views, significantly, were formulated at the time of the Hyde Park riots; as Hobbes's views were also formulated at a time of political chaos and instability.) Similarly, it does not seem too far-fetched to associate Pavlov's hierarchic views – he speaks of 'the blind force' of the subcortex as requiring regulation and 'restraint' by the superior powers of the cortex – with the political ferment of Russia at this time. In a similar fashion, I think that the moral deterioration of Mount Carmel in the sixties, culminating in the authoritarianism and absolutism instituted in 1969, reflected, in miniature, the moral/political deterioration of America at this time, its steady movement towards a Hobbesian state.

est, and perhaps the only, such group remaining in the United States, and one of the very few such groups remaining in the world. Almost half of these patients were immersed in states of pathological 'sleep', virtually speechless and motionless, and requiring total nursing-care; the remainder were less disabled, less dependent, less isolated and less depressed, could look after many of their own basic needs, and maintain a modicum of personal and social life. Sexuality, of course, was forbidden in Mount Carmel.

Between 1966 and 1969, we brought the majority of our post-encephalitic patients (many of whom had been immured in remote, unnoticed bays of the hospital) into a single, organic, and self-governing community; we did what we could to give them the sense of being *people*, and not condemned prisoners in a vast Institution; we instituted a search for missing relatives and friends, hoping that some relationships – broken by time and indolence, rather than hostility and guilt – might thus be re-forged; and I myself formed with them such relationships as I could.

These years, then, saw a certain establishment of sympathies and kinships, and a certain melting-away of the rigid staff/inmate dichotomy; and with these, and all other forms of treatment, a certain – but pitifully limited – improvement in their overall condition, neurological and otherwise. Opposing all forms of therapeutic endeavour, and setting a low ceiling on what could be achieved, was the crushing weight of their illness, the Saturnian gravity of their Parkinsonism, etc; and behind this, and mingling with it, all the dilapidations, impoverishments, and perversions of long isolation and immurement.[24]

24. It is of the greatest interest to compare the state of these patients at Mount Carmel with that of the only existing post-encephalitic community in England (at the Highlands Hospital). Conditions at Highlands – where there are large grounds, free access to and from a neighbouring community, devoted attention, and a much

Some of these patients had achieved a state of icy hopelessness akin to serenity: a realistic hopelessness, in those pre-DOPA days: they *knew* they were doomed, and they accepted this with all the courage and equanimity they could muster. Other patients (and, perhaps, to some extent, all of these patients, whatever their surface serenity) had a fierce and impotent sense of outrage: they had been *swindled* out of the best years of life; they were consumed by the sense of time lost, time *wasted*; and they yearned incessantly for a twofold miracle – not only a cure for their sickness, but an indemnification for the loss of their lives. They wanted to be given back the time they had lost, to be magically replaced in their youth and their prime.

These were their expectations before the coming of L-DOPA.

---

freer and easier atmosphere – are akin to those which obtained at Mount Carmel in its early days. The patients at Highlands (most of whom have been there since the 1920s), although they have severe post-encephalitic syndromes, convey an altogether different appearance from the patients at Mount Carmel. They tend, by and large, to be mercurial, sprightly, impetuous and hyper-active – with vivid and ardent emotional reactions. This is in the greatest contrast to the deeply Parkinsonian, entranced, gravē or withdrawn appearance of so many patients at Mount Carmel. It is clear that both groups of patients have the same disease, and it is equally clear that the *form* and evolution of illness have been quite different in the two groups. My visits to Highlands have always given me the strangest double sense of mixed familiarity and unfamiliarity, as I saw a large group of patients so similar, yet so dissimilar, to ours at Mount Carmel. Nothing has brought home to me so clearly the overwhelming effect which life-style and life-circumstances may have on the development of post-encephalitic illness.

THE COMING OF L-DOPA[25]

L-DOPA is a 'miracle-drug' – the term is used everywhere; and this, perhaps, is scarcely surprising, for the physician who pioneered its use – Dr Cotzias – himself calls L-DOPA 'a true miracle-drug ... of our age'. It is curious to hear sober physicians, and others, in the twentieth century, speaking of 'miracles', and describing a drug in millennial terms. And the fervid enthusiasm aroused by reports of L-DOPA, both in the world at large and among physicians who give it and patients who take it – this too is amazing, and suggests that feelings and phantasies of an extraordinary nature are being excited and indulged. The L-DOPA 'story' has been intimately interwoven, for the last six years, with fervours and feelings of a mystical type; it cannot be understood without reference to these; and it would be quite misleading to present it in purely literal and historical terms.

25. One of the great surprises (or should one say providences?) of nature is that the plant world contains so many substances which have a profound effect upon animals – and yet, apparently, are of no obvious 'use' to the plant. Thus the foxglove (*Digitalis*) contains digitalis glycosides, which are invaluable in the treatment of heart-failure; the autumn crocus (*Colchicum*) contains colchicine, invaluable in the treatment of gout, etc., etc. It is again characteristic that many such 'natural remedies' are discovered at a very early stage of human history, and may form part-and-parcel of a folk-medicine long before their efficacy is allowed by conventional or established medical science. It has recently been established, by chemical analysis, that several species of bean contain large amounts of L-DOPA (of the order of 25 gm. L-DOPA in a pound of beans). There is also a suggestion (which requires careful examination) that such L-DOPA-rich beans may have constituted a 'folk-remedy' for Parkinsonians for many centuries, if not longer. Thus although we ascribe 'The Coming of L-DOPA' to A.D. 1967, it may well have 'come' by 1967 B.C.

We rationalize, we dissimilate, we pretend: we pretend that Modern Medicine is a Rational Science, all facts, no nonsense, and just what it seems. But we have only to tap its glossy veneer for it to split wide open, and reveal to us its roots and foundations, its old dark heart of metaphysics, mysticism, magic and myth. Medicine is the oldest of the arts, and the oldest of the sciences: would one not expect it to spring from the deepest knowledge and feelings we have?

There is, of course, an ordinary medicine, an everyday medicine, humdrum, prosaic, a medicine for stubbed toes, quinsies, bunions and boils; but all of us entertain the idea of *another* sort of medicine, of a wholly different kind: something deeper, older, extraordinary, almost sacred, which will restore to us our lost health and wholeness, and give us a sense of perfect well-being.

For all of us have a basic, intuitive feeling that once we *were* whole and well; at ease, at peace, at home in the world; totally united with the grounds of our being; and that then we lost this primal, happy, innocent state, and fell into our present sickness and suffering. We had something of infinite beauty and preciousness – and we lost it; we spend our lives searching for what we have lost; and one day, perhaps, we will suddenly find it. And this will be the miracle, the millennium!

We may expect to find such ideas most intense in those who are enduring extremities of suffering, sickness, and anguish, in those who are consumed by the sense of what they have lost, or wasted, and by the urgency of recouping before it is too late. Such people, or patients, come to priests or physicians in desperations of yearning, prepared to believe anything for a reprieve, a rescue, a regeneration, a redemption. They are credulous in proportion to their desperation – the predestined victims of quacks and enthusiasts.

This sense of what is lost, and what must be found, is essentially a metaphysical one. If we arrest the patient in his metaphysical search, and ask him *what it is* that he wishes or seeks, he will not give us a tabulated list of items, but will say, simply, 'My happiness', 'My lost health', 'My former condition', 'A sense of reality', 'Feeling fully alive', etc. He does not long for this thing or that; he longs for a *general* change in the complexion of things for everything to be *all right* once again, unblemished, the way it once was. And it is at this point, when he is searching, here and there, with so painful an urgency, that he may be led into a sudden, grotesque mistake; that he may (in Donne's words) mistake 'the Apothecaryes shop' for 'the Metaphoricall Deity': a mistake which the apothecary or physician may be tempted to encourage.

It is at this point that he, ingenuously, and his apothecary and doctor, perhaps disingenuously, together depart from reality, and that the basic metaphysical truth is suddenly twisted (and replaced by a fantastic, mechanical corruption or falsehood). The chimerical concept which now takes its place is one of the delusions of vitalism or materialism, the notion that 'health', 'well-being', 'happiness', etc. can be reduced to certain 'factors' or 'elements' – principles, fluids, humours, commodities – *things* which can be measured and weighed, bought and sold. Health, thus conceived, is reduced to a *level*, something to be titrated or topped-up in a mechanical way. Metaphysics in itself makes no such reductions: its terms are those of organization or design. The fraudulent reduction comes from alchemists, witch-doctors, and their modern equivalents, and from patients who long *at all costs* to be well.

It is from this debased metaphysics that there arises the notion of a mystical substance, a miraculous drug, something which will assuage all our hungers and ills, and deliver us instantly from our miserable state: metaphorical equivalents of the Elixir of Life.[26] Such notions and hopes fully retain today their ancient, magical, mythical force, and – however we may disavow them – show themselves in the very words we use: 'vitamins' (vital amines), and the vitamin-

26. The notion of 'mystical substances' arises from a *reductio ad absurdum* of two world-views which, legitimately employed, have great elegance and power: one is the mosaic or topist view, associated with the philosophies of empiricism and positivism, and the other is a holist or monist view. These derive, respectively, from Aristotelian and Platonic metaphysics. Used with mastery, and a full understanding of their powers and limits, these two world-views have provided a groundwork for fundamental discoveries in physiology and psychology during the past two hundred years.

Mysticism arises by taking analogy for identity – turning similes and metaphors (or 'as' statements) into absolutes (or 'is' statements), converting a useful epistemology into 'absolute truth'. A mystical topism asserts that the world consists of a multitude of points, places, particles or pieces, without intrinsic relation to each other, but 'extrinsically' related by a 'causal nexus': it asserts this both exclusively and conclusively – it is 'the truth', 'the whole truth', and excludes any other 'truth'. Given such a view, one can conceive the possibility of affecting a single point or particle, without the least effect on those surrounding it: one would, for example, be able to *knock out* one point with absolute accuracy and specificity. The therapeutic correlate of such a mysticism is the notion of a *perfect Specific*, which has exactly the effect one wants, and no possibility of any other effects. A famous example of such a supposed Specific is the drug arsephenamine, devised by Ehrlich for the treatment of syphilis. Ehrlich's own modest and realistic claims were immediately distorted by absolutist wishes and tendencies – and arsephenamine was soon dubbed 'The Magic Bullet'. This sort of mystical medicine, then, is dedicated to the search for more and more 'magic bullets'.

A mystical holism, conversely, asserts that the world is an entirely uniform and undifferentiated mass of 'world-stuff', 'primal matter', or plasm. A famous example of such a mystical-holist physiology is exemplified by a dictum ascribed to Flourens: 'The brain is homogeneous like the liver; the brain secretes thought as the liver secretes bile.' The therapeutic correlate of such a monist mysticism is the notion of an all-purpose drug, a Panacea or Catholicon, a Quintessential extract of World-Stuff or Brain-Stuff, absolutely pure bottled Goodness or Godness (or Guinness) – de Quincey's 'portable

cult; or 'biogenic amines' (life-giving amines) – of which dopamine (the biologically active substance into which L-DOPA is converted) is itself an example.

The notion of such mystical, life-giving, sacramental remedies gives rise to innumerable cults and fads, and to enthusiasms of a particularly extravagant and intransigent type. One sees this in Freud's espousal of the drug cocaine;[27] in the first wild reactions to the appearance of cortisone, when some medical conferences, in the words of a contemporary observer, 'more closely resembled revivalist meetings'; in the present world-wide 'drug-scene';[28] and, not

---

ecstasy corked up in a pink-bottle' (*Confessions*, Everyman edition, p. 179).

It should be added that both of these mystical reductions finally boil down to the same thing (nothing), and this is scarcely surprising because they form opposite faces of a two-faced mistake. There is an essential difference between the legitimate, epistemological form of Topism and Holism, and their illegitimate, mystical forms. In the former there is a clear knowledge and acknowledgement of the *episteme* itself – the mode of knowledge, the grounds of conception, and how these lie with respect to the world. The mystical forms resemble delusions or *agnosias*, with overlooking of what they overlook, and denial that they deny: they represent incurable forms of epistemological disease. Such deteriorated epistemologies – as Wittgenstein noted – are like ladders with rotten rungs; one tries to climb up to the 'Truth' with their aid, but the ladder continually gives way beneath one.

27. See Appendix.

28. William James (*Varieties*, pp. 304–8; see Appendix) suggests that one of the primary reasons why people turn to alcohol is to achieve a sense of mystic at-oneness, a return to elemental and primal bliss, and that in this partly metaphysical and partly regressive use it exemplifies the deeply felt need for 'mystagogue' drugs; he quotes with approval the familiar maxim that 'the best cure for dipsomania is religiomania'.

We see from history and anthropology that the craving for mystagogues is universal and ancient, and that a wide knowledge of mystagogues is possessed by all races. The use of mystagogues, in the last century, constituted a literary pastime (and at times a necessity),

least, in our present enthusiasm for the drug L-DOPA. It is impossible to avoid the feeling that here, over and above all legitimate enthusiasms, there is this special enthusiasm, this mysticism, of a magical sort.[29]

We may now pass on to the 'straight' story of L-DOPA, remembering the mystical thread which always winds through it. Parkinson himself looked in vain for the 'seat' or substrate of Parkinsonism, although he tentatively located it in the 'pith' of the lower or medullary parts of the brain. Nor was there any real success in defining the location and nature of the pathological process until a century after the publication of Parkinson's 'Essay'.[30] In 1917 von Economo described the findings of severe damage to the *substantia nigra* (a nucleus in the midbrain, consisting of large

---

and was part-and-parcel of the development of the Romantic Imagination. In our own century, especially in the last twenty years, the use of mystagogues has again become widespread and explicit, Huxley taking mescal to 'cleanse the doors of perception', and Leary promoting LSD as a 'sacramental' drug. Here – as with L-DOPA – one sees the amalgamation of genuine needs with mystical means, the mistaking of an infinite, metaphorical symbol for a finite, ingestible drug.

29. An entertaining, instructive yet pernicious example of this came to my attention when a medical letter of mine ('Incontinent nostalgia due to L-DOPA', *Lancet*, 27 June 1970, p. 1394) was released to the Press, and appeared in more and more garbled and extravagant versions: one paper put into my mouth the amazing claim that I could revive the dead by the use of L-DOPA.

30. There had, in fact, been tentative earlier localizations of a prescient sort, e.g. a famous case, in the 1890s, in which the development of a one-sided Parkinsonism was correlated with the growth of a tuberculoma of one cerebral peduncle; several cases of syphilitic disease of the midbrain, associated with Parkinsonism, etc. The organization of Parkinsonism, indeed, was appreciated, both theoretically and practically, *before* the finding of specific cell-damage: thus two operations for Parkinsonism – cutting the posterior spinal roots, and excising portions of the cerebral cortex – were performed, and found useful, before 1910.

pigmented cells) in a number of patients with *encephalitis lethargica* who had shown severe Parkinsonian symptoms. The following year Greenfield, in England, and pathologists elsewhere, were able to define similar, but milder, changes in these cells in patients who had had ordinary Parkinson's disease. These findings, in company with other pathological and physiological work, suggested the existence of a clearly defined *system*, linking the *substantia nigra* to other parts of the brain: a system whose malfunctioning or destruction might give rise to Parkinsonian symptoms. In Greenfield's words:

... A general survey has shown *paralysis agitans* in its classical form to be a systemic degeneration of a special type affecting a neuronal system whose nodal point is the *substantia nigra*.

In 1920 the Vogts, with remarkable insight, suggested that this anatomically and functionally distinct system might correspond with a *chemically distinct* system, and that a specific treatment for Parkinsonism, and related disorders, might become possible if this hypothetical chemical substance could be identified and administered.

Studies should answer the question [they wrote], whether the striatal system or parts of it do or do not possess a special disposition towards certain injuring agents ... Such a positive or negative tendency to react can be assumed to be ultimately due to the specific chemistry of the corresponding centre. The disclosure of the existence of such specific chemistry represents, in turn, at least the first step towards elucidation of its true nature, thereby initiating the development of a biochemical approach to treatment ...

Thus in the 1920s, there was not merely a vague notion of 'something missing' in Parkinsonism patients (such as Charcot had entertained), but a clear path of research stretching out, pointing towards a prospect of ultimate success.

The most astute clinical neurologists, however, had reservations about this: was there not *structural* damage in the *substantia nigra*, and perhaps elsewhere, damage to nerve-cells and their connections? Could *this* be reversed? Would the administration of the missing chemical substrate be sufficient, or safe, given a marked degree of structural disorganization? Might there not be some danger of over-stimulating or over-loading such cells as were left? These reservations were expressed, with great pungency, by Kinnier Wilson:

Paralysis agitans seems at present an incurable malady *par excellence*; the antidote to the 'local death' of cell-fibre systems would be the equally elusive 'elixir of life' ... It is worse than useless to administer to the Parkinsonian any kind of nerve tonic to 'whip up' his decaying cells; rather must some form of readily assimilable pabulum be sought, in the hope of supplying from without what the cell itself cannot obtain from within.

Neurochemistry, as a science, scarcely existed in the 1920s, and the project envisaged by the Vogts had to await its slow development. The intermediate stages of this research form a fascinating story in themselves, but will be omitted from consideration here. Suffice it that in 1960 Hornykiewicz, in Vienna, and Barbeau, in Montreal, using different approaches, but almost simultaneously, provided clear evidence that the affected parts of the brain in Parkinsonian patients were defective in the nerve-transmitter *dopamine*, and that the transfer and metabolism of dopamine in these areas was also disturbed. Immediate efforts were made to replenish the brain-dopamine in Parkinsonian patients by giving them the natural precursor of dopamine – laevodihydroxyphenylalanine, or L-DOPA (dopamine itself could not pass into the brain). The results of these early therapeutic efforts were encouraging but inconclusive, and seven more years of arduous research had to be undertaken. Early in 1967, Dr Cotzias and his colleagues, in their now-classic paper, were able to report a resounding therapeutic success

in the treatment of Parkinsonism, giving massive doses of
L-DOPA by mouth.[31]

The impact of Dr Cotzias's work was immediate and astounding in the neurological world. The good news spread
quickly. By March 1967, the post-encephalitic and Parkinsonian patients at Mount Carmel had already heard of L-
DOPA: some of them were eager to try it at once; some had
reservations and doubts, and wished to see its effects on
others before they tried it themselves; some expressed total
indifference: and some of course were unable to signal any
reaction.

The cost of L-DOPA in 1967 and 1968 was exceedingly
high (more than £2,000 a pound), and it was impossible for
Mount Carmel – a charity hospital, impoverished, unknown, unattached to any university or foundation, beneath
the notice of drug-firms, industrial, or government sponsors
– to buy L-DOPA at this time. Towards the end of 1968, the
cost of L-DOPA started a sharp decline, and in March 1969
it was first used at Mount Carmel. The cases that follow are
a sample of the stories of more than 200 patients to whom I
administered L-DOPA during the next three years.

31. Dr Cotzias's first work used DL-DOPA, a mixture of the biologically active L-DOPA with its inactive isomer D-DOPA. The
separation of these two isomers, in 1966–7, was not easily accomplished, and was exceedingly costly.

AWAKENINGS

1. FRANCES D.

Miss D. was born in New York in 1904, the youngest and brightest of four children. She was a brilliant student at High School until her life was cut across, in her fifteenth year, by a severe attack of *encephalitis lethargica* of the relatively rare hyperkinetic form. During the six months of her acute illness she suffered intense insomnia (she would remain very wakeful until four in the morning, and then secure at most two or three hours' sleep), marked restlessness (fidgeting, distractible and hyperkinetic throughout her waking hours, tossing-and-turning throughout her sleeping hours) and impulsiveness (sudden urges to perform actions which seemed to her senseless, which for the most part she could restrain by conscious effort). This acute syndrome was considered to be 'neurotic', despite clear evidence of her previously well-integrated personality and harmonious family life.

By the end of 1919, restlessness and sleep-disorder had subsided sufficiently to allow resumption and finishing of High School, although they continued to affect Miss D. more mildly for a further two years. Shortly after the end of her acute illness, Miss D. started to have 'panting attacks', at first coming on two or three times a week, apparently spontaneously, and lasting many hours; subsequently becoming rarer, briefer, milder, and more clearly periodic (they would usually occur on Fridays) or circumstantial (they were especially prone to occur in circumstances of anger and frustration). These respiratory crises (as they clearly were, although they also were termed 'neurotic' at the time) became rarer and rarer, and ceased to occur entirely after 1924. Miss D., indeed, made no spontaneous mention of these attacks when first seen by me, and it was only later, when being questioned in greater detail before the administration of L-DOPA, that she recollected these attacks of half a century previously.

Following the last of her respiratory crises, Miss D. had the first of her oculogyric crises, and these indeed continued to be her sole post-encephalitic symptom for twenty-five years (1924–49), during which time Miss D. followed a varied and successful career as a legal secretary, as an active committee-woman in social and civic affairs, etc. She led a full life, with many friends, and frequent entertaining; she was fond of theatre, an avid reader, a collector of old china, etc. Talented, popular, energetic, well-integrated emotionally, Miss D. thus showed no sign of the 'deterioration' said to be so common after severe encephalitis of the hyperkinetic type.

About twenty years ago, Miss D. started to develop a more sinister set of symptoms; in particular a tendency to freeze in her movements and speech, and a contrary tendency to hurry in her walking, speech, and handwriting. When in 1969 I first asked Miss D. about her symptoms she gave me the following answer: 'I have various banal symptoms which you can see for yourself. But my *essential* symptom is that I cannot start and I cannot stop. Either I am held still, or I am forced to accelerate. I no longer seem to have any in-between states.' This statement sums up the paradoxical symptoms of Parkinsonism with perfect precision. It is instructive, therefore, that in the absence of 'banal' symptoms (e.g. rigidity, tremor, etc., which only became evident in 1963), the diagnosis of Parkinsonism failed to be made, but that a large variety of other diagnoses (such as 'catatonia', 'hysteria') were offered. Miss D. was finally labelled Parkinsonian in 1964.

Her oculogyric crises, to return to this cardinal symptom, were originally of great severity, coming many times a month and lasting up to fifteen hours each. Within a few months of their onset they had settled down to a fairly strict periodicity, coming 'like clockwork' every fifth day, so much so that Miss D. could plan a calendar for months in advance, knowing that she would inevitably have a crisis every five days, and only very occasionally at other times. The rare departures from this schedule which occurred were usually associated with circumstances of great annoyance or distress. The crisis would occur abruptly, without warning, her gaze being forced first downwards or to either side for several minutes, and then suddenly upwards, where it would stay for the remainder of the attack. Miss D. stated that her face would assume 'a fixed angry or scared expression' during these attacks, although she experienced neither rage nor fear while they lasted. Movement would be difficult during a crisis, her voice would be abnormally soft, and her thoughts seemed to 'stick'; she would always experience a 'feeling of resistance', a force which opposed movement, speech and thought, during the attack. She would also feel intensely wakeful in each attack, and find it impossible to sleep; as the crises neared their termination, she would start to yawn and become intensely drowsy; the attack would finally end quite suddenly, with restoration of normal movement, speech, and thought (this sudden restoration of normal consciousness Miss D. – a crossword addict – would call 'resipiscence'). In addition to these classical oculogyric crises, Miss D. started to experience a number of variant crises after 1955: forced deviation of gaze became exceptional, being replaced by a fixed and stony stare; some of these staring attacks were of overwhelming severity, completely depriving her of movement and speech, and lasting up to three days. She was admitted to a municipal hospital on several occasions during the 1960s when neighbours had discovered her in these attacks, and she was displayed at staff meetings as a striking case of 'periodic catatonia'. Since 1962, Miss D. has also had brief staring attacks, lasting only a few minutes, in which she is arrested and feels 'entranced'. Yet another paroxysmal symptom has been attacks of flushing and sweating, coming on at irregular intervals, and lasting fifteen to thirty minutes. (Miss D. had completed her menopause in the mid 1940s.) Since 1965, staring and oculogyric crises had become mild and infrequent, and when admitted to Mount Carmel Hospital at the start of 1969, Miss D. had been free of them for more than a year, and continued to be exempt from them until given L-DOPA in June 1969.

Although, as mentioned, rigidity and tremor had appeared in 1963, the most disabling of Miss D.'s symptoms, and the ones which finally necessitated her admission to a chronic disease hospital, were threefold: a progressive flexion-dystonia of the neck and trunk, uncontrollable festination and forced running, backwards or forwards, and uncontrollable 'freezing' which would sometimes arrest her in awkward positions for hours on end. A further symptom of relatively recent onset, for which no local infective aetiology could be found, was urinary frequency and urge; sometimes this urge would coexist with or call forth a 'block' or 'reluctance' of micturition – an intolerable coupling of opposing symptoms.

On admission to Mount Carmel Hospital, in January 1969, Miss D. was able to walk freely using two sticks, or for short distances alone; by June 1969, she had become virtually unable to walk by herself alone. Her posture, which was bent on admission, had become almost doubled-up over the course of the following six months. Transferring from bed to chair had become impossible, as had turning over in bed, or cutting up food. In view of this rather rapid deterioration, and the uselessness of all conventional anti-Parkinson drugs, the advent of L-DOPA came at a critical time for Miss D.,

who seemed about to slip into an accelerating and irrevocable
decline.

Before L-DOPA

Miss D. was a tiny, bent woman, so kyphotic that, on standing, her face was forced to gaze at the ground. She was able
to raise her head briefly, but it would return within seconds
to its habitual position of extreme emprosthotonos, with the
chin wedged down on the sternum. This habitual posture
could not be accounted for by rigidity of the cervical muscles:
rigidity was not more than slightly increased in the neck,
and in oculogyric crises her head would be forced backwards
to an equally extreme degree.

There was quite severe masking of the face, alertness and
emotional expression being conveyed almost exclusively by
Miss D.'s quick-glancing, humorous eyes – anomalously mobile in her mask-like face. Spontaneous blinking was rare.
Her voice was clear and intelligible, although it was monotonous in volume and timbre, lacked 'personal' intonations
and inflections, and could only momentarily be raised above
a whispering and hushed hypophonic intensity; at intervals
there would be sudden vocal hurries and festinations, accelerated rushes of words sometimes terminating in a verbal
'crash' at the end of a sentence.

Voluntary movement elsewhere, like speech, was characterized by the contradictory features of akinesia and hyper-
kinesis, either alternating or in paradoxical simultaneity.
Most hand movements were marked by akinesia – with
feebleness, parsimony, excessive effort, and decay on repetition of the movement. Her handwriting, once started, was
large, effortless and rapid; but if Miss D. became over-excited,
her writing would slip out of control, either becoming larger
and faster and more violent until it covered the entire paper
with eddies and scrawls, or smaller and slower and stickier
until it became a motionless point. She could rise from her

chair without impediment, but having risen would tend to 'freeze', often for many minutes, unable to take the first step. At such times she would display an almost cataleptic fixity of posture, almost doubled-over, and resembling a film which had come to a stop. Once a first step was taken – and walking could be inaugurated by a little push from behind, a verbal command from the examiner, or a visual command in the form of a stick, a piece of paper, or something definite to step over on the floor – Miss D. would teeter forward in tiny rapid steps. Six months previously, on her admission, when walking had been altogether easier, festination had represented a most serious problem, always tending to end (like her verbal stampedes and accelerating scrawls) in catastrophe. In remarkable contrast was her excellent ability to climb stairs stably and steadily, each stair providing a stimulus to a step; having reached the top of the stairs, however, Miss D. would again find herself 'frozen' and unable to proceed. She often remarked that 'if the world consisted entirely of stairs', she would have no difficulty getting around whatever.[1] Pulsion in all directions (propulsion, lateropul-

1. Miss D.'s ability to climb stairs in a regular and controlled fashion, which stood in the most dramatic contrast with her irregular and uncontrollable tendencies to hurry or freeze in her walking, furnishes us with our first example of the use, and indeed the necessity, of *external means* to activate Parkinsonian patients, and to regulate or control their activity. Such direct methods of activation and regulation – direct in that they concern themselves directly with the actual behavioural and experiential disorders of Parkinsonism, and not with its chemical or anatomical substrate – are of fundamental importance, both theoretically and practically, in helping us to understand, and through understanding to help, Parkinsonian patients. Such direct methods are discovered, or can be learned (and *should* be learned!) by all Parkinsonian patients, by their friends and relatives, by their physicians and nurses, by all who come into close contact with them; they are easy, and often delightful, to learn; they can make a literally vital difference to the lives of Parkinsonian patients; and they form an essential complement to the use of L-DOPA.

sion, retropulsion) could all be elicited with dangerous ease. Severe and protracted freezing would also tend to occur when any switch of activity was necessitated: this was most obvious in her walking, when she had to turn, but also

---

This is a theme which will be touched on again and again in the course of this book (see, especially, the footnotes to p. 85 and p. 323).

We have noted (p. 32 *et seq.*) that Parkinsonian patients suffer from both 'negative' and 'positive' troubles (a particular and profound form of 'negative phenomenon' is not adequately described in the classical literature, and is described for the first time on p. 141 of this book). We have noted too – a point which will require amplification later – that the problems of Parkinsonism are not 'purely motor' (as is usually taught), any more than they are 'purely mental' (both sets of terms are nonsensical); we have started to realize, and will see more and more clearly, that Parkinsonism affects the very basis of action and perception, *being itself*, in absolutely characteristic ways; that the 'negative' phenomena of Parkinsonism are peculiar deficiencies of being ('unbeing'), and the 'positive' phenomena peculiar distortions of being ('misbeing'), – and that these ontological deficits and distortions are profoundly akin to those of psychoneurosis in some ways, and profoundly different in others.

The central problem in all Parkinsonian disorders is *passivity* – passivity *and* pulsivity, i.e. inertia – as the central cure for them all is *activity* (of the right kind). The essence of this passivity lies in peculiar difficulties of self-stimulation, and initiation, not in the capacity to respond to stimulation. This means, in the severest cases, that the patient is totally unable to help himself, although he can very easily be helped by other people, or other means, outside himself; in less severe cases (as Luria has never ceased to stress) the Parkinsonian patient *can* help himself in a limited fashion, by using his normal and active powers to regulate his pathological or 'de-activated' ones. Thus a Parkinsonian patient may be totally mute unless spoken to, when he may be able to reply with perfect facility; he may be motionless unless motioned to, when he immediately makes a motor reply (waving, gesticulating, rising to meet one); he may be mute and motionless in a silent environment, but sing and dance perfectly if music is provided; he may (like Frances D.) remain frozen in one spot, or helplessly festinant, unless steps are provided, or regular marks, in which case he may use them with perfect facility.

This problem of passivity, of needing a continuing stimulus to

showed itself, on occasion, when she had to shift her glance from one place to another, or her attention from one idea to another.

Rigidity and tremor were not particularly prominent in

---

follow, affects all Parkinsonian patients, irrespective of the origin or severity of their illness. It is currently being studied by Richard Gregory, who has shown, with great simplicity and elegance, that while a Parkinsonian patient can track a moving stimulus with perfect accuracy, he immediately comes to a stop if the stimulus stops, and cannot resume until the stimulus resumes. This occurs even if the stimulus is of a highly predictable sort, e.g. a simple sinusoidal wave. The patient *understands* what he has to do perfectly well, but despite understanding he cannot *undertake* – he needs the continuous presence of the stimulus-wave. Frequently, and deplorably, Parkinsonian patients may be regarded as 'stupid', in view of their peculiar difficulties in undertaking simple tasks; but we see from these experiments, and from clinical observations, that this is in no sense a real stupidity or lack of ideas (as happens with the apraxias of cortical injury, or with lack of specific training or skills), but a pseudostupidity – a loss of initiative.

The problem, then, is to provide a continual stimulus of the appropriate kind – and if we can achieve this we can recall Parkinsonians from inactivity (or abnormal activity) into normal activity, and from the abyss of unbeing into normal being. '*Qui non agit non existit*': when the Parkinsonian is not active he does not exist – when we recall him to activity we recall him to life.

We may use alternative terms, and say that the problem of activation is one of *order* or *organization*, of finding forms of order or organization which will combat the specific *disorders* and *disorganizations* which constitute Parkinsonism. We observe of Parkinsonians that either they fail to move at all, or they move wrongly, and that the wrongness of their movements is a wrongness of *scale* – their movements are too large or too small, too fast or too slow. Thus what the Parkinsonian needs, and what we must give him, is *measure* (or metric), so that he can overcome his peculiar deficiencies or distortions of measuring (his '*ametria*' and '*dysmetria*').

What is a measure – and how do we measure? We create and use two sorts of measure: measures that are abstract, absolute and formal (measuring-sticks and pendulums, rulers and clocks, the C.G.S. measures of engineering and physics); or measures that are concrete,

the clinical picture. A coarse (flapping) tremor of the right hand would occur, rather rarely, in response to physical or emotional tension: it tended to come on, most characteristically, with the futile effort and distress of freezing. There was mild hypertonia of the left arm and marked ('hemiplegic') hypertonia of the legs. There was also a suggestion of hyper-reflexia and spasticity on the left side of the body. The clinical picture was completed by a number of spontaneous movements and hyperkineses. The muscles about the mouth exhibited puckering movements and occasional pursings and poutings of the lips. There was occasional grinding of the teeth and masticatory movements. Her head was never held quite still, but bobbed and nodded in an irregular fashion. These mouth and head movements were aggravated,

---

actual, and active – measures that relate to our environment and ourselves. ('Man is the measure of all things,' said da Vinci.) Both come together, for example, in the concept of 'a foot', which was at first a living, practical measure, based on the size of a human foot, and then a precise and abstract measure, the distance between two marks on a rigid, lifeless rod.

So, in the most general terms, we find that ametric-dysmetric Parkinsonian patients can be activated and regulated, ordered and organized, by either sort of measure: by regular marks in a conventional, formal (and linear) space-time, e.g. stairs, steps painted on the ground, clocks, metronomes, and devices that *count* in a simple, regular and orderly manner; or by co-action and co-ordination with a concrete, living activity or agent. Thus, in the case of Miss D., the chalking of regular lines on the ground enabled her to walk stably, but like a puppet or robot; but taking her arm, and strolling with her, enabled her to stroll like a normal human being. The first form of treatment is *kinetic*, the second *mimetic*. The first is directed to *the scale of motion*, the second to *the shape of action*. Parkinsonism, at its severest, presents itself as an akinetic amimia (as opposed to certain cortical disorders which are amimic akinesias). Since right mimesis *entails* right kinesis, whereas kinesia *per se* entails only itself, the best form of therapy is mimetic, kinetic therapy constituting a second best – a prosthetic or algorithmic substitute (like a wooden leg, or an artificial pace-maker).

synkinetically, during effort. Every so often, perhaps five or six times an hour, Miss D. would be impelled to take a sudden, deep, tic-like inspiration. A residue of the original restlessness and akathisia could be observed in the incessant fidgeting shown by her right hand, a local restlessness which was stilled only when the hands were otherwise occupied.

Miss D. was exceedingly alert and observant of all that went on about her, but not pathologically vigilant or insomniac. She was clearly of superior intelligence, witty and precise in her speech, and without significant stereotypy or stickiness of thought save, as indicated, in her crises. She was notably exact, orderly, punctual, and methodical in all her activities, but showed no severe obsessional symptoms such as fixed compulsions or phobias.

She had continued to maintain, despite being institutionalized, a healthy self-respect, many interests and a close attention to her environment, providing a focus of stability and humour and compassion on a large ward of disabled and sometimes very disturbed post-encephalitic patients.

She was started on L-DOPA on 25 June 1969.

Course on L-DOPA

30 June. Although this was only five days after the start of treatment, and Miss D. was receiving no more than 0·5 gm. of L-DOPA daily, she exhibited some general restlessness, increased fidgeting of the right hand, and masticatory movements. The puckering of circumoral muscles had become more pronounced and now showed itself to be a form of compulsive grimace, or tic. There was already an obvious increase of general activity: Miss D. was now always, but always, doing something – crocheting (which had been slow and difficult before administration of the drug), washing clothes, writing letters, etc. She seemed somewhat *driven*, and unable to tolerate inactivity. Miss D. also complained even at this very early stage of 'difficulty in catching the breath', and showed a tachypnoea of forty breaths to the minute, without variation in the force or rhythm of breathing.

6 *July*. On the eleventh day of drug-trial, and receiving 2 gm. L-DOPA daily, Miss D. now exhibited a complex mixture of desirable and adverse effects. Among the good effects she showed a sense of well-being and abounding energy, a much stronger voice, less freezing, less postural flexion, and stabler walking with longer strides. Among the adverse effects she showed aggravation of her former mild chewing and biting movements, so that she incessantly chewed on her gums, which had become very sore; increased fidgeting of her right hand, to which was now added a tic-like flexion and extension of the forefinger; finally, and most distressing to her, a disintegration of the normal automatic controls of breathing. Her breathing had now become rapid, shallow, and irregular, and was broken up by sudden violent inspirations two or three times a minute, each of which would follow a sudden, powerful, and fully conscious though uncontrollable *urge* to breathe. Miss D. remarked at this time: 'My breathing is no longer automatic. I have to think about each breath, and every so often I am *forced* to gasp.'

In view of these adverse symptoms, the dosage was reduced on this day. Over the ensuing ten days, on a dose of 1·5 gm. L-DOPA daily, Miss D. maintained the desirable effects of the drug and showed less restlessness, chewing, and pressure of activity. Her respiratory symptoms, however, persisted, growing more pronounced daily, finally differentiating, around 10 July, into clear-cut respiratory crises. These attacks would start, without any warning whatever, with a sudden inspiratory gasp; followed by forced breath-holding for ten to fifteen seconds, then a violent expiration, and finally an apnoeic pause for ten to fifteen seconds. In these early and relatively mild attacks there were no associated symptoms or autonomic disturbances (e.g. tachycardia, hyperten-

sion, sweating, trembling, apprehension, etc.). This strange
and distorted form of breathing could be interrupted for a
minute or two by a strong effort of will, but would then resume its bizarre and imperative character. Her crises would
last between one and three hours, finally subsiding over a
period of about five minutes, with resumption of normal,
automatic, unconscious breathing of even rate, rhythm, and
force. The timing of these attacks was of interest, for it bore
no constant relationship to the times at which L-DOPA was
administered. Thus, for the first five days of respiratory
crises, attacks occurred invariably in the evening and at no
other times. On 15 July, for the first time, an attack occurred
in the afternoon (at 1 p.m., an hour after L-DOPA had been
given): on 16 July, for the first time, an attack occurred very
early in the morning, before the first daily dose of L-DOPA
had been taken. Subsequently, two or three attacks would
occur every day, although the evening attacks continued to
be the longest and severest.

On 16 July, I observed that the attacks were now assum-
ing a most frightening intensity. A violent and protracted
gasp (which looked and sounded as desperate as that of a
nearly drowned man finally coming to the surface for a lung-
ful of air) would be followed by forced breath-holding for
up to fifty seconds, during which time Miss D. would struggle to expel breath through a closed glottis, in so doing becoming purple and congested from the futile effort; finally
the breath would be expelled with tremendous violence,
making a noise like the boom of a gun. No voluntary control
whatever was possible at this time; in Miss D.'s words: 'I can
no more control it than I could control a spring tide. I just
ride it out, and wait for the storm to clear.' During this crisis
speech was, of course, quite impossible, and there was a clear
increase of rigidity throughout the body. The pulse-rate was
raised to 120, and the blood-pressure rose from its normal
130/75 to 170/100. Twenty mg. of benadryl, given intra-

venously, failed to alter the course of this attack. Despite
what I would have imagined was a terrifying experience, and
an expression of terror on her face, Miss D. denied that any
alteration of thinking or special apprehension had been experienced during the crisis. Greatly concerned about the possible effects of so violent an attack in an elderly patient, I was
disposed at this time to discontinue the L-DOPA. But, at Miss
D.'s insistence, in view of the real benefits she was obtaining
from the drug, and in the hope that her respiratory instability might decrease, I contented myself with reducing its dosage to 1·0 gm. daily.

Despite this small dosage, Miss D. continued to have respiratory crises of varying severity, two or more commonly
three times a day. Within two or three days, these had established a routine – a crisis at 9 a.m., a crisis at noon, and
a crisis at 7.30 p.m. – which remained fixed despite chance
and systematic alterations of the times at which she would
receive L-DOPA. We had also come to suspect, by 21 July,
that her respiratory crises were readily conditionable: on
this day our speech-therapist stopped to talk to Miss D. at
five in the afternoon (normally a crisis-free time), and inquired whether she had had any crises recently; before Miss
D. could begin to frame an answer, she was impelled to
gasp violently and launch into an unexpected crisis which
seemed suspiciously like an answer to the question.

By now a therapeutic dilemma was becoming clear. There
was no doubt of the enormous benefit derived from L-DOPA:
Miss D. was looking, feeling and moving far better than
she had done in twenty years; but she had also become over-
excitable and odd in her behaviour, and in particular seemed
to be experiencing a revival or revocation of an idiosyncratic
respiratory sensitivity (or behaviour) which had lain dormant in her for forty-five years. There was also, even in her
first month of treatment, a number of minor 'side-effects'
(a term which I found it increasingly difficult to give any

meaning to), with the promise (or threat) of others lurking
in posse – as I imagined it – in an as-yet unactualized state.
Could we find a happy medium, an in-between state and
dosage which would greatly assist Miss D. *without* calling
forth her respiratory symptoms and other 'side-effects'?

Once more (on 19 July) the dosage was reduced – to a
mere 0·9 gm. of L-DOPA daily. This reduction was promptly
followed, that very day, by the occurrence of an oculogyric
crisis – Miss D.'s first such in almost three years. This was
disconcerting, because we had already observed, in several
other post-encephalitic patients, a situation in which any
given therapeutic dose of L-DOPA evoked respiratory crises,
and any lessening of this dose oculogyric crises, and we
feared that Miss D., too, might have to walk a tightrope
between these two disagreeable alternatives.

Although the reported experience of others encouraged
us to suppose that one could 'balance' or 'titrate' patients
by finding exactly the right dose of L-DOPA, our experience with Miss D. – at this time – suggested that she could
no more be 'balanced' than a pin on its point. Her oculogyric crisis, which was severe, was at once followed by a second
and third oculogyric crises; with increase of the L-DOPA to
0·95 gm. a day, *these* crises ceased, but respiratory crises returned; with diminution of L-DOPA to 0·925 gm. a day
(we were forced, at this stage, to encapsulate L-DOPA ourselves, in order to allow these infinitesimal increments and
decrements of dose), the reverse switch occurred; and at a
dose of 0·9375 gm. a day, she experienced *both* forms of
crisis, in alternation, or simultaneously.

It became clear, at this time, that Miss D.'s crises, which
were now occurring several times a day, showed a close association not only with overall psycho-physiological state,
mood, and circumstance, but with certain specific dynamics,
and in this way acted like migraines, and even like hysterical symptoms. If Miss D. had had a poor night and was tired,

crises were more likely; if she was in pain (an ingrown toe-nail was troubling her at this time), she tended to have a crisis; if she became excited, she was especially prone to have a crisis, whether the excitement was fearful, angry or hilarious in character; when she became frustrated, she exhibited crises; and when she desired attention from the nursing staff, she developed a crisis. I was slow to realize, while noting the causes of Miss D.'s crises, that the most potent 'trigger' of all was me, myself: I had indeed observed that as soon as I entered her room, or as soon as she caught sight of me, she usually had a crisis, but assumed that this was due to some other cause I had failed to notice, and it was only when an observant nurse giggled and remarked to me, 'Dr Sacks, *you* are the object of Miss D.'s crises!', that I belatedly tumbled to the truth. When I asked Miss D. if this could be the case, she indignantly denied the very possibility, but blushed an affirmative crimson. There was, finally, one other neurotic cause of her crises which I could not have known of had Miss D. not mentioned it to me: 'As soon as I *think of getting a crisis,*' she confessed, 'I am apt to get one. And if I try to think of not getting a crisis, I get one. And if I try to think about not thinking about my crises, I get one. Do you suppose they are becoming an obsession?'

In the final week of July, Miss D.'s well-being was compromised not only by these crises, but by a number of other symptoms and signs, which increased in number and variety from day to day, and almost from hour to hour – a pathological blossoming, or ebullience, which could not be stopped and which could scarcely be modified, however we subdivided or timed the daily dose. Her respiratory crises, in their most florid form, became quite frightening to watch. Her breath-holding increased in duration to almost a minute; her expirations became complicated by stridor, forced retching, and forced phonations ('Oouuggh!'). At times, the rhythm would be broken by a run of forty or fifty quick dog-like pants. Now, for the first time, Miss D. started to experience some apprehension during these attacks, and maintained that it was 'not a normal fear', but 'a special, strange sort of fear' which seemed to flood over her, and which was wholly unlike anything she had ever experienced before. I repeatedly suggested to her that the L-DOPA should be stopped, but Miss D. fiercely insisted that it must not be stopped, that everything would 'work itself out', and – on one occasion – that stopping the drug would be 'like a death-penalty'. In this way, and in others, Miss D. indicated that she was no longer (or, at least, not always) her usual, reasonable self, but that she was moving towards a state of passion, intransigence, obstinacy and obsession.

On 23 July, she experienced a new symptom. She had just washed her hands (she now felt a 'need' to wash them thirty times daily), and was about to walk to supper, when she suddenly found that she could not lift her feet from the ground, and that the more she fought to do so, the more they 'attached themselves' to the ground. Her feet were 're-leased', quite suddenly and spontaneously, after about ten minutes. Miss D. was alarmed, annoyed and amused at this novel experience: 'It's like my feet rebelled against me,' she said. 'It's like they had a will of their own. I was glued there, you know. I felt like a fly caught on a strip of fly-paper.' And later that evening she added, musingly: 'I have often read about people being *rooted to the spot*, but I never knew what it meant – not until today.'

Other impulses and transfixions appeared in the ensu-ing days, usually quite abruptly, and without the slightest warning. Miss D. would lift a tea-cup to her mouth, and find herself unable to put it down; she would reach for the sugar-bowl, and find her hand 'stuck' to the bowl; when doing crosswords, she would find herself staring at a particular word, and be unable to shift either her gaze or her attention from it; and, most disquietingly (not only for herself but for others), she would at times feel 'compelled' to gaze into someone else's eyes: 'Whenever I do this,' she explained, disarmingly, 'it stops me getting an oculogyric crisis.' Her inclination to munch and gnaw grew greater and greater: she would chew and over-chew her food, with a growling noise, like a dog with a bone, and in the absence of food would bite her lips, or gnash her teeth. It was extraordinary to see such activity in this refined and elderly lady, and Miss D. herself was very conscious of the incongruity: 'I am a quiet person,' she expostulated on one occasion. 'I could be a distinguished maiden-aunt. And now look at me! I bite and chew like a ravenous animal, and there's nothing I can do about it.' It seemed, indeed, during these last days of July, that Miss D. was being 'possessed' or taken over by a mass of strange and almost sub-human compulsions; and she herself confided this dark thought to her diary, although she forbore to express it aloud.

And yet – there were good days, or at least one good day. On 28 July, during an eagerly awaited and greatly enjoyed day-trip to the country, Miss D. spent the entire day without so much as a hint of respiratory abnormality, oculogyria, or any other of her myriad abnormalities. She returned from this in a most radiant mood, and exclaimed: 'What a perfect day – so peaceful – I shall never forget it! It's a joy to be alive on a day like this. And I do feel alive, more truly alive than I've felt in twenty years. If this is what L-DOPA can do, it's an absolute blessing!'

The following day saw the onset of the worst and most protracted crisis of Miss D.'s entire life. Sixty hours were spent in a state of virtually continuous respiratory crisis. This was accompanied, not only by her 'usual' spasms and compulsions, but by a host of other symptoms never before experienced. Her limbs and trunk repeatedly became 'jammed' in peculiar postures, and fiercely resisted both active and passive attempts to dislodge them. This absolute con-

straint was accompanied by a most intense, and almost frenzied, urge to move, so that Miss D., though motionless, was
locked in a violent struggle with herself. She could not tolerate the idea of bed, and screamed incessantly unless left in
her chair. Every so often she would burst loose from her
'jammed' state, and catapult forwards for a few steps only
to 'jam' once more, as if she had suddenly run into an invisible wall. She exhibited extreme pressure of speech, and
now showed, for the first time, an uncontrollable tendency
to repeat words and phrases again and again (palilalia). Her
voice, normally low-pitched and soft, rose to a shrill and pier-
cing scream. When she was jammed in awkward positions
she would scream: 'My arms, my arms, my arms, my arms,
please move my arms, my arms, move my arms . . .' Her excitement seemed to come in waves, each wave rising higher
and higher towards some limitless climax, and with these
waves a mixture of anguish and terror and shame overwhelmed her, to which she gave voice in palilalic screamings:
'Oh, oh, oh, oh ! . . . please don't . . . I'm not myself, not myself . . . It's not me, not me, not me at all.'

This crescendo of excitement responded only to massive
doses of parenteral barbiturates, and these would allow only
a few minutes of exhausted sleep, with resumption of all
symptoms immediately on waking. Her L-DOPA, of course,
had been stopped with the inauguration of this monstrous
crisis.

Finally, on 31 July, Miss D. sank naturally into a deep
and almost comatose sleep, from which she awoke after
twenty-four hours. She had no crises on 2 and 3 August, but
was intensely Parkinsonian (far more than she had ever
been before the administration of L-DOPA), and painfully
depressed, although she still showed a ghost of her old pluck
and humour: 'That L-DOPA,' she whispered (for she was
now almost voiceless), 'that stuff should be given its proper
name – Hell-DOPA !'

1969–72

During August 1969 Miss D. remained in a subterranean state: 'She looks almost dazed at times,' our speech-pathologist, Miss Kohl, wrote to me, 'like someone who has come back from the front line, like a soldier with shell-shock.' During this shock-like period, which lasted about ten days, Miss D. continued to show an exacerbation of her Parkinsonism so extreme that she could perform none of the elementary activity of daily life without help from the nursing staff. For the remainder of the month, she was less Parkinsonian (though still far more so than she had been before the administration of L-DOPA), but quite deeply and painfully depressed. She had little appetite ('She seems to have no appetite for *anything*,' wrote Miss Kohl; 'really no appetite for living. She was like a blow-torch before, and now she's like a candle guttering out. You would never believe the difference'), and lost twenty pounds, and when I returned to New York in September – having been away for a month – I did in fact momentarily fail to recognize the pale, shrunken, and somehow caved-in figure of Miss D.

Before the summer, Miss D., despite her half-century of illness, had always been active and perky, and had seemed considerably younger than her sixty-five years; now she was not only wasted and far more Parkinsonian than I had ever seen her, but frighteningly *aged*, as if she had fallen through another half-century in the month I was away. She looked like an escapee from Shangri-La.

In the months following my return Miss D. spoke to me at length about this month; her candour, courage and insight provided a convincing analysis of how and *why* she felt as she did; and since her state (I believe) shares essential qualities and determinants with the 'post-DOPA' states experienced by many other Parkinsonian patients (though, of course, it was notably more severe than the majority of

patients experience or can expect to experience) I shall interrupt her 'story' for her analysis of the situation.

Miss D. stressed, first, the extreme feeling of 'let-down'
produced by the sudden withdrawal of the drugs: 'I'd done a
vertical take-off,' she said. 'I had gone higher and higher on
L-DOPA – to an impossible height. I felt I was on a pinnacle
a million miles high ... And then, with the boost taken
away, I crashed, and I didn't just crash to the ground, I shot
way in the other direction, until I was buried a million miles
deep in the ground.'

Secondly, Miss D. spoke (as has every patient of mine
who has been through a comparable experience) of the
bewilderment, uncertainty, anxiety, anger and disappointment which assailed her when the L-DOPA 'started to go
wrong'; when it produced more and more 'side-effects'
which I – we, her doctors – seemed powerless to prevent, despite all our reassurances, and all our fiddlings and manipulations with the dosage; and finally, the extremity of her
hopelessness when the L-DOPA was stopped, an act which she
saw as a final verdict or decree: something which said in
effect, 'This patient has had her chance and lost it. We gave
her the magic and it failed. We now wash our hands of
her, and consign her to her fate.'

A third aspect of the L-DOPA 'situation' was alluded to
again and again by Miss D. (especially in a remarkable diary
she kept at this time and of which she showed me portions).
This was an acute, an almost intolerable exacerbation of certain feelings which had haunted her at intervals throughout
her illness,[2] and which rose to a climax during the final days
of L-DOPA administration and the period immediately fol-

2. I think such feelings haunt *all* patients who find themselves,
their very sense of 'self', grotesquely changed by illness or other
circumstances, but perhaps post-encephalitic and schizophrenic
patients most of all, for they suffer the greatest ontological outrage,
the most intense and 'inexplicable' assaults on the citadel of the
self.

lowing withdrawal of the drug. These were feelings of astonishment, rage, and terror that *such things could happen to
her*, and feelings of impotent outrage that she, Miss D., could
do nothing about these things. But deeper and still more
threatening feelings were involved: some of the 'things'
which gripped her under the influence of L-DOPA – in particular, her gnawing and biting compulsions,[3] certain violent
appetites and passions, and certain obsessive ideas and images – could not be dismissed by her as 'purely physical' or
completely 'alien' to her 'real self', but, on the contrary,
were felt to be in some sense *releases* or *exposures* or *disclo-
sures* or *confessions* of very deep and ancient parts of herself, monstrous creatures from her unconscious and from
unimaginable physiological depths below the unconscious,
pre-historic and perhaps pre-human landscapes whose features were at once utterly strange to her, yet mysteriously
familiar, in the manner of certain dreams. And she could
not look upon these suddenly exposed parts of herself with
detachment; they called to her with Siren voices, they enticed
her, they thrilled her, they terrified her, they filled her with
feelings of guilt and punishment, they possessed her with the
consuming, ravishing power of nightmare.

3. Such gnawing and biting compulsions, along with gnashing and
grinding of the teeth, and a great variety of other abnormal or abnormally perseverative mouth-movements, are among the commonest
'side-effects' of L-DOPA. Such movements may be quite irresistible,
of great violence, and liable to inflict considerable damage upon the
gums, tongue, teeth, etc. (See 'Abnormal Mouth-Movements and
Oral Damage Associated with L-DOPA Treatment', by Sacks *et al.*,
Annals of Dentistry, 29, 1970, pp. 130–44). In addition to local damage, such compulsions – like other forms of compulsive scratching,
hurting, tickling and 'titillation' generally – may evoke an intense
and ambivalent mixture of pleasure and pain, and thus form the
nucleus of ever more complex hedonic, algolagnic and sado-masochistic
perversions: this vicious process is akin to that seen in some patients
with Gilles de la Tourette syndrome, and in self-mutilating children
with Lesch-Nyhan syndrome.

Connected with all of these feelings and reactions were her feelings towards me – the equivocal figure who had offered her a drug so wonderful and so terrible in its effects; the devious and Janus-faced physician who had prescribed for her a revivifying, life-enhancing drug, on the one hand, and a horror-producing, life-destroying drug, on the other hand. I had first seemed a Redeemer, promising health and life with my sacramental medicine; and then a Devil, confiscating health and life, or forcing on her something worse than death. In my first role – as the 'good' doctor – she necessarily loved me; in my second role – as the 'wicked' doctor – she necessarily hated and feared me. And yet she dared not express the hate and fear; she locked it within herself, where it coiled and recoiled upon itself, coagulating into the thickness and darkness of guilt and depression. L-DOPA, by virtue of its amazing effects, invested me – its giver, the physician held 'responsible' for these effects – with all too much power over her life and well-being. Invested with these holy and unholy powers, I assumed, in Miss D.'s eyes, an absolute, and absolutely contradictory, sovereignty; the sovereignty of parents, authorities, God. Thus Miss D. found herself entangled in the labyrinth of a torturing transference-neurosis, a labyrinth from which there seemed to be no exit, no imaginable exit, whatsoever.

My own disappearance from the scene (on 3 August) at the height of her anguish was experienced both as an enormous relief and as an irretrievable loss. I had placed her in the labyrinth in the first place; yet was I not the thread to lead her from it?

This, then, was Miss D.'s situation when I returned in September.[4] I felt what was happening with her, in a very fragmentary and inchoate way, the moment I laid eyes on

4. And not only Miss D.'s situation but more or less the situation of some twenty or thirty other Parkinsonian patients under my care who had been 'running the gauntlet' of L-DOPA that summer.

her again, but it was, of course, months and even years before my own intuitions, and hers, reached the more conscious and explicit formulations which I have sketched above.

Summer 1972

Three years have passed since these events. Miss D. is still alive and well, and living – living a sort of life. The dramatic quality of summer 1969 is a thing of the past; the violent vicissitudes of that time have never been repeated with her, and in retrospect have some of the unreality and nostalgia of a dream, or of a unique, never-repeated, unrepeatable and now almost unimaginable Historical Event. Despite her ambivalences, Miss D. greeted my return with pleasure, and with a gentle, qualified request that the use of L-DOPA should be considered again. The insistence and intransigence had gone out of her manner; I felt that her seemingly subterranean month without L-DOPA had also been a month of deep reflection, and of inner changes and accommodations of great complexity. It had been, I was subsequently to realize, a sort of Purgatory, a period in which Miss D. struggled with her divided and manifold impulses, using all her recently acquired knowledge of herself (and her propensities of response to L-DOPA), and all her strength of mind and character, to achieve a new unification and stability, deeper and stronger than anything preceding it. She had, so to speak, been forged and tempered by the extremities she had passed through, not broken by them (as were so many of my patients). Miss D. was a superior individual; she had lived and fought with herself and for herself through half a century of illness, and had (against innumerable odds) been able to maintain a life of her own, outside an institution, until her sixty-sixth year. Her disease and her pathological potentials I had already seen; her mysterious reserves of health and sanity only became apparent to me *after* the summer of 1969, and in the ensuing three years.

The rest of Miss D.'s story is more easily told. I put her back on L-DOPA in September 1969 and she has remained on this, more or less continually, ever since. We observed in Miss D. (as in several other patients) that the concurrent use of amantadine ('Symmetrel') could ameliorate some of the responses to L-DOPA, although these benign effects might become reversed after a few weeks, and we have therefore maintained Miss D. on an intermittent regimen of amantadine added to L-DOPA. We tried, as recommended in the literature, to reduce abnormal excitements and movements by the use of phenothiazides, butyrophenones and other major tranquillizers, but found in Miss D. (as with all our other patients) that these drugs could only reduce or exacerbate the *total* effects of L-DOPA, i.e. that they did not distinguish between the 'good effects' and the 'side-effects' of L-DOPA – as so many enthusiastic physicians do. We found minor tranquillizers and anti-histamines, etc., virtually without any effect on Miss D., but barbiturates – especially the parenteral use of sodium amytal – a valuable mainstay for severe crises of one sort or another.

The responses to L-DOPA (or rather to L-DOPA–amantadine combinations) have been in every sense *milder* than those of summer 1969: Miss D. has never again been as sensationally well as she was then, nor as sensationally ill. Her Parkinsonism is always present, but considerably less severe than it was in the days before L-DOPA; although every few weeks, however, when the effects of the amantadine–L-DOPA mixture become less benign, she shows disabling exacerbations of Parkinsonism (and other symptoms), followed by disabling 'withdrawal symptoms' (similar to, though milder than, those of August 1969) during the week or so she is taken off amantadine. This cycle of improvements – exacerbation – withdrawal symptoms is repeated about ten times a year. Miss D. dislikes the cycle, but has grown to accept it. She has, indeed, lost all choice in the matter, for if her L-

DOPA is stopped altogether she moves into a state which is far more distressing and disabling than her original 'pre-DOPA' state. Her position is therefore this: that *she needs* L-DOPA, *but cannot tolerate it* – fully, or indefinitely.[5]

Miss D.'s crises have become rarer and less severe – occurring now only once or twice a week – but, perhaps more remarkably, they have quite changed their character. In the summer of 1969 (as in the summer of 1919), her crises were at first purely respiratory in character, and only subsequently drew to themselves the innumerable other phenomena described earlier. When, however, Miss D. resumed her crises, in the autumn of 1969, it was only these other phenomena which occurred; their respiratory components (or aspects) had mysteriously vanished, and have never shown themselves again. Her 'new' crises were usually marked by the most extreme palilalia, the same word or phrase sometimes being uttered hundreds of times in succession, variously accompanied by intense excitement, sundry urges, compulsions, exacerbated Parkinsonism, and peculiar states of 'block' or 'prohibition' of movement, etc. One must stress the words 'usually', 'variously', and 'etc.', for though every crisis was unmistakably a crisis, no two crises were exactly the same. Moreover the particular character and course of each crises, as well as its occurrence-as-a-whole, could be extraordinarily modified by suggestion or circumstance: thus the intense affect, which was usually angry or

5. Miss D. has been a relatively fortunate patient in both these regards. Her need and her intolerance for L-DOPA are both moderate in degree. In other patients – some of whose histories are given later in this book – the need and the intolerance for L-DOPA were both overwhelming, precluding the possibility of any compromise or position of satisfaction whatever. Miss D. was never off L-DOPA long enough to determine the duration of her 'post-DOPA' state; in other patients (to be described later), there is no doubt that L-DOPA led to profound disturbances of reaction and behaviour which lasted for well over a year following its withdrawal.

fearful, would become one of merriment and hilarity if Miss
D. happened to be watching a funny film or TV show, while
her 'block', so to speak, could be *drawn out* of one limb and
transferred to another.[6] By far the best treatment of her

6. The astonishing variability of such crises, and their openness to
suggestion, were even better shown in another patient, L. W., whose
history is not in this book. L.W. had at least a hundred clearly different forms of crisis: hiccoughs; panting attacks; oculogyrias; sniffing attacks; sweating attacks; attacks in which her left shoulder
would grow flushed and warm; chattering of the teeth; paroxysmal
ticcing attacks; ritualized iterative attacks, in which she would tap
one foot in three different positions, or dab her forehead in four set
places; counting attacks; verbigerative attacks, in which certain set
phrases were said a certain number of times; fear attacks; giggling
attacks, etc., etc. Any allusion (verbal or otherwise) to any given
type of crisis would infallibly call it forth in this patient.
L.W. would also have bizarre 'miscellaneous' crises, in which a
great variety of phenomena (sniffing, oculogyria, panting, counting,
etc., etc.) would be thrown together in unexpected (and seemingly
senseless) combinations; indeed new and strange combinations were
continually appearing. Although I observed dozens of these complex
crises I was almost never able to perceive any physiological or symbolic unity in them, and after a while I ceased to look for any such
unity, and accepted them as absurd juxtapositions of physiological
oddments, or, on occasion, improvised collages of physiological bric-
à-brac. This was also how Mrs W., a talented woman with a sense of
humour, regarded her own miscellaneous crises: 'They are just a
mess,' she would say, 'like a junk shop, or a jumble-sale, or the sort
of stuff you just throw in the attic.' *Sometimes*, however, one could see
patterns which were clear-cut but unintelligible, or patterns which
seemed to hint, tantalizingly, at some scarcely imaginable unity or
significance; and of these crises Mrs W. would say: 'This one's a
humdinger, a surrealistic attack – I *think* it's saying something, but
I don't know what it is, nor do I know what language it's in.' Some
of my students who happened to witness such attacks also received
a surrealistic impression: 'That's absolutely wild,' one of them once
said. 'It's just like a Salvador Dali !' Another student, fantastically
inclined, compared her crises to uncanny, unearthly buildings or
music ('Martian churches or Arcturan polyphonies'). Although
none of us could agree on the 'interpretation' of L. W.'s crises, we

crises was music, the effects of which were almost uncanny. One minute would see Miss D. compressed, clenched and blocked, or jerking, ticcing and jabbering – like a sort of human bomb; the next, with the sound of music from a wireless or a gramophone, the complete disappearance of all these obstructive-explosive phenomena and their replacement by a blissful ease and flow of movement as Miss D., suddenly freed of her automatisms, smilingly 'conducted' the music, or rose and danced to it. It was necessary only that the music be *legato*; *staccato* music (and especially percussion bands) sometimes had a bizarre effect, causing Miss D. to jump and jerk with the beat – like a mechanical doll or marionette.

By the end of 1970, Miss D. had run the gauntlet of L-DOPA, amantadine, DOPA-decarboxylases, apomorphine (all variously divided and sub-divided), alone or in combination with anti-cholinergics, anti-adrenergics, anti-histamines, and every other adjuvant or blocker which ingenuity could devise. She had been through them all, and she had *had it*. 'That's it !' she said. 'You've thrown the whole pharmacy at me. I've been up, down, sideways, inside-out, and everything else. I've been pushed, pulled, squeezed and twisted. I've gone faster, and slower, as well as *so* fast I actually stayed in one place. And I keep opening up and closing down, like a human concertina ...' Miss D. paused for breath. Her words irresistibly depicted a Parkinsonian 'Alice' in a post-encephalitic Wonderland.

By this time, then, Miss D. clearly saw that L-DOPA had become a necessity to her, and equally clearly that her responses to it had become limited and unspectacular, and

---

all felt them as having a strange fascination – the fascination of dreams, or peculiar art-forms; and, in this sense, if I sometimes thought of Parkinsonism as a relatively simple and coherent dream of the midbrain, I thought of L. W.'s crises as surrealistic deliria concocted by the forebrain.

would stay this way; she realized that this was now unalterably the case. This decision marked the completion of her 'dis-investment' in L-DOPA, her renunciation of the passionate hopes and yearnings which had dominated her life for more than a year. Thus, denying nothing, pretending nothing, and expecting nothing (though in her diary she continued to express, from time to time, half-serious, half-joking hopes that things might be different), Miss D. turned *away* from her phantasies, and *towards* her reality – a double turning-point which marked her release from the labyrinth which had trapped her for a year. All her relationships, from this point onwards, assumed a much easier and saner and pleasanter quality. Her attitude to L-DOPA became one of detached and humorous resignation, as did her attitude to her own symptoms and disabilities; she ceased to envy the patients who were flying aloft on L-DOPA, or to view with identificatory terror those patients who had done badly on the drug; and, above all, she ceased to see me as a Redeemer/ Destroyer holding her fate in my drug-giving hands. The denials, the projections, the identifications, the transferences, the postures and the impostures of the L-DOPA 'situation' fell away like a carapace, revealing 'the old Miss D.' – the real self – underneath.

In the second half of 1970, then, Miss D. became ready and eager to address herself to what could be done with regard to her Parkinsonism, her relationships, and the business of staying alive and human in a Total Institution.[7] These problems – perhaps – might have been by-passed had L-DOPA been and remained the Perfect Remedy, had it sustained its first promise; but it had not – for Miss D. She now saw L-DOPA divested of its glamour: as a most useful, and indispensible, adjunct, but no longer as Salvation. Now she could be face-to-face with her own resources, and mine, and

7. This term, and many of the concepts embodied in it, I owe to Goffman's remarkable book *Asylums*.

those of the institution, to make the best of what remained.[8]

In these ways, then, Miss D. acclimatized herself to the vagaries of L-DOPA, and actively modified the morbid

---

8. A brief allusion to some of Miss D.'s 'methods' may be made. In her long years of illness, she had observed her own propensities and symptoms with a minute curiosity, and had devised many ingenious ways of reducing, overcoming, or circumventing these. Thus, she had various ways of 'defreezing' herself if she chanced to freeze in her walking: she would carry in one hand a supply of minute paper balls of which she would now let one drop to the ground: its tiny whiteness immediately 'incited' or 'commanded' her to take a step, and thus allowed her to break loose from the freeze and resume her normal walking-pattern. Miss D. had found that regular blinking, or a loud-ticking watch, or horizontal lines or marks on the ground, etc., similarly served to *pace* her, and to prevent the incontinent hastenings and retardations which otherwise marred her ambulation. Similarly in reading, or talking, she learned to emphasize certain words at set intervals, which would serve to prevent verbal hurry, stuttering, impaction or freezing. In these and a thousand and one other ways, Miss D. – by herself, with me, with other patients, and with an increasingly intrigued staff of nurses, physiotherapists, speech-therapists, etc. – filled many productive and enjoyable hours exploring and playing with endless possibilities of self – and mutual help. Such methods are discovered or devised by *all* gifted post-encephalitic and Parkinsonian patients, and I have learned more from such patients than from a library of volumes. Miss D. (like half a dozen other highly articulate post-encephalitic patients under my care) has often depicted for me the strange and deeply paradoxical world in which she lives. These patients describe a fantastical-mathematical world remarkably similar to that which faced 'Alice'. Miss D. lays stress on the fundamental distortions of Parkinsonian *space*, on her peculiar difficulties with angles, circles, sets, and limits. She once said of her 'freezing': 'It's not as simple as it looks. I don't just come to a halt, I am still going, but I *have run out of space to move in* ... You see, *my* space, *our* space, is nothing like *your* space: our space gets bigger and smaller, it bounces back on itself, and it loops itself round till it runs into itself.'

ADDITIONAL COMMENTS

Since the publication of my original *Listener* article in 1972, of *Awakenings* itself in June of 1973, and the exhibition of the television

phenomena of her Parkinsonism, catatonia, impulsiveness, etc. But there were other problems, not stemming from herself, which were beyond her power to modify directly: these,

film based on the book in 1974, the most persistent and penetrating questions directed at me have had reference to the radical sense in which I have spoken of 'personal space', 'action-space', 'actual space', etc., and of my insistence, in the original *Listener* article, that Parkinsonism and allied disorders could not be comprehended unless fundamental relativistic concepts were used. In view of these questions, and the crucial importance of the topic – an importance no less practical than theoretical – I feel I must amplify and clarify what I mean. The gist of what here follows has an organic connection with the whole of this book, but it should especially be read in relation to a number of other scattered footnotes (viz. those on pp. 62, 128, 143, and 301 and 302).

We may first take a brief historical look at notions of 'space'. An essential difference (one might almost say, *the* essential difference) between the philosophies of Newton and of Liebniz hinges on their differing notions and uses of the word 'space' – the Newtonian concept of 'motion' versus the Leibnizian one of 'action'. For Newton space and time were *absolutes* – absolute media in which motion occurred; they were *not* hypotheses ('*Hypotheses non fingo*'), or, as we would say now, frames-of-reference. For Leibniz, in contrast, 'space' and 'time', and all such notions of continuity and extension, were simply ways of speaking, ways of picturing and measuring *the size of actions*: they were concrete and actual, not absolute and abstract, i.e. they were convenient (or conventional) constructions or 'models', figurative language (albeit of a very special sort). (These essentially relativistic concepts of Leibniz are fully spelled out in his correspondence with Clark – a correspondence interrupted by Leibniz's death, and not published until many years after his death.) The notion of 'space' as a way of speaking and looking at the world, rather than as a Euclidean or Newtonian absolute, was revived by Gauss in his famous papers on the possible curvatures of possible spaces, and then by the great Russian geometers in their 'alternative geometries'. These, then, combined with Maxwellian dynamics, were the intellectual antecedents of Einstein's thought, his notions of coordinate-systems in motion relative to each other, of the possibility of countless, individual, variable space–times . . .

Let us now come to practical examples, familiar and unfamiliar, of 'personal space' and 'personal time', which indicate how our

essentially, were the problems of living in a Total Institution.

These problems, in their most general terms, were epito-

---

judgements and our actions may be at variance with the abstract measure of clocks and rulers, or the judgements and actions of other human beings. First, a familiar and universal example, which all of us have experienced when impatient, hurried, or 'pressed for time': 'a watched pot never boils,' as the old saying has it – if we are impatiently awaiting its boiling, it seems to take 'unduly long', and we may feel that the very watches we wear have become unreliable; again, if we are hurrying to catch a bus or train, the distance we must traverse seems 'unduly long', and the time we have 'unduly short'.

Thus we may experience illusions (or misleading conjectures) about space–time when we are hurried or festinant; and equally we may have illusions when dawdling or procrastinant. Now let us examine Parkinsonian behaviour in this light, concerning ourselves especially with *illusions of scale*. I have had letters from Frances D., and other Parkinsonian patients, which showed singular (and often comic) disparities of scale; I remember one such letter from Frances D., of which the first page was in a perfectly formed but microscopic hand (so small I needed a magnifying-glass to decipher it), while at the start of the second page (which was in normally sized script) she had written: 'I see that what I wrote yesterday was far too small, although I didn't see this at the time. Today I have borrowed a ruler and ruled lines on this page, and I will use the lines to guide my writing, so that I don't inadvertently make it tiny again.' Other letters from Frances D., and certain other patients, were sometimes marked by enormous (though perfectly shaped and formed) writing, and this too would be done in seeming ignorance of its abnormal magnitude. Similar disturbances were common in speech: most Parkinsonian patients tend to speak softly, and often to do so without knowing they are doing so; but if asked to 'speak up', they may find no difficulty in raising their voices; on the other hand Cecil M., who had 'megaphonia', habitually spoke in a Brobdingnagian voice, and felt everyone round him was speaking too softly (I should add that his hearing was perfectly normal – it was his *judgement* of sounds which showed aberrations). Again, in walking, one may see 'microambulation' ('*marche à petits pas*') in Parkinsonian patients; if such patients measure themselves against regular marks or clocks, or the framework of dimensions around them, or against the move-

mized in the Pascalian antimonies which echoed through her diary : the sense of isolation and the sense of confinement; the sense of emptiness and the sense of pettiness; the sense of

_____

ments of other persons whom they take to be 'normal', they may perceive (and perhaps correct) their own tiny steps; but this may not happen, or may be prevented from happening – the patient may be engrossed in his own scale of walking, and fail to realize that either the walking or the scale is 'wrong'. Parkinsonian patients often make 'macro-' or 'micro-gestures' – gestures of the right *sort*, but on the wrong *scale* (too large, too small, too fast, too slow . . .); these they may perform completely unwittingly, unaware that the gesture is inappropriate in scale. I am often able to show a beautiful example of such 'kinetic illusions' when I demonstrate Aaron E. (a deeply Parkinsonian, but not post-encephalitic, patient) to my students: 'Mr. E.,' I say, 'would you be kind enough to clap your hands steadily and regularly – *thus*?' 'Sure, doc.,' he replies, and after a few steady claps is apt to proceed into an incontinent festination of clapping, culminating in an apparent 'freezing' of motion. 'There, doc.!' he says, turning to me with a pleased smile. 'Didn't I do it nice and regular, just like you asked me?' 'Gentlemen!' I say to the students. 'You be the judges. Did Mr E. clap his hands steadily and regularly, as he says?' 'Why, of course not!' exclaims one of the students. 'His movements kept getting faster and faster, and smaller and smaller – like *this*!' At this point Mr E. leaps to his feet in indignation: 'What do you mean?' he cries to the student. 'What do you mean by saying my movements got faster and smaller – in that crazy way you did it yourself? My movements were perfectly regular and stable – like *this*!' And, concentrating fiercely, totally absorbed in his own activity, he falls once again into the grossest festination. This demonstration (when it works! and this depends on how much Mr E. is enclosed in his own frame-of-reference, versus how much he can stand outside it and make comparisons and corrections) is – in the charming idiom of my New York students – 'mind blowing', 'mind boggling', 'wild!', 'out of sight!' It is, indeed, literally *shocking*, because of the clarity with which it shows that what Aaron E. clearly perceives in others, he cannot perceive in himself; that he may use a frame-of-reference (or coordinate-system, or way of judging space-time) which departs from 'the normal' in an ever-increasing and accelerating way; and that he may be so enclosed within his own (contracting) frame-of-reference, that he is unable to perceive the contracting scale in his own movements. Thus, the curious 'dialogue'

being an inmate – put inside by society, cut off from society
. . . subjected to innumerable, degrading rules and regulations;
the sense of having been reduced to the status of a child or

---

between Mr E. and the students comes to resemble an imaginary
Einsteinian dialogue between people in lifts (or frames-of-reference)
which are moving or accelerating relative to each other; and the
entire demonstration provides the clearest manifestation of relativity
in action, the clearest vindication of Frances D.'s insights when she
speaks of different 'spaces', and says: '. . . *my* space, *our* space, is
nothing like *your* space'.

Such a demonstration certainly establishes that individuals may
have varying experiences of space and time – and (a point continually
stressed by Richard Gregory) that their experiences are themselves
hypotheses or conjectures. It does not, by itself, show that the false
conjectures of Aaron E. are of a relativistic kind, rather than of a
simpler kind, involving simple visual or kinaesthetic or motor illusions.
We are all subject to the latter – as shown by the 'queer feeling' (or
continually violated delusion of motion) we may experience if we
walk on an escalator which has stopped. Patients with cortical
apraxias and agnosias are especially liable to misperceptions (miscon-
jectures) of this sort, and so too, for a while, are patients who have
sustained peripheral injuries (e.g. an injury which has de-activated,
hence de-realized, a leg or a foot): such patients may make *individual* misjudgements, or a series of these, with regard to the size of
individual objects, especially meaningless, geometrical objects like
steps (see the footnote on p. 62), because of an uncertainty or deficiency in their own inner scales, secondary to a mutilation or
distortion in part of their body image, of their own biological meas-
uring-apparatus . . . But such errors, which all of us are prone to when
faced with new motor tasks (skiing, pole-vaulting, riding bicycles, etc.)
are different in kind from Parkinsonian misjudgement. The Parkinsonian – unlike the cortical apraxic-agnosic – *understands* perfectly
well what is meant by a 'foot'; he has in no sense lost his *ideas* of
dimension. What we observe, however, is that all his space–time
judgements are *pushed out of shape*, that his entire coordinate-
system is subject to expansions, contractions, torsions and warps; and
that such generalized distortions of his metrical field are produced by
pulling, pushing, and twisting forces – by the tractions, pulsions and
torsions of being which constitute the very essence of his illness. The
apraxic-agnosic patient may make errors of action or cognition, but
he is not *driven* into misperformance or miscognition through being

prisoner, of having been lost or ground up in a Machine; the sense of enduring frustration, desolation and impotence.

These inhuman, institutional qualities, though present

the subject of violent deforming forces; he may, so to speak, have forgotten his tape-measure or pocket-watch, but he has not had all his measuring devices, his metrical judgements, warped by forces which he may be unable to recognize, because the judgement by which he might judge his judgements is itself warped, and so on ... The Parkinsonian engrossed in his Parkinsonism can no more judge the 'abnormality' of his own state than could a self-conscious rod, accelerated towards the velocity of light, which had itself undergone a Lorentz contraction. It is for reasons of this sort that it is insufficient to speak of Parkinsonism as a simple '*dyskinesia*' (motor disorder). One must speak of it as a systematic disorder of space–time parameters, a systematic warping of coordinate-systems; indeed one must go further, and say that this misjudgement or warping is secondary to a systematic disorder of 'will' or *force*, which has the effect of warping Parkinsonian 'space' and making it a dynamic, field, or relativistic disorder. It was such considerations as these which led me to write, in my original *Listener* article: 'The qualities of dynamic being (or disorder) ... are relativistic ... being those of a highly structured, anisotropic continuum, in which the space-deforming curvatures are determined by Parkinsonian or other ontological "forces" which take the place of gravitational potentials.'

I noted also, in this original article, that such relativistic disorders may not only be evident in the behaviour (or procedures) of Parkinsonian patients, but in their perceptions (or conjectures), and this most dramatically in post-encephalitic patients intensely excited by L-DOPA: '... in such states', I wrote, 'the visual field can assume an exaggerated perspective, which culminates in a sort of "fish-eye" vision ... There may be hallucinations of wind-like forces and swirls and eddies ... in which case patients "see" space as an intensely structured (and distorted) dynamic continuum.'

A final point in this extremely long but crucial footnote. I have intimated, time and time again, that there are profound analogies between the nature of Parkinsonism and that of psychosis, but also profound dissimilarities. They are alike in that both are experienced and enacted as *systematic disorders of judgement*; they are wholly unalike in that the Parkinsonian misrepresents or misjudges space and time, so that his 'dimensions' and models are pulled awry – whereas the psychotic misjudges intention and expression, so that

to some degree from the founding of the hospital, grew suddenly harsher and more absolute in September 1969.[9] One could clearly perceive, in many other patients, how this grim transition greatly modified the clinical state, not simply in terms of mood and attitude, but also in terms of crises, tics, impulsions, catalepsies, Parkinsonian phenomena, etc., and, of course, their reactions to L-DOPA.

There is no doubt that Miss D. herself was greatly affected by these changes in her environment; I cannot, however, make any definite judgement as to how much her course on L-DOPA was an inevitable consequence of the drug's action and her individual, built-in reactivity, and how much it may have been modified by the increasingly adverse conditions of her life. I can only represent the total picture, as fairly and fully as I can, and leave such judgements to my readers.

Three things, however, have been unmistakably clear. First, that whenever Miss D. succeeds in expressing her feelings and achieving some change in her environment, *all* her pathological phenomena decrease. Secondly, that whenever Miss D. leaves the hospital for a day's outing (such outings have become increasingly rare since the easy-going days of 1969) *all* her symptoms and signs decrease. Lastly, that since Miss D. has forged a deep and affectionate relationship with two other patients on the ward – i.e. since the early part of 1971 – she has been visibly better in *all* possible ways.

So, finally, we come to the present time, the summer of 1972. Miss D. continues on a modest, intermittent dosage of L-DOPA and amantadine. She is pretty active and can look

---

his 'histrions' and metaphors are pulled awry. Thus the Parkinsonian dynamically misjudges extensional reality, the psychotic moral and affective reality.

9. During this time of acute institutional deterioration, Miss D. would sometimes exclaim: 'My God, they call this place a *sanatorium*? If you ask me, it's becoming a *thanatorium*!'

after her basic needs for nine months in the year, the other three months being occupied with exacerbations of illness and withdrawal symptoms. She has a small crisis perhaps twice a month, which no longer really disturbs her or anyone else. She reads a good deal, crochets like a professional, and does innumerable crosswords far faster than I can. She is most herself when she talks to her friends. She has put most of her petulancies, obstinacies, dependencies and insistencies quite firmly behind her. She is now very genial (except when she shuts herself up with her diary in her blacker, private moods), and well-liked by everyone round her. One often sees her by the window, a mild old lady approaching seventy, somewhat bowed and fixed in her attitude, crocheting rapidly, and looking at the traffic which roars through Bexley.

She is not one of our Star Patients, one of those who did fabulously well on L-DOPA, and stayed well. But she has survived the pressures of an almost life-long, character-deforming disease; of a strong cerebral stimulant; and of confinement in a chronic hospital from which very few patients emerge alive. Deeply rooted in reality, she has triumphantly survived illness, intoxication, isolation and institutionalization, and has remained what she always was – a totally human, a prime, human being.

2. MAGDA B.

Mrs B. was born in Austria in 1900, and came to the United States as a child. Her childhood was free of any serious illnesses, and her academic and athletic progress at High School was exemplary. In 1918–19, while working as a secretary, she contracted a severe somnolent-opthalmoplegic form of *encephalitis lethargica*, recovered from this after a few months, but started to show Parkinsonism and other sequelae around 1923.

The course of her illness over the following forty-five years was at first known to me only from exiguous hospital notes, for Mrs B. had been quite unable to speak for many years. In addition to the ophthalmoplegia which failed to resolve after her acute encephalitis, Mrs B.'s chief problems were profound akinesia and apathy, and a variety of autonomic disturbances (profuse salivation, sweating, and repeated peptic ulcerations). She had not been prone to oculogyric or other crises. She showed occasional 'flapping' tremor, but virtually no rigidity, dystonia or resting ('pill-rolling') tremor.

A note dated 1964 remarks on the 'curious absence of anger or frustration in circumstances which would seem to warrant these reactions'. A note written in 1966, when Mrs B. was seriously ill from concurrent illness, commented upon the absence of any anxiety or fear in response to her situation. During 1968, she was repeatedly subjected to verbal and physical abuses by a mad, hostile dement placed next to her in the ward (the latter would insult and curse her, and occasionally struck her): Mrs B. showed neither motor nor emotional reaction to such intolerable goading. Many other notes, which need not be quoted in detail, similarly attested to her abnormal passivity and calmness. On the other hand, there was no suggestion of depressive or paranoid tendencies, and no evidence of eccentric ideation or behaviour: Mrs B. seemed amiable and appreciative of help, but docile, bland, and perhaps incapable of emotional reaction.

Before L-DOPA

Mrs B. was seated, motionless, in her wheel chair, when first seen by me: akinesia was so extreme at this time that she would sit without blinking, or change of facial expression, or any hint of bodily movement, for the greater part of the day. She showed a habitual dropped posture of the head, but was able to combat this for brief periods. There was little or no cervical rigidity. She appeared to have a bilateral nuclear and internuclear ophthalmoplegia, with alternating exotropia. Mrs B. was sweating very freely, showed a greasy sebarrhoeic skin, and moderately increased lacrimation and salivation. There were rare attacks of spontaneous lid-clonus or closure, but no spontaneous blinking at all. Mrs B. was virtually aphonic – able to produce a faint 'Ah!' with great effort, but not to articulate a single word audibly : she had been speechless for more than ten years, and severely hypophonic for at least fifteen years before this.

She showed profound facial masking – at no time during the initial examinations did any hint of facial expression appear – was scarcely able to open the mouth, to protrude the tongue beyond the lip-margin, or to move it at all within the mouth from side to side. Chewing and swallowing were feeble and slowly performed – the consumption of even a small meal would take more than an hour – but there were no signs of bulbar or pseudo-bulbar palsy.

All voluntary movements were distinguished by extreme slowness and feebleness, with almost no involvement of 'background' musculature, and a tendency to premature arrest of movements in mid-posture. When raised from her chair – for Mrs B. was quite unable even to inaugurate the act of rising by herself – she stood as motionless as a statue, although she was unable to maintain her balance, due to an irresistible tendency to fall backwards. Stepping was not only impossible, but somehow seemed *unthinkable*. If she closed her eyes, while standing or sitting, she at once dropped forward like a wilted flower.

Mrs B. was thus profoundly incapacitated, unable to speak and almost unable to initiate any voluntary motion, and in need of total nursing care. Added to the motor problems were a striking apathy and apparent incapacity for emotional response, and considerable drowsiness and torpor for much of the day. Conventional anti-Parkinsonian drugs had been of very little use to her, and surgery had never been considered. She had been regarded for many years as a 'hopeless' backward post-encephalitic, with no capacity for rehabilitation. She was started on L-DOPA on 25 June.

Course on L-DOPA

2 July. After one week of treatment (and on a dose of 2 gm. L-DOPA daily), Mrs B. started *talking* – quite audibly – for the first time in many years, although her vocal force would decay after two or three short sentences, and her new-found voice was low-pitched, monotonous and uninflected.

8 July. With raising of the dose to 3 gm. L-DOPA daily, Mrs B. became nauseated, and insomniac, and showed striking dilation of the pupils, but no tachycardia, lability of blood-pressure, or akathisia. She now showed considerable spontaneous activity – ability to shift positions in her chair, to turn in bed, etc. She was much more alert, and had ceased to show any drowsiness or 'dullness' in the course of the day. Her voice had acquired further strength, and the beginnings of intonation and inflection: thus one could now realize that this patient had a strong Viennese accent, where a few days previously her voice had been monotonous in timbre, and, as it were, *anonymously* Parkinsonian.

Mrs B. was now able to hold a pencil in her right hand, and to make a first entry in her diary: her name, followed by the comment, 'It is twenty years since I have written. I'm afraid I have almost forgotten how to write my name.'

She also showed emotional reaction – anxiety at her sleeplessness and vomiting – and requested me to reduce the new drug, but by no means to stop it. The dose was reduced to 2 gm. daily.

Reduction of the dose alleviated the nausea, insomnia and mydriasis, but led to a partial loss of vocal and motor power.

A week later (15 July), it was possible to restore the larger (3 gm. daily) dose, without causing any adverse effects whatever, and she was subsequently maintained on this dose. On this, Mrs B. had shown a stable and continued improvement. By the end of July, she was able to rise to her feet and stand unaided for thirty seconds, and to walk twenty steps between parallel bars. She could adjust her position in chair or bed to her own comfort. She had become able to feed herself. Diminishing flexion of the trunk and neck could be observed with each passing week, so that by mid-August a striking normalization of posture had occurred.

Previously indifferent, inattentive, and unresponsive to her surroundings, Mrs B. became, with each week, more alert, more attentive, and more interested in what was taking place around her.

At least as dramatic as the motor improvement, and infinitely moving to observe, was the recovery of emotional responsiveness in this patient who had been so withdrawn and apathetic for so many years. With continued improvement of her voice, Mrs B. became quite talkative, and showed an intelligence, a charm, and a humour, which had been almost totally concealed by her disease. She particularly enjoyed talking of her childhood in Vienna, of her parents and family, of schooldays, of rambles and excursions in the country nearby, and as she did so would often laugh with pleasure at the recollection, or shed nostalgic tears – normal emotional responses which she had not shown in more than twenty years. Little by little Mrs B. emerged as a *person*, and as she did so was able to communicate to us, in vivid and frightening terms, what an *unperson* she had felt before receiving L-DOPA. She described her feelings of impotent anger and mounting depression in the early years of her illness, and the succeeding of these feelings by apathy and indifference: 'I ceased to have any moods,' she said. 'I ceased to care about anything. Nothing *moved* me – not even the death of my parents. I forgot what it felt like to be happy or unhappy. Was it good or bad? It was neither. It was nothing.'[10]

1969–71

Mrs B.'s course on L-DOPA, by and large, was the smoothest and most satisfactory I have seen in *any* patient.[11] Throughout her two years on the drug, she maintained an altogether admirable degree of activity, sanity, and general fullness of living. There was, it is true, some small dropping-off in her level of energy and motility towards the end of the second year, and there were brief outcroppings of morbid activity: these latter will be described in the context they occurred in.

Much of this was associated with her renewal of emotional contact with, and obvious delight in, her daughters and sons-in-law, her grandchildren, and the many other relatives who came to her now she was well, and, so to speak, restored to reality. She remembered every birthday and anniversary, and never forget to mark them with a letter; she showed herself agreeable and eager to be taken out on car-rides, to restaurants, to theatres, and above all, to the homes of her family, without ever becoming demanding or importunate. She renewed contact with the Rabbi and other orthodox patients in the hospital, went to all the religious services, and loved nothing so much as lighting the Shabbas candles. In short, she donned again her former identity, as a 'frum' Viennese lady of good family and strong character. More remarkably, she assumed, with apparent ease, the mantle of old age and 'Grannie-hood', 'bubishkeit', despite having

10. 'Thus when God forsakes us, Satan also leaves us' – Sir Thomas Browne.

11. It is curious that the *only* two patients I have ever seen who showed an almost unqualified excellence of response for the entire two years they were taking L-DOPA (M.B. and N.G.) were not, as might be thought, minimally involved patients with Parkinson's disease, but two of the most profoundly involved post-encephalitics I have ever seen.

dropped, as through a vacuum, from her mid-twenties to her late sixties.[12]

She had not, apparently become bitter or virulent in the decades of her illness, and this, perhaps, was connected with her apathy: 'I often felt', said one of her daughters, 'that Mother *felt* nothing, although she seemed to notice and remember everything. I used to feel terribly sad at her state, without getting too angry – after all, how can you blame or get mad at a *ghost*?'

Mrs B. did develop two brief psychotic reactions while on L-DOPA. The first of these was in relation to her husband, who failed to visit her with the rest of the family. 'Where is he?' she would ask her daughters. 'Why doesn't he come to see me?' Her daughters temporized, explaining he was ill, indisposed, out of town, on a trip, etc. (He had in fact died some five years before.) These many discrepancies alarmed Mrs B., and precipitated a brief delusional episode. During

12. It is of much interest and significance that Magda B. seemed to have little or no difficulty in accommodating to the immense time-lapse, the immense 'loss' of time, entailed by her illness. This is in absolute contrast to the following patient (Rose R.), who on 'awakening' after forty-three years, found herself faced with 'a time-gap beyond comprehension or bearing', 'an intolerable and insoluble anachronism' to which accommodation was completely impossible (see p. 114). Why such a difference? I think this reflects the absolute contrast (discussed in the Introduction) between 'negative' and 'positive' disorders of being. Magda B., engulfed in non-activity, non-being, nothingness, situationlessness, was not, I think, frustrated or tormented like Rose R.; she was becalmed, asleep, on the ocean of life. When Being and activity were given to her, she accepted it as a pure gift, with gratitude and joy; but their absence, prior to her Awakening, was *also* accepted, with a placid indifference (and so too, conceivably, might have been a return to inactivity and inexistence, had the L-DOPA lost its effect). However, it is possible that Magda B., once awakened to life and hope, could not have borne its loss again; and that *this* was the reason why she died when she did, while still enjoying the gift of life, and before its anticipated, cruel *re-confiscation.*

this time, she heard her husband's voice in the corridors, saw his name in the papers, and 'understood' he was having innumerable *affaires*. Seeing what was happening, I asked her daughters to tell her the truth. Mrs B.'s response to this was: 'Ach! you sillies, why didn't you tell me?' followed by a period of mourning, and complete dissipation of her psychotic ideas.

Her other psychosis had reference to a rapidly advancing deterioration of eyesight, which had been 'accepted' with indifference before the L-DOPA. This was especially severe in her second year on the drug, when the faces of her children, the face of the *world*, were rapidly becoming dim and ungraspable. Mrs B. rebelled against the diagnosis of 'senile macular degeneration, progressive and incurable', the more so as this was delivered to her by a specialist she had never seen before, with a curt finality and a marked lack of sympathy, and for some weeks implored us pitifully to restore her sight, and experienced dreams and hallucinations of seeing again perfectly. During this painful period, Mrs B. developed a curious 'touching tic', continually touching the rails, the furniture, and – above all – various people as they passed in the corridor. I once asked her about this: 'Can you blame me?' she cried. 'I can hardly see anything. If I touch and keep touching, it is to keep me in touch!' As Mrs B. adjusted to her increasing blindness, and as she started to learn Braille (an enterprise *she* had thought of and insisted upon), her anguish grew less, her dreams and demands and hallucinations ceased, and her compulsive touching grew less marked, and *much* less importunate.[13] It should be

13. I am not suggesting that this touching tic was entirely 'psychogenic' or *created* by circumstance. I have seen somewhat similar touching tics in impulse-ridden post-encephalitic patients who were *not* in Mrs B.'s position. But I *do* think that a mild, or latent, propensity to tic was 'brought out' by her excitement, and given shape by her circumstances, so that it *became* a reflection or expression of her feelings.

stressed, perhaps, that the dosage of L-DOPA was not altered in these psychoses, for it was clear that they were reflections of an alterable reality.

In July 1971, Mrs B., who was in good general health and not given to 'hunches', had a sudden premonition of death, so clear and peremptory she phoned up her daughters. 'Come and see me today,' she said. 'There'll be no tomorrow ... No, I feel quite well ... Nothing is bothering me, but I *know* I shall die in my sleep tonight.'

Her tone was quite sober and factual, wholly unexcited, and it carried such conviction that *we* started wondering, and obtained blood-counts, cardiograms, etc., etc. (which were all quite normal). In the evening Mrs B. went round the ward, with a laughter-silencing dignity, shaking hands and saying 'Good-bye' to everyone there.

She went to bed and she died in the night.

3. ROSE R.

Miss R. was born in New York City in 1905, the youngest child of a large, wealthy and talented family. Her childhood and school days were free of serious illness, and were marked, from their earliest days, by love of merriment, games and jokes. High-spirited, talented, full of interests and hobbies, sustained by deep family affection and love, and a sure sense of who and what and why she was, Miss R. steered clear of significant neurotic problems or 'identity-crises' in her growing-up period.

On leaving school, Miss R. threw herself ardently into a social and peripatetic life. Aeroplanes, above all, appealed to her eager, volant and irrepressible spirit; she flew to Pittsburgh and Denver, New Orleans and Chicago, and twice to the California of Hearst and Hollywood (no mean feat in the planes of those days). She went to innumerable parties and shows, was toasted and fêted, and rolled home drunk at night. And between parties and flights she dashed off sketches of the bridges and waterfronts with which New York abounded. Between 1922 and 1926, Miss R. lived in the blaze of her own vitality, and lived more than most other people in the whole of their lives. And this was as well, for at the age of twenty-one she was suddenly struck down by a virulent form of *encephalitis lethargica* – one of its last victims before the epidemic vanished. 1926, then, was the last year in which Miss R. really *lived*.

The night of the sleeping-sickness, and the days which followed it, can be reconstructed in great detail from Miss R.'s relatives, and Miss R. herself. The acute phase announced itself (as sometimes happened : compare Maria G.) by nightmares of a grotesque and terrifying and premonitory nature. Miss R. had a series of dreams about one central theme : she dreamed she was imprisoned in an inaccessible castle, but the castle had the form and shape of herself; she dreamed of enchantments, bewitchments, entrancements; she dreamed that she had become a living, sentient statue of stone; she dreamed that the world had come to a stop; she dreamed that she had fallen into a sleep so deep that nothing could wake her; she dreamed of a death which was different from death. Her family had difficulty waking her the next morning, and when she awoke there was intense consternation : 'Rose,' they cried 'wake up ! What's the matter? Your expression, your position ... You're so still and so strange.' Miss R. could not answer, but turned her eyes to the wardrobe-mirror, and there she saw that her dreams had come true. The local doctor was brisk and unhelpful : 'Catatonia,' he said; '*Flexibilitas cerea*. What can you expect with the life she's been leading? She's broken her heart over one of these bums. Keep her quiet and feed her – she'll be fine in a week.'

But Miss R. was not to recover for a week, or a year, or forty-three years. She recovered the ability to speak in short sentences, or to make sudden movements before she froze up again. She showed, increasingly, a forced retraction of her neck and her eyes – a state of almost continuous oculogyric crisis, broken only by sleep, meals and occasional 'releases'. She was alert, and seemed to notice what went on around her; she lost none of her affection for her numerous family – and they lost none of their affection for her; but she seemed absorbed and preoccupied in some unimaginable state. For the most part, she showed no sign of distress, and no sign of anything save intense *concentration*: 'She looked', said one of her sisters, 'as if she were trying her hardest to remember something – or, maybe, doing her damnedest to forget something. Whatever it was, it took all her attention.' In her years at home, and subsequently in hospital, her family did their utmost to penetrate this absorption, to learn what was going on with their beloved 'kid' sister. With them – and, much later, with me – Miss R. was exceedingly candid, but whatever she said seemed cryptic and gnomic, and yet at the same time disquietingly clear.[14]

14. The following are typical of some of the 'dialogues' I had with Miss R.
'What are you thinking about, Rosie?'
'Nothing, just nothing.'
'But how can you possibly be thinking of nothing?'
'It's dead easy, once you know how.'
'How exactly do you think about nothing?'
'One way is to think about the same thing again and again. Like $2=2=2=2$; or, I am what I am what I am what I am ... It's the same thing with my posture. My posture continually leads to itself. Whatever I do or whatever I think leads deeper and deeper into itself ... And then there are maps.'
'Maps? What do you mean?'
'Everything I do is a map of itself, everything I do is a part of itself. Every part leads into itself ... I've got a thought in my mind, and then I see something in it, like a dot on the skyline. It comes nearer

When there was only this state, and no other problems, Miss R.'s family could keep her at home: she was no trouble, they loved her, she was simply – elsewhere (or nowhere). But three or four years after her trance-state had started, she started to become rigid on the left side of her body, to lose her balance when walking, and to develop other signs of Parkinsonism. Gradually these symptoms grew worse and worse, until full-time nursing became a necessity. Her siblings left home, and her parents were ageing, and it was increasingly difficult to keep her at home. Finally, in 1935, she was admitted to Mount Carmel.

Her state changed little after the age of thirty, and when I first saw her in 1966, my findings coincided with the original notes from her admission. Indeed, the old staff-nurse on her ward, who had known her throughout, said: 'It's uncanny, that woman hasn't aged a day in the thirty years I've known her. The rest of us get older – but Rosie's the same.' It was true: Miss R. at sixty-one looked thirty years younger;

---

and nearer, and then I see what it is – it's just the same thought I was thinking before. And then I see another dot, and another, and so on . . . Or I think of a map; then a map of that map; then a map of that map of that map, and each map perfect, though smaller and smaller . . . Worlds within worlds within worlds within worlds . . . Once I get going I can't possibly stop. It's like being caught between mirrors, or echoes, or something. Or being caught on a merry-go-round which won't come to a stop.'

'And do you have any *other* ways of thinking about nothing?'

'Oh yes! The dots and maps are *positive* nothings, but I also think of *negative* nothings.'

'And what are those like, Rosie?'

'That's impossible to say, because they're takings-away. I think of a thought, and it's suddenly gone – like having a picture whipped out of its frame. Or I try to picture something in my mind, but the picture dissolves as fast as I can make it. I have a particular idea, but can't keep it in mind; and then I lose the *general* idea; and then the general idea of a general idea; and in two or three jumps my mind is a blank – all my thoughts gone, blanked out or erased.'

she had raven-black hair, and her face was unlined, as if she had been magically preserved by her trance or her stupor.

She sat upright and motionless in her wheelchair, with little or no spontaneous movement for hours on end. There was no spontaneous blinking, and her eyes stared straight ahead, seemingly indifferent to her environment but completely absorbed. Her gaze, when requested to look in different directions, was full, save for complete inability to converge the eyes. Fixation of gaze lacked smooth and subtle modulation, and was accomplished by sudden, gross movements which seemed to cost her considerable effort. Her face was completely masked and expressionless. The tongue could not be protruded beyond the lip-margins, and its movements, on request, were exceedingly slow and small. Her voice was virtually inaudible, though Miss R. could whisper quite well with considerable effort. Drooling was profuse, saturating a cloth bib within an hour, and the entire skin was oily, sebarrhoeic, and sweating intensely. Akinesia was global, although rigidity and dystonia were strikingly unilateral in distribution. There was intense axial rigidity, no movement of the neck or trunk muscles being possible. There was equally intense rigidity in the left arm, and a very severe dystonic contracture of the left hand. No voluntary movement of this limb was possible. The right arm was much less rigid, but showed great akinesia, all movements being minimal, and decaying to zero after two or three repetitions. Both legs were hypertonic, the left much more so. The left foot was bent inwards in dystonic inversion. Miss R. could not rise to her feet unaided, but when assisted to do so could maintain her balance and take a few small, shuffling, precarious steps, although the tendency to backward-falling and pulsion was very great.

She was in a state of near-continuous oculogyric crisis, although this varied a good deal in severity. When it became more severe, her Parkinsonian 'background' was increased

in intensity, and an intermittent coarse tremor appeared in
her right arm. Prominent tremor of the head, lips and tongue
also became evident at these times, and rhythmic movement
of buccinators and corrugators. Her breathing would become
somewhat stertorous at such times, and would be accompanied by a guttural phonation reminiscent of a pig grunting. Severe crises would always be accompanied by tachycardia and hypertension. Her neck would be thrown back in
an intense and sometimes agonizing opisthotonic posture.
Her eyes would generally stare directly ahead, and could not
be moved by voluntary effort: in the severest crises they were
forced upwards and fixed on the ceiling.

Miss R.'s capacity to speak or move, minimal at the best of
times, would disappear almost entirely during her severer
crises, although in her greatest extremity she would sometimes call out, in a strange high-pitched voice, perseverative
and palilalic, utterly unlike her husky 'normal' whisper:
'Doctor, doctor, doctor, doctor ... help me, help, help, h'lp,
h'lp ... I am in terrible pain, I'm so frightened, so frightened,
so frightened ... I'm going to die, I know it, I know it, I
know it, I know it ...' And at other times, if nobody was
near, she would whimper softly to herself, like some small
animal caught in a trap. The nature of Miss R.'s pain during
her crises was only elucidated later, when speech had become
easy: some of it was a local pain associated with extreme
opisthotonos, but a large component seemed to be central –
diffuse, unlocalizable, of sudden onset and offset, and inseparably coalesced with feelings of dread and threat, in the
severest crises a true *angor animi*. During exceptionally severe attacks, Miss R.'s face would become flushed, her
eyes reddened and protruding, and she would repeat, 'It'll
kill me, it'll kill me, it'll kill me ...' hundreds of times in
succession.[15]

15. Compare cases cited by Jelliffe (1932): the patient who would
cry out in 'anguish' during her attacks, but could give no reason for

Miss R.'s state scarcely changed between 1966 and 1969, and when L-DOPA became available I was in two minds about using it. She was, it was true, intensely disabled, and had been virtually helpless for over forty years. It was her *strangeness* above all which made me hesitate and wonder – fearing what might happen if I gave her L-DOPA. I had never seen a patient whose regard was so turned away from the world, and so immured in a private, inaccessible world of her own.

I kept thinking of something Joyce wrote about his mad daughter: '... fervently as I desire her cure, I ask myself what then will happen when and if she finally withdraws her regard from the lightning-lit revery of her clairvoyance and turns it upon that battered cabman's face, the world ...'

Course on L-DOPA

But I started her on L-DOPA, despite my misgivings, on 18 June 1969. The following is an extract from my diary.

25 June. The first therapeutic responses have already occurred, even though the dosage has only been raised to 1·5 gm. a day. Miss R. has experienced two entire days unprecedentedly free of oculogyric crises, and her eyes, so still and preoccupied before, are brighter and more mobile and attentive to her surroundings.

1 July. Very real improvements are evident by this date: Miss R. is able to walk unaided down the passage, shows a distinct reduction of rigidity in the left arm and elsewhere, and has become able to speak at a normal conversational volume. Her mood is cheerful, and she has had no oculogyric crises for three days. In view of this propitious response, and the absence of any adverse effects, I am increasing the dosage of L-DOPA to 4 gm. daily.

6 July. Now receiving 4 gm. L-DOPA. Miss R. has con-

---

her fear (p.36), or the patient who would feel every attack to be 'a calamity' (p. 42).

tinued to improve in almost every way. When I saw her at lunchtime, she was delighted with everything: 'Dr Sacks!' she called out, 'I walked to and from the New Building today' (this is a distance of about six hundred yards). 'It's fabulous, it's gorgeous!' Miss R. has now been free from oculogyric crises for eight days, and has shown no akathisia or undue excitement. I too feel delighted at her progress, but for some reason am conscious of obscure forebodings.

7 *July*. Today Miss R. has shown her first signs of unstable and abrupt responses to L-DOPA. Seeing her 3½ hours after her early-morning dose, I was shocked to find her very 'down' – hypophonic, somewhat depressed, rigid and akinetic, with extremely small pupils and profuse salivation. Fifteen minutes after receiving her medication she was 'up' again – her voice and walking fully restored, cheerful, smiling, talkative, her eyes alert and shining, and her pupils somewhat dilated. I was further disquieted by observing an occasional impulsion to run, although this was easily checked by her.

8 *July*. Following an insomniac night ('I didn't feel in the least sleepy: thoughts just kept rushing through my head'), Miss R. is extremely active, cheerful and affectionate. She seems to be very busy, constantly flying from one place to another, and all her thoughts too are concerned with movement; 'Dr Sacks,' she exclaimed breathlessly, 'I feel great today. I feel I want to fly. I love you, Dr Sacks, I love you, I love you. You know, you're the kindest doctor in the world ... You know I always liked to travel around: I used to fly to Pittsburgh, Chicago, Miami, California ...' etc. Her skin is warm and flushed, her pupils are again very widely dilated, and her eyes constantly glancing to and fro. Her energy seems limitless and untiring, although I get the impression of exhaustion somewhere beneath the pressured surface. An entirely new symptom has also appeared today, a sudden quick movement of the right hand to the chin, which is

repeated two or three times an hour. When I questioned Miss R. about this she said: 'It's new, it's odd, it's strange, I never did it before. God knows why I do it. I just suddenly get an *urge*, like you suddenly got to sneeze or scratch yourself.' Fearing the onset of akathisia or excessive emotional excitement, I have reduced the dosage of L-DOPA to 3 gm. daily.

9 *July*. Today Miss R.'s energy and excitement are unabated, but her mood has veered from elation to anxiety. She is impatient, touchy and extremely demanding. She became much agitated in the middle of the day, asserting that seven dresses had been stolen from her closet, and that her purse had been stolen. She entertained dark suspicions of various fellow patients: no doubt they had been plotting this for weeks before. Later in the day, she discovered that her dresses were in fact in her closet in their usual position. Her paranoid recriminations instantly vanished: 'Wow!' she said, 'I must have imagined it all. I guess I better take myself in hand.'

14 *July*. Following the excitements and changing moods of 9 July, Miss R.'s state has become less pressured and hyperactive. She has been able to sleep, and has lost the tic-like 'wiping' movements of her right hand. Unfortunately, after a two-week remission, her old enemy has re-emerged, and she has experienced two severe oculogyric crises. I observed in these not only the usual staring, but a more bizarre symptom – captivation or enthralment of gaze: in one of these crises she had been forced to stare at one of her fellow-patients, and had felt her eyes 'drawn' this way and that, following the movements of this patient around the ward. 'It was uncanny,' Miss R. said later. 'My eyes were spellbound. I felt like I was bewitched or something, like a rabbit with a snake.' During the periods of 'bewitchment' or fascination, Miss R. had the feeling that her 'thoughts had stopped', and that she could only think of one thing, the object of her gaze. If, on the other hand, her attention was distracted,

the quality of thinking would suddenly change, the motionless fascination would be broken up, and she would experience instead 'an absolute torrent of thoughts', rushing through her mind: these thoughts did not seem to be 'her' thoughts, they were not what she wanted to think, they were 'peculiar thoughts' which appeared 'by themselves'. Miss R. could not or would not specify the nature of these intrusive thoughts, but she was greatly frightened by the whole business: 'These crises are different to the ones I used to get,' she said. 'They are worse. They are completely *mad!*'[16]

25 July. Miss R. has had an astonishing ten days, and has shown phenomena I never thought possible. Her mood has been joyous and elated, and very salacious. Her social behaviour has remained impeccable, but she has developed an insatiable urge to sing songs and tell jokes, and has made very full use of our portable tape-recorder. In the past few days, she has recorded innumerable songs of an astonishing lewdness, and reams of 'light' verse all dating from the twenties. She is also full of anecdotes and allusions to 'current' figures – to figures who were current in the mid-1920s. We have been forced to do some archival research, looking at old newspaper-files in the New York Library. We have found that almost all of Miss R.'s allusions date to 1926, her last year of real life before her illness closed round her. Her memory is uncanny, considering she is speaking of so long ago. Miss R. wants the tape-recorder, and nobody around; she

16. Jelliffe (1932) cites many cases of oculogyric crises with fixation of gaze and attention, and also of crises with reiterative 'autochthonous' thinking. Miss R. never vouchsafed the nature of the 'mad' thoughts which came to her during her crises at this time, and one would suspect from the reticence that these thoughts were of an inadmissible nature, either sexual or hostile. Jelliffe refers to several patients who were compelled to think of 'dirty things' during their crises (pp. 37–8), and to another patient (p. 39) who experienced during his crises 'ideas of reference to which he pays no attention'.

stays in her room, alone with the tape-recorder; she is looking
at everyone as if they didn't exist. She is completely engrossed
in her memories of the twenties, and is doing her best to
not-notice anything later. I suppose one calls this 'forced
reminiscence', or incontinent nostalgia.[17] *But I also have the
feeling that she feels her 'past' as present, and that, perhaps
it has never felt 'past' for her. Is it possible that Miss R.
has never, in fact, moved on from the 'past'? Could she still
be 'in' 1926 forty-three years later? Is 1926 'now'?*[18]

28 July. Miss R. sought me out this morning – the first
time she had done so in almost two weeks. Her face has lost
its jubilant look, and she looks anxious and shadowed and
slightly bewildered: 'Things can't last,' she said. 'Something awful is coming. God knows what it is, but it's bad
as they come.' I tried to find out more, but Miss R. shook her
head: 'It's just a feeling, I can't tell you more . . .'

1 August. A few hours after stating her prediction, Miss
R. ran straight into a barrage of difficulties. Suddenly she
was ticcing, jammed and blocked; the beautiful smooth flow
which had borne her along seemed to break up, and dam,
and crash back on itself. Her walking and talking are gravely affected. She is impelled to rush forward for five or six
steps, and then suddenly freezes or jams without warning;

17. See 'Incontinent Nostalgia Induced by L-DOPA', Sacks *et al.*
Lancet, June 1970, p. 1394.

18. Our earth in 1969
      Is not the planet I call mine,
      The world, I mean, that gives me strength
      To hold off chaos at arm's length.

     My Eden landscapes and their climes
     Are constructs from Edwardian times . . .

     Me alienated? Bosh! It's just
                              . . . that I feel
     Most at home with what is Real.
                                          W. H. AUDEN

she continually gets more excited and frustrated, and with increasing excitement the jamming grows worse. If she can moderate her excitement or her impulsion to run, she can still walk the corridor without freezing or jamming. Analogous problems are affecting her speech: she can only speak softly, if she is to speak at all, for with increased vocal impetus she stutters and stops. I have the feeling that Miss R.'s 'motor space' is becoming confined, so that she rebounds internally if she moves with too much speed or force. Reducing her L-DOPA to 3 gm. a day reduced the dangerous hurry and block, but led to an intensely severe oculogyric crisis – the worst Miss R. has had since starting L-DOPA. Moreover, her 'wiping' tic – which re-appeared on the 28th – has grown more severe and more *complex* with each passing hour. From a harmless feather-light brush of the chin, the movement has become a deep circular gouging, her right index-finger scratching incessantly in tight little circles, abrading the skin and making it bleed. Miss R. has been quite unable to stop this compulsion *directly*, but she can override it by thrusting her tic-hand deep in her pocket and clutching its lining with all of her force. The moment she forgets to do this, the hand flies up and scratches her face.

August 1969[19]
During the first week of August, Miss R. continued to have oculogyric crises every day of extreme severity, during which she would be intensely rigid and opisthotonic, anguished, whimpering and bathed in sweat. Her tics of the right hand became almost too fast for the eye to follow, their rate having increased to almost 300 per minute (an estimate confirmed by a slow-motion film). On 6 August, Miss R. showed very obvious palilalia repeating entire sentences and strings of words again and again: 'I'm going round like

19. The following is based on notes provided by our speech-pathologist, Miss Marjorie Kohl. I myself was away during August.

a record', she said, 'which gets stuck in the groove ...'
During the second week of August, her tics became more
complex, and were conflated with defensive manoeuvres,
counter-tics and elaborate rituals. Thus Miss R. would clutch
someone's hand, release her grip, touch something near by,
put her hand in her pocket, withdraw it, slap the pocket
three times, put it back in the pocket, wipe her chin *five*
times, clutch someone's hand ... and move again and again
through this stereotyped sequence.

The evening of 15 August provided the only pleasant in-
terlude in a month otherwise full of disability and suffering.
On this evening, quite unexpectedly, Miss R. emerged from
her crises and blocking and ticcing, and had a brief return of
joyous salacity, accompanied with free-flowing singing and
movement. For an hour this evening, she improvised a variety of coprolalic limericks to the tune of 'The Sheikh of
Araby', accompanying herself on the piano with her uncon-
tractured right hand.

Later this week, her motor and vocal block became absolute. She would suddenly call out to Miss Kohl: 'Margie,
I ... Margie, I want ... Margie! ...', completely unable to
proceed beyond the first word or two of what she so desperately wanted to say. When she tried to write, similarly,
her hand (and thoughts) suddenly stopped after a couple
of words. If one asked her to try and say what she wanted,
softly and slowly, her face would go blank, and her eyes
would shift in a tantalized manner, indicating, perhaps
her frantic inner search for the dislimning thought. Walking
became impossible at this time, for Miss R. would find her
feet completely stuck to the ground, but the impulse to move
would throw her flat on her face. During the last ten days of
August, Miss R. seemed to be totally blocked in all spheres
of activity; everything about her showed an extremity of
tension, which was entirely prevented from finding any out-

let. Her face at this time was continually clenched in a horrified, tortured and anguished expression. Her prediction of a month earlier was completely fulfilled: something awful *had* come, and it was as bad as they came.

1969–72

Miss R.'s reactions to L-DOPA since the summer of 1969 have been almost non-existent compared with her dramatic initial reaction. She has been placed on L-DOPA five further times, each with an increase of dose by degrees to about 3·0 gm. per day. Each time the L-DOPA has procured *some* reduction in her rigidity, oculogyria and general entrancement, but less and less on each succeeding occasion. It has *never* called forth anything resembling the amazing mobility and mood change of July 1969, and in particular has never recalled the extraordinary sense of 1926-ness which she had at that time. When Miss R. has been on L-DOPA for several weeks its advantages invariably become over-weighted by its disadvantages, and she returns to a state of intense 'block', crises, and tic-like impulsions. The form of her tics has varied a good deal on different occasions: in one of her periods on L-DOPA her crises were always accompanied by a palilalic verbigeration of the word 'Honeybunch!' which she would repeat twenty or thirty times a minute for the entire day.

However deep and strange her pathological state, Miss R. can invariably be 'awakened' for a few seconds or minutes by external stimuli, although she is obviously quite unable to generate any such stimuli or calls-to-action for herself. If Miss A. – a fellow-patient with dipsomania – drinks more than twenty times an hour at the water fountain, Miss R. cries, 'Get away from that fountain, Margaret, or I'll clobber you!' or 'Stop sucking that spout, Margaret, we all know what you really want to suck!' Whenever she hears my name being paged she yells out, 'Dr Sacks! Dr Sacks!! They're after you again!' and continues to yell this until I have answered the page.

Miss R. is at her best when she is visited – as she frequently is – by any of her devoted family who fly in from all over the country to see her. At such time she is all agog with excitement, her blank masked face cracks into a smile, and she shows a great hunger for family gossip, though no interest at all in political events or other current 'news'; at such times she is able to say a certain amount quite intelligibly, and in particular shows her fondness for jokes and mildly salacious indiscretions. Seeing Miss R. at this time one realizes what a 'normal' and charming and alive personality is imprisoned or suspended by her ridiculous illness.

On a number of occasions I have asked Miss R. about the strange 'nostalgia' which she showed in July 1969, and how she experiences the world generally. She usually becomes distressed and 'blocked' when I ask such questions, but on a few occasions she has given me enough information for me to perceive the almost incredible truth about her. She indicates that in her 'nostalgic' state she *knew* perfectly well that it was 1969 and that she was sixty-four years old, but that she *felt* that it was 1926 and she was twenty-one; she adds that she can't really imagine what it's like being older than twenty-one, because she has never really experienced it. For most of the time, however, there is 'nothing, absolutely nothing, no thoughts at all' in her head, as if she is forced to block off an intolerable and insoluble anachronism – the almost half-century gap between her age as felt and experienced (her *ontological* age) and her actual or *official* age. It seems, in retrospect, as if the L-DOPA must have 'de-blocked' her for a few days, and revealed to her a time-gap beyond comprehension or bearing, and that she has subsequently been forced to 're-block' herself and the possibility of any similar reaction to L-DOPA ever happening again.

She continues to look much younger than her years; indeed, in a fundamental sense, she *is* much younger than her age. But she is a Sleeping Beauty whose 'awakening' was unbearable to her, and who will never be awoken again.

4. ROBERT O.

Mr O. was born in Russia in 1905, but came to the United States as an infant. He enjoyed excellent health, and showed unusual scholastic ability (graduating from High School at the age of fifteen), until his seventeenth year, when he developed a somnolent form of *encephalitis lethargica* concomitantly with the flu. He was intensely drowsy, although not stuporous, for six months, but shortly after recovering from this acute illness became aware of abnormalities in his sleeping, mind and mood.

Between 1922 and 1930, reversal of sleep-rhythm was perhaps the major problem, Mr O. tending to be very sleepy and torpid by day, and very restless and insomniac by night. Other sleep disorders, at this time, included sudden fits of yawning, narcolepsy, somnambulism, somnoloquy, sleep-paralyses and nightmares.

Emotionally equable before his encephalitis, Mr O. subsequently showed a tendency to rather marked mood-swings (with frequent sudden depressions and occasional elations) which seemed to him to 'come out of the blue', and to show no obvious connection with the actual circumstances of his external or emotional life. There were also short periods of restlessness and impulsiveness, when he would feel 'driven to move around, or do something', which again he could not connect with the day-to-day circumstances of living. He also observed, in these early days, that 'something had happened' to his mind. He retained his memory, his love of reading, his accurate vocabulary, his keenness, his wit, but found that he could no longer concentrate for long periods, because 'thoughts would dart into my mind, not my own, not intended if you know what I mean', or, alternatively, because 'thoughts would suddenly vanish, smack in the middle of a sentence ... They'd drop out, leaving a *space* like a frame minus a picture.' Usually, Mr O. was content to ascribe his erratic thinking to the sleeping-sickness, but at other times became convinced that 'influences' of various sorts were 'fiddling' with his thoughts.

In 1926, or thereabouts, he started to develop twitching and shaking of both arms, and observed that he had ceased to swing the left arm when walking. He presented himself for examination at Pennsylvania Hospital in 1928, at which time the following features were noted: 'Fine tremor of the fingers and tongue ... fibrillary twitchings of the forearm muscles ... mask-like expression ... constant blinking of both eyes.' During the four years of his outpatient attendance at this hospital, he appeared mentally clear at all times, but was observed to suffer from periods of depression and occasionally of euphoria.

Despite these symptoms, Mr O. was able to work as a salesman until 1936, and subsequently to maintain himself independently, on a small disability pension, until his admission to Mount Carmel Hospital in 1956. In the years immediately preceding his admission here, Mr O. had become somewhat solitary and seclusive in his habits, rather eccentric in his speech and thinking, obsessive almost to stereotypy in his daily activities, and religious.

On admission, Mr O. was able to walk independently, but showed a mildly flexed posture of the trunk. He showed a coarse intermittent tremor of the left arm and leg, rigidity and cog-wheeling in all limbs, masking of the face and inability to look upwards. He asserted, firmly, but pleasantly, that his moods were dictated by the interactions of protons and neutrons in the atmosphere, and that his neurological problems were the result of a spinal tap performed in 1930.

In the early 1960s, Mr O. developed two new symptoms, which his fellow-patients termed 'pulling faces' and 'talking to 'isself'. The grimacing scarcely resembled any normal expression, but looked more like a man being sick, with retching, protrusion of the tongue, and agonized-looking clenching of the eyes. The 'talking to 'isself' was not really talking either, but a sort of murmuring-purring sound emitted with each expiration, rather pleasing to the ear, like the sound of a distant sawmill, or bees swarming, or a contented lion after a satisfactory meal. It is interesting that Mr O. had experienced the 'impulse' to make noises and faces for at least thirty years, but had controlled these successfully until 1960. These symptoms were most marked if he was tired, excited, frustrated or ill; they *also* became more striking if they excited attention, which led, of course, to the usual vicious circle.

These years also saw the gradual worsening of his rigid-dystonic symptoms, and his hurrying and festination. I saw Mr O. several times between 1966 and 1968 (i.e. before his receiving L-DOPA), and got to know him quite well. He was an odd, charming, rather gnome-like man, full of surprising turns and twists of phrase, some of these very droll, and some of them quite irrelevant to the mainstream of his thought; his 'thought-disorder', his very original and sometimes shocking views, and his mocking sense of humour, were all inseparably combined – as in many gifted schizophrenics – and all of these joined to give a curiously Gogolian flavour to his thought and conversation. He showed very little affect of any kind as he spoke, and I never saw him 'put out' in any way during the course of these three years. He was, it seemed, never angry, never belligerent, never anxious, never demanding, but he was assuredly not apathetic in the sense of Mrs B. I had the impression, rather, that his affects had been splintered and displaced and dispersed, in some unimaginably complex but clearly protective fashion. He was a very narcissistic man, not too concerned with the world.

His voice was rapid, soft, low-pitched and gibbering, as if he were very pressed for time and had a secret to confide. He showed extreme rigidity of the trunk, with a rather disabling flexion-dystonia which forced the trunk forward at a sharp angle to his legs. Mr O. was quite unable to straighten up voluntarily – the effort, if anything, increased the dystonia – but did straighten up when he was in bed and asleep. He showed a marked plastic rigidity of the limbs, without dystonic components, and occasional 'flapping' tremor. He was able to rise to his feet easily, and to walk rather swiftly; he had difficulty coming to a halt, and he could not walk slowly. Propulsion and retropulsion were readily called forth. In addition to his grimacing and humming, Mr O. showed a variety of smaller movements of the ears, the eyebrows, the platysma, or chin. He showed a rather unblinking, lizard-like stare, except when grimacing, or during his rare paroxysms of blepharoclonus. But, all-in-all, Mr O. was one of our most active and independent patients, able to look after himself in every way, to walk round the neighbourhood, and to carry out his singular social activities, which were confined to feeding pigeons, giving candies to children, and nattering by the hour with the hoboes down the road.

Hyoscine and other anti-cholinergics helped his rigidity a little; surgery had never been considered. In view of the fact that he could already get around sufficiently, and that he showed tendencies which might be worsened by L-DOPA, I was somewhat hesitant at first to try this with him. But his bent back was 'killing him', he said, so we felt it was worth trying the L-DOPA for *this*.

Course on L-DOPA

The administration of L-DOPA was started on 7 May. During the first ten days of the trial, with the daily dosage of L-DOPA being progressively raised to 4 gm. daily, neither therapeutic nor adverse effects were observed.

On 19 May (while he was receiving 4 gm. L-DOPA daily), I noticed for the first time some adverse effects of the drug. Grimacing, which had been sporadic previously, had become frequent, and severe in intensity. Mr O.'s voice was more hurried and showed some tendency to block : this was vividly described by Mr O. himself : 'The words clash together : they interrupt one another : they jam the exit.' His walking also had become more hurried, and had developed an urgent, impatient quality : this too was memorably described by Mr O. 'I feel forced to hurry,' he said, 'as if Satan was chasing me.'

On the evening of 21 May, while performing late rounds, I observed Mr O., fast asleep, pursing his lips during sleep and every so often waving his arms or talking during his sleep.

In the hope of reducing his axial rigidity and flexure, I increased the dose of L-DOPA to 6 gm. daily. This did lead to reduction of rigidity in the limbs, and to a lesser extent in the trunk and neck-muscles, but any advantage this might have been to the patient was offset by a further and intolerable increase in forced and involuntary movements. In particular, forced protrusion and propulsion of the tongue now became violent and practically continuous, and was associated with forced gagging and retching. Speech was rendered impossible by continued tongue-pulsions. Other forms of grimacing – especially forced closures of the eyes – had also become incessant; so much so that Mr O. was virtually blind. In view of these intolerable effects, I felt that L-DOPA should be discontinued, and it was accordingly reduced over the course of a week. By 10 June, the L-DOPA had been cut out, and Mr O. had returned to his pre-DOPA status.

1969–72

Mr O. never *voiced* any disappointment as such, or anger, or envy of those round him who had done well on L-DOPA, but he *showed* his feelings in a change of behaviour. He went out less, and stopped feeding the pigeons. He started reading much more – especially Cabbala – and spent hours making 'diagrams' which he kept locked in a drawer. He was never disagreeable, but he became less accessible. And his thinking seemed more scattered, and less benign than before; his wit had always been sharp, but now became mordant, and once in a while it became vitriolic. And yet, there were pleasant times, especially on fine Sunday mornings, when the protons and neutrons were behaving themselves. At such times Mr O. would walk round the block and once in a while he would drop in to see me (my apartment was only a few yards from the hospital); I would give him some cocoa, and he would look through my books, which he handled with scholarly ease and absorption; he seemed, at such times, to enjoy my presence, provided I said nothing and asked him no questions; he too would be silent, exempt from the nagging and pressure of thought.

But his physical state was going downhill, and it seemed to do so much faster than before. He 'deteriorated' much more in 1970 than in the preceding decade. His axial dystonia became almost unbearable, forcing his trunk forwards at right angles to his legs. Most disquietingly, he started to lose weight – muscle-bulk and strength which he desperately needed. We gave him custards and milk-shakes and second helpings and egg-nogs, until he protested he was being stuffed like a goose; we gave him injections of anabolic steroids; we did inumerable tests to see whether he had hidden cancer or infection – all of which were entirely negative.

His urine was full of creatinine, but this was no more than a reflection of his clinical state. He was wasting away in front of our eyes and nothing we could do seemed to stay his cachexia.[20]

Having observed repeatedly that the effects of L-DOPA were extremely variable, even in the same patient, and that its actions on a second trial might be quite different from those originally seen, we decided in 1971 to try it again. Its actions *were* different this time, whether 'better' or 'worse' it is impossible to say. On its second trial, L-DOPA caused none of the grimacing and respiratory difficulties which were so intolerable the first time: these, if anything, rather declined in severity. The plastic rigidity of his limbs was reduced, so much indeed that they became almost flaccid; but the axial dystonia was unchanged or increased.

L-DOPA, the first time, had scarcely affected his *thinking*, but it did so the second time in a disastrous sort of way. Mr O.'s thoughts became faster, more pressured, less controlled, and fragmented. He had shown occasional 'slippages' and odd associations for fifty years past, but now these burst forth in incontinent fashion.

His thinking and speaking became more and more splintered, and full of neologisms; words and even fragments of words broke up, re-assorted, and were given new mean-

20. It is well known (and was remarked by Parkinson himself) that progressive weight-loss is a most ominous and usually terminal symptom in Parkinsonian patients. In some patients, this is clearly attributable to reduced intake, difficulties in eating, etc. In a number of post-encephalitic patients, on the other hand, one may see the most extreme weight-loss despite normal and even voracious eating, which suggests the possibility of a central cachexia, of patients being consumed in their own metabolic furnace. The opposite – a mysterious fattening and increase of bulk – may also be seen in some of these patients. In a number of cases, the sudden onset of cachexia or its opposite comes on with L-DOPA, and seems to reflect a central effect of this drug. Whether Mr O.'s cachexia had been set off by L-DOPA is open to question.

ings; he now spoke in a very accelerated Bleulerian 'word salad', brilliant in a way, but very difficult to follow – like *Finnegans Wake* run backwards on tape.

The L-DOPA, of course, was once again stopped, but Mr O.'s acute thought-disorder continued unabated. It continued, in fact, for another twelve months. Yet there was, clearly, a part of him which was not fragmented, but 'together' and vigilant, for he recognized everybody, and the routine of the ward. He was never, for a moment, confused or disoriented, like someone who is demented or in a delirium. The former Mr O., one couldn't help feeling, was still present somewhere, watching and controlling, somewhere *behind* the broken-up ravings. (See footnote to p. 279.)

His weight-loss, throughout this, continued unabated. He lost seventy pounds over a period of two years, and finally became almost too weak to move. He shrivelled to death in front of our eyes.

One other circumstance, perhaps, deserves recording. The week before he died, Mr O. suddenly became quite lucid in his speech and thought; and more than this, he 're-found' feelings which had been scattered and suppressed for fifty years; he ceased to be 'schizophrenic', and became a simple and direct human being. We had several talks in those final days, the tone of which was set by Mr O. 'Don't give me any guff,' he said. 'I *know* the score. Bob's down to skin and bone. He's *ready* to go.' In his last few days he joked with the nurses, and he asked the Rabbi to read him a psalm. A few hours before his death he said: 'I was going to kill myself, in '22 ... I'm glad I didn't ... It's been a good game, encephalitis and all.'

5. HESTER Y.

Mrs Y. was born in Brooklyn, the elder child of an immigrant couple. She had no illnesses of note in her growing-up years, certainly nothing which suggested *encephalitis lethargica.*

She showed from the first an active intelligence, and an unusually independent and equable character. Her warmth, her courage, and her acute sense of humour are affectionately remembered by her younger brother: 'Hester' (he said to me, forty years later) 'was always a good sport and a wonderful sister. She had strong likes and dislikes, but she was never unfair. She was always in scrapes, like the rest of us kids, but she was as tough as they come – she took everything in her stride. And she could laugh at everything, especially herself.'

After finishing High School, and a lightning courtship, Mrs Y. married at the age of nineteen. She gave birth to a son the following year, and to a daughter three years after her marriage. She enjoyed ten years of family life before being struck by illness in her thirtieth year. It is clear that Mrs Y. was the fulcrum of her family, giving it balance and stability with her own strength of character, and that when *she* became ill, its foundations were rocked. Her symptoms, at first, were paroxysmal and bizarre. She would be walking or talking with a normal pattern and flow, and then *suddenly*, without warning, would come to a stop – in mid-stride, mid-gesture, or the middle of a word; after a few seconds she would resume speech and movement, apparently unaware that any interruption had occurred. She was considered, at this time, to have a form of epilepsy, so-called 'absences' or '*petit mal* variants'. In the months that followed, these standstills grew longer, and would occasionally last for several hours; she would often be discovered quite motionless, in a room, with a completely blank and vacuous face. The merest touch, at such times, served to dissipate these states, and to permit immediate resumption of movement and speech. The diagnosis, at this period, had been changed to 'hysteria'.

After two years of these paroxysmal and mysterious standstills, unmistakable signs of Parkinsonism appeared, accompanied by indications of catatonia or trance, impeding all movement and speech and thought. As her Parkinsonism and entrancement grew rapidly worse, Mrs Y. became 'strange' and difficult of access – and it was this, more than her physical difficulties, which disquieted, alarmed and angered her family. This change is described by her brother as follows: 'Hester was vivid in all her reactions, until her thirties when her illness took hold of her. She didn't lose any of her feelings, and she didn't become hostile or cold, but she seemed to get more remote all the time. One could see her being carried away by the illness, like a swimmer sucked out by the tide. She was being sucked away right out of our reach ...' By her thirty-fifth year, Mrs Y. was virtually immobile and speechless, and totally immured in a deep, far-off state. Her husband and children felt tortured and helpless, and had no idea which way they should turn. It was Mrs Y. herself who finally decided that it would be best for everybody if she were admitted to hospital; she said, 'I'm finished. There's nothing else to do.'

She entered Mount Carmel in her thirty-sixth year. Her entry to hospital, the finality implied, broke the morale and coherence of her husband and children. Her husband visited her twice in hospital, and found it unbearable; he never came again, and finally divorced her; her daughter became acutely psychotic, and had to be institutionalized in a local state hospital; her son left home and fled 'somewhere out West'. The Y.s – as a family – had ceased to exist.

Mrs Y.'s life in Mount Carmel was eventless and placid. She was well liked by other patients and nurses and staff, for her humour and character somehow 'showed through' her dense immobility. She was virtually motionless and speechless at all times, and when I first met her, in 1966, I suddenly realized – with a profound sense of shock – that it was possible for Parkinsonism and catatonia to reach an *infinite* degree of severity.[21] She certainly gave no impression

21. When I speak of 'a profound sense of shock' in regard to my first glimpse of Hester, I do not use the phrase lightly or loosely. Although it is now seven years ago, I sharply recall the stunned feeling, the sense of amazement which came over me, as I suddenly realized the *infinite* nature, the *qualitative* infinity, of the phenomenon which faced me ... One speaks of infinite anguishes, poignancies, desires, and joys – and one does so naturally, with no sense of paradox: one thinks of them as infinities, in the infinitude of the soul, i.e. one conceives them in a metaphysical sense. But *Parkinsonism* – was this not something categorically different? Was it not a simple, mechanical disorder of function – a mere excess or deficiency – something essentially finite, something which could be measured in the divisions or units of a suitable scale? Was it not, as it were, a commodity or *thing*, to be weighed and assayed as a grocer weighs butter? This is what I had been taught, what I had read, what I thought. And then I saw Hester, and experienced a sudden jarring of my thinking, a sudden wrenching from a way of seeing, a frame of reference, to one which was deeply and shockingly different. When I saw Hester, I suddenly realized that all I had thought about the finite, ponderable, numerable nature of Parkinsonism was nonsense. I suddenly realized, at this moment, that Parkinsonism could in no sense be seen as a thing, which increased or decreased by finite increments. It suddenly came to me that Parkinsonism was a propensity, a tendency – which had no minimum, no maximum, and no finite units; that it was anumerical; that from its first, infinitesimal, intimation or twinge, it could proceed by an infinite multitude of infinitesimal increments to an infinite, and then more infinite, and still more infinite, degree of severity. And that its 'least part', so to speak, possessed (in infinitesimal form) the entire, indivisible nature of the whole. Given such a concept we would also have to envisage it as irrational (surd), immeasurable and incommensurable, and also as illimitable and *insatiable* (like greed). Such thoughts carried a

of deadness or apathy (like Magda B.); no impression of veto or 'block' (like Lucy K.); no impression of aloofness or withdrawal (like Leonard L. and Miron V.); but she did give the impression of an infinite remoteness. She seemed to dwell in some unimaginably strange, inaccessible ultimity, in some bottomlessly deep hole or abyss of being; she seemed crushed into an infinitely dense, inescapable state, or held motionless in the motionless 'eye' of a vortex. This impression was accentuated by her slow rhythmic humming, and by her slowly rotating palilalic responses.[22] She showed an infinite coercion or *consent* of behaviour — a circular, effortless, ceaseless movement, which seemed still because its locus was infinitesimal in size. She was utterly still, intensely still, yet perpetually moving, in an ontological orbit contracted to zero.

One thing, and one only, could slightly reduce the depth of her state, and allow some emergence from the abyss of Parkinsonism. Every afternoon, in physiotherapy, Mrs Y. would be suspended in a warm pool of water, and after an hour of attempted active and passive movement, she would be stirred a little from her infinite akinesia and show a brief ability to move her right arm, and to make small pedalling motions with her legs in the water. But within half an hour, even this capacity would have faded, and she would be totally reverted to entranced akinesia.

In addition to her akinesia, Mrs Y. had developed, over

---

disquieting implication, viz. that if Parkinsonism *per se* was immeasurable, it would never be possible to find an exact countermeasure, to counter it, cancel it out, or 'titrate' it (in more than a limited and temporary fashion). This dark thought, which I endeavoured to banish, first came to me when I saw Hester in 1966, and recurred to me in the winter of 1967, when I first read of the amazing effects of L-DOPA in patients, and of the appearance of 'side-effects' despite the exactest 'titrations' of dosage.

22. '. . . magnetized by some words of his own speech, his mind was slowly circling round and round in the same orbit.' James Joyce, 'An Encounter'.

the years, a severe dystonic contracture of the left arm, and a flexion-dystonia of the neck, which almost impacted the chin on the sternum. This, added to her profound akinesia of chewing and swallowing, had made feeding almost insuperably difficult. Akinesia of chewing and swallowing had become so severe, by May of 1969, that Mrs Y. was being fed on a liquid diet, and the necessity of tube-feeding had become imminent. She was started on L-DOPA as a life-saving measure, for we feared she would die from aphagia or starvation. L-DOPA was first administered in orange-juice, on 7 May.

Course on L-DOPA

During the first ten days of L-DOPA administration (7–16 May), during which the daily dosage was gradually increased to 4 gm., no change whatever was to be observed in Mrs Y. Fearing that some or all of the drug was being decomposed by the acid orange-juice in which it was being given, I requested, on 16 May, that it be given in apple sauce instead. The next day Mrs Y. 'exploded' – as the nursing-staff put it. There was no subjective or objective 'warning' whatever. On Saturday 17 May, about half an hour after receiving her morning gram of L-DOPA, Mrs Y. suddenly jumped to her feet, and before incredulous eyes walked the length of the ward. 'What do you think of that, eh?' she exclaimed in a loud, excited voice. 'What do you think of that, what do you think of that, what do you think of that?' When I spoke to an awed staff-nurse, a couple of days later, she told me what she thought of it: 'I've never seen anything like it. Hester's wonderful, it's just like a miracle.'

Throughout the course of this amazing weekend, Mrs Y. walked excitedly all round the hospital, starting conversations with fellow-patients who had never heard her talk before, rejoicing ebulliently in her new-found freedom. Her capacity to chew and swallow were suddenly increased, and so too was her appetite: 'Don't give me any of that slush!'

she exclaimed, when presented at lunch-time with her usual thin soup. 'I want a steak, well done!' The steak, duly procured and grilled, was devoured with great relish, and with no sign of difficulty in chewing or swallowing. With her right hand suddenly released from its decades-long constraint, Mrs Y. made the first entries in a notebook I had left with her, and which I had not seriously imagined that she would ever find a use for.

19 *May.* Having left Mrs Y., on Friday evening, in her usual state of profound immobility, I was awed at the change which had occurred over the weekend. I had, at this time, had relatively little experience of the dramatic responses to L-DOPA which occur in some post-encephalitic patients, and such responses as I had seen had always been preceded by *some* 'warming-up' period of increasing activity; but Mrs Y.'s 'awakening' had commenced and been completed in a matter of seconds.[23] Entering her room on Monday morning,

23. Her sudden mobilization and 'normalization', after years of virtually total immobility, seemed incredible, and indeed impossible, to all who saw it – hence my awe, and the awe of the staff, our feeling that it was '. . . just like a miracle'. I have said that I had 'a profound sense of shock' when I first saw Hester in 1966, and realized that she had reached a virtual standstill, physically and mentally; but this was as nothing compared with the shock I received in 1969, when I saw her moving and talking with ease and fluency, with all her original patterns of action perfectly preserved and intact. This sense of shock deepened the more I pondered upon it, until I realised that almost all my ideas on the nature of Parkinsonism, of activity, of existence, and of time itself, would have to be completely revised . . .

For if a *normal* person is 'de-activated' for even a short time, he meets profound and peculiar difficulties in re-activation, that is, in resuming his previous patterns of activity. Thus if one breaks a leg or ruptures one's quadriceps (and has one's leg further de-activated by enclosure and immobilization in plaster) one finds that one is *functionally disabled* even when one is anatomically healed : thus, after such an experience (or, more accurately, after such a hiatus in normal experience and activity) one finds that one has 'forgotten'

I was loudly greeted by a transformed Mrs Y. sitting on the edge of her bed, perfectly balanced, with wide-open shining eyes, a somewhat flushed complexion, and a smile going from one ear to the other. Loudly, delightedly, and somewhat pali-

---

how to use the de-activated limb, and that one must *re-learn* (or re-discover) how to use it all over again, a process which may take many weeks or months. Indeed, if a limb is severely de-activated for any length of time, one will lose all sense of its existence. Such observations show us the truth of Leibniz's dictum '*Qui non agit non existit*' – he who does not act does not exist. Normally, then, we see that a hiatus in activity leads to a hiatus in existence – we are critically dependent on a continual flow of impulses and information to and from all the sensory and motor organs of the body. *We must be active or we cease to exist: activity and actuality are one and the same* ...

What, then, of Hester, who after being totally motionless, and (presumably) de-activated, for many years, jumped up and walked in the twinkling of an eye? We might suppose, as I did at first, that she was not really de-activated during her motionless state; but this hypothesis is refutable on several grounds – clinical observations on the absoluteness of her standstill, her own descriptions of the quality of her experience during standstill (see p. 141), and the electrical silence found in attempts to record electrical activity in her muscles during periods of standstill; all of these observations indicate that she was truly and completely de-activated during her standstills. But it was also apparent that her standstills had *no subjective duration whatever*. There was no 'elapsing of time' for Hester during her standstills; at such times she would be (if the logical and semantic paradox may be allowed) at once action-less, being-less, and time-less ... Only through such considerations, fantastic as they seemed to me at first, could I comprehend how Hester was able to resume normal activity after years of inactivity, in contrast to an 'ontologically normal' person who would lose or 'forget' action-patterns over a length of time, and would then require a further, and perhaps very considerable length of time before being able to 'remember' or re-learn the lost action-patterns. In Hester, by contrast, it was as if the ontological current, the current of being, could be suddenly 'switched off' and as suddenly 'switched on', with no loss of action-patterns in between, nor any need to re-learn them subsequently – and this because *for her no time had elapsed.*

lalically, she poured into my ears the events of the weekend; her speech was very rapid, slightly pressured, and exultant: 'Wonderful, wonderful, wonderful!' she repeated. 'I'm a new person, I feel it, I feel it inside, I'm a brand-new person. I feel so much, I can't tell you what I feel. Everything's changed, it's going to be a new life now ...' etc. Similar sentiments were expressed in the diary which Mrs Y. had now started to keep. The first entry, made on Saturday 17 May, read: 'I feel very good. My speech is getting louder and clearer. My hands and fingers move more freely. I can even take the paper off a piece of candy, which I haven't done for years.' The following day she wrote: 'Anyone who reads this diary will have to excuse my spelling and my writing – they must remember that I haven't done any writing for years and years.' And to this she added, very poignantly: 'I would like to express my feelings fully. It is so long since I had any feelings. I can't find the words for my feelings. I would like to have a dictionary to find words for my feelings ...' One

---

We often say that 'Procrastination is the thief of time,' and the same is true of haste or festination. Hastening and dawdling, festination and cunctation, whether neurotic or Parkinsonian, are not proper activities (one might call them 'pseudo-activities'), and form one way of 'wasting' or 'losing' time. But it is the 'negative' phenomena of Parkinsonism, in particular the phenomena of *nothingness*, *eventlessness* and 'standstill', which are the absolute thieves of time. Thus, in the cases of Hester and similar patients, there had been an intermittent or progressive taking-away of 'true time' – of 'ontological time', experimental time, activity time, as opposed to the 'formal time' of clocks and calendars – since the start of their illnesses. In this way, her situation (or, rather, her 'situationlessness') was somewhat akin to that of Rose R., who avowed (and showed) that she had been practically devoid of experience for forty-three years, and that during this period there had been 'nothing, absolutely nothing, no thoughts at all' for her. Both of these patients, then, had been deprived of time, deprived of being, in a fundamental and almost incredible way; but whereas Rose R. found this confiscation unendurable, Hester Y., after a torturing interim, managed to accommodate to her loss with courage and humour.

feeling at least was straightforward: 'I am *enjoying* my food,
I feel ravenous for food. Before I simply ate what was put in
my mouth.' Concluding her entries for the weekend, Mrs Y.
summed up: 'I feel full of pep, vigour and vitality. Is it the
medicine I am taking, or just my new state of mind?' Her
handwriting, sustained over three pages of her diary, was
large, fluent, and highly legible.

Completely motionless and submerged for over twenty
years, she had surfaced and shot into the air like a cork released from great depth; she had exploded with a vengeance
from the shackles which held her. I thought of prisoners released from gaol; I thought of children released from school;
I thought of spring-awakenings after winter-sleeps; I thought
of the Sleeping Beauty; and I also thought, with some fore-
boding, of catatonics, suddenly frenzied.

Examining Mrs Y. on 19 May, I found a remarkable
loosening in her previously locked neck and right arm, while
in the left arm and legs tone seemed to be, if anything, even
less than normal. Salivation was much reduced, and drooling had ceased. The expiratory hum was no longer evident.
She seemed extremely alert, and her eye-movements, swift
and frequent, were now accompanied by appropriate head-
movements. When asked to clap, an action which had been
not only impossible but unthinkable before she received
L-DOPA, Mrs Y. could now clap with an exuberant force,
although the clapping was performed with her right arm
predominantly. She became excited with the act of clapping,
and after about fifteen claps, suddenly switched to an alternation of clapping and slapping her thighs, and then to an
alternation of clapping and touching her hands behind her
head. I was disquieted by these unsolicited variations, not
knowing whether to ascribe them to high spirits, or to something more driven and compulsive than this.

20 *May*. Compulsive tic-like movements made their appearance yesterday. Mrs Y.'s right hand now shows exceed-

ingly quick darting motions, suddenly touching her nose, her ear, her cheek, her mouth. When I asked her why she made these movements, she said: 'It's nothing, it's nothing. They don't mean a thing. It's just a habit, a habit – like my humming's a habit.' Her movements were extraordinarily quick and forceful, and her speech seemed two or three times quicker than normal speech; if she had previously resembled a slow-motion film, or a persistent film-frame stuck in the projector, she now gave the impression of a speeded-up film – so much so that my colleagues, looking at a film of Mrs Y. which I took at this time, insisted the projector was running too fast. Her threshold of reaction was now almost zero, and all her actions were instantaneous, precipitate and excessively forceful.[24] Mrs Y. had slept poorly the night before, and was to have no sleep at all the following night.

21 *May*. I was informed by the nursing staff, when I came on the ward, that Mrs Y. had 'flipped' and had become 'terribly excitable' and 'hysterical'. When I entered her room, I found her intensely agitated and akathisic, constantly kicking and crossing her legs, banging her hands, and uttering sudden high-pitched screams. She could be calmed, to

24. If Mrs Y., before L-DOPA, was the most *impeded* person I have ever seen, she became, on L-DOPA, the most *accelerated* person I have ever seen. I have known a number of Olympic athletes, but Mrs Y. could have beaten them all in terms of reaction-time; under other circumstances she could have been the fastest gun in the West. Such velocity and alacrity and impetuosity of movement can only be achieved in pathological states. It is seen, above all, in Gilles de la Tourette (multiple tic) syndrome; in certain hyperkinetic children; and in states of 'amok' and hyperkinetic catatonia, where movements (according to Bleuler) '... are often executed with great strength, and nearly always involve unnecessary muscle-groups ... All actions may be executed with far too much power and energy for the purpose.' And, of course, by a number of drugs. The subject of pharmacological retardation and acceleration was treated by H. G. Wells in an entertaining and prophetic story ('The New Accelerator'), written at the close of the last century.

a remarkable extent, by speaking to her in a soft soothing voice, or holding her hands, or by a very *gentle* pressure on her frenzied limbs. A constraint, in contrast, caused intense frustration, and heightened her agitation and frenzy : thus if one tried to prevent her kicking her legs, an unbearable tension developed which sought discharge in pounding of the arms; if *these* were constrained, she would lunge with her now-mobilized head from side to side; and if *this* was constrained she would scream.

For much of this day, Mrs Y. wrote in her diary, covering page after page in a rapid scrawl full of paligraphic repetitions, puns, clangs, and violent, perseverative crossings-out – a script (and mode of thought) as different from her calm, freely flowing writing of the weekend as this had been from the agonizingly obstructed, virtually impossible lettering which was all she could do before L-DOPA had been given. I was at first astonished that Mrs Y. *could* write in face of such emotional and motor agitation, but it was soon evident that writing was a *necessity* to her at this juncture, and that the ability to express and record her thoughts in this way allowed a vital act of catharsis and self-communion. It also allowed an indirect form of communication with *me*, for she was prepared to express herself in writing, and show her writings to me, but not to vouchsafe her most intimate thoughts directly to me.

Her writings, at this time, were almost entirely expressions of blame, rage, and terror, mingled with feelings of grief and loss. There were long paranoid tirades against various nurses and nursing-aides who had 'persecuted' and 'tormented' her since she entered the hospital, and vengeful phantasies as to how she would now 'get back' at them. She reverted, again and again, to a former neighbour in the hospital, a hostile dement who two years before had thrown a glass of water all over her. And there were innumerable pages blotted with tears, which bore witness to her grief and her merciless conscience: 'Look at me now,' she wrote in her diary. 'I'm fifty-five, bent double ... a cripple ... a hag ... I used to be so pretty, Dr Sacks; you'd never believe it now ... I've lost my husband and son ... I drove them away ... My daughter's crazy ... It's all my fault. It must be a punishment for something I did ... I've been asleep for twenty years and grown old in my sleep.'

What she did *not* express in her diary, and which was perhaps still repressed, were sexual feelings and libidinous substitutes – the *voracities* which so many other patients showed during climactic excitements induced by L-DOPA. That she was consumed by such feelings, *under the surface*, was shown by her lascivious-nightmarish dreams at this time, and the quality of her hallucinations later this day. I was called to see Mrs Y. around eight in the evening, because she was constantly screaming with ear-splitting intensity. When I entered her room she flew into a panic, mistook my fountain-pen for a syringe, and started screaming: 'It's a needle, a needle, a needle, a needle ... take it away, take it away ... don't stick me, don't stick me!', her screams becoming louder and louder all the time, while she thrashed her legs and her trunk in an absolute frenzy. She had written in her diary: 'I don't *think* I am in a concentration-camp??????', the queries growing larger and more numerous till they covered the entire page; and on the following page, in huge capital letters, 'PLEASE I AM NOT MAD, NOT MAD.' Her face was flushed, her pupils dilated, and her pulse was bounding and exceedingly rapid. When she was not screaming at this time, she showed gasping and panting, and violent out-thrustings of her tongue and her lips.

I requested the nurses to give her 10 mg. of thorazine, intramuscularly, and within fifteen minutes her frenzy subsided, and was replaced by exhaustion, contrition and sobbing. The terror, suspicion and rage went out of her eyes, and were replaced by a look of affection and trust: 'Don't let it happen again, Dr Sacks,' she whispered. 'That was like a nightmare, but worse. Must never happen again, never, never, never ... never again.' Mrs Y. now consented to my lowering the dose of L-DOPA, which she had strenuously and violently opposed before: 'It'll be a death sentence, if you lower it,' she had said in the morning.

22–5 *May*. I lowered the L-DOPA from 3 gm. to 2 gm. to 1 gm. a day, but Mrs Y. continued to show excessive arousal, although there was no return of the intense paranoia which occurred on the 21st. She decided, on the 22nd, to settle her scores with her former neighbour, and on the morning of this day threw a jug of water at her, and came back from this chuckling, in a much better mood. When I asked her whether she had been brooding over the matter for the entire two years, she said: 'No, of course not. I didn't care at the time. I didn't give it a thought till I started L-DOPA. And then I got mad, and couldn't stop thinking about it.' She continued, at this time, to write in her diary – indeed she scarcely did anything else at this time, and the moment she stopped writing her agitation and akathisia immediately recurred. There were no more tirades or phantasies of vengeance after she had secured her token-revenge on her token-persecutor, and her writings on the 22nd and 23rd were entirely concerned with the questions of illness and family and sadness and guilt, and by the increasing recognition that 'Fate' – not herself – was responsible for everything. On the 24th she said to me: 'Please stop the L-DOPA. It's too much to handle. Everything has happened far too fast these few days ... I need to cool off and think everything over.' I stopped her L-DOPA on this day, as requested. Seeing her on the 25th rigid, motionless, speechless again, her eyes lustreless and her head on her chest – I could hardly believe that the entire cycle of triumphant emergence, 'complications', and withdrawal, had all taken place in the span of a week.

1969–72

It is now forty months since the above notes were written, forty months in which Mrs Y. has continued to take L-DOPA (except on rare occasions, described below), to react to it violently and hyperbolically, and yet to maintain for herself a fuller and more active life than the great majority of our patients at Mount Carmel. Of all the patients I have ever known, Mrs Y. is the most extravagant and unstable in her physiological activity and reactions to L-DOPA; yet she is the 'coolest' and sanest in her emotional attitudes and accommodations to these, and the most resourceful and ingenious in diverting, circumventing or otherwise 'managing' her preposterous reactions to L-DOPA. With consummate skill and ease Mrs Y. pilots herself through physiological storms of an incredible ferocity and unpredictability, continually negotiating problems which would cause most patients to founder on the spot. Although, in other case histories, I have avoided lists and tabulations, I will here make use of them in order to avoid diffuseness and prolixity.

1. *Sensitivity to* L-DOPA *and oscillations of response.* Like all post-encephalitic (and Parkinsonian) patients who have been maintained on L-DOPA for any length of time, Mrs Y. has become exceedingly sensitive to it, her average maintenance-dose now being no more than 750 mg. a day. Her reactions to it have become (indeed, they were almost so from the start) entirely all-or-none in character – she either reacts totally, or not at all: she is no more capable of graduated reaction than one is capable of a graduated sneeze. Her reactions, which were very rapid to begin with, have now become virtually instantaneous – she leaps from one physiological extreme to another in the twinkling of an eye, in a flash, in a fraction of a second: she jumps from one state to another as quickly as one jumps from one

thought to another. Such transitions – or, more accurately, transiliences – are no longer 'correlated' in any predictable way with the timing of her L-DOPA doses – indeed, she is apt to make somewhere between 30 and 200 abrupt physiological reversals a day. Of all our patients who are 'swingers' or 'yo-yos', Mrs Y. is the most profound, abrupt and frequent in her oscillations. The abruptness and totality of these reversals scarcely give one an impression of a gradual, graduated process, but of sudden reorganizations or transformations of *phase*. If her L-DOPA is stopped, she immediately goes into a coma.

2.   *Proliferation of responses to* L-DOPA. It has been indicated that within three days of her 'awakening' on L-DOPA, Mrs Y. showed the onset of clear-cut *tics*. These have continually proliferated in number, so much so that I can now recognize more than 300 distinct and individual patterns of tic. Every two or three days, so to speak, a new tic is 'invented' – sometimes, seemingly, *de novo*, sometimes as an elaboration of an already-existing tic, sometimes as an amalgam or 'conflation' of two or more pre-existing tics, sometimes as a defensive manoeuvre or counter-tic. These tics affect every aspect of action and behaviour, and one may often perceive a dozen or two proceeding *simultaneously*, apparently independently controlled and in complete functional isolation from one another. All of these tics have distinctive styles and rhythms or movements – 'kinetic melodies' (in Luria's term) – and when Mrs Y. is merrily ticcing, she gives the impression of a clock-shop gone mad, with innumerable clocks all ticking and chiming in their own time and tune.[25]

25. Thus, when looking at (or 'listening to') Hester's tics, of which a dozen might be proceeding simultaneously, one received no impression of synchrony or symphony, but an impression of polyphony, of many unrelated *tempi* and melodies proceeding independ-

3. *Mutual transformations (or phase-relations) of tics.*
Mrs Y. shows several basic phases of tic, the relationships of
which are most clearly shown when they are demonstrated
with one and the same basic tic-form. Thus a given tic may
take an abrupt, precipitate, darting form; a rhythmical clon-
ic form (like her original humming-tic); or a tonic (or catatonic) form – a so-called 'tic of immobility'. The changes
between these phases may be quite instantaneous : thus Mrs
Y. may be suddenly arrested in 'mid-tic', i.e. transformed to
a cataleptic perseveration of the tic; again one of her 'favourite' tonic tics – a bizarre flexion of the right arm, so that its
fingers rest between the shoulder-blades – may immediately
'break up' into precipitate tics.

4. *No reversion to psychosis.* She becomes immensely excited, emotionally as well as motorically, many times a day,
and her excitement, at such times, will assume any form
which suggests itself or is appropriate : her 'favourite' and
most typical excitement is a hilarious excitement ('*titillatio
et hilaritas*'), and she loves to be told jokes, to be tickled, or
to be put in front of comedy-shows on the television at these
times. Anguish, rage and terror are alternatives to hilarity,
but shown much less often. She does *not* display voracities
and greeds like a number of patients (Rolando P., Margaret
A., Maria G., etc.), nor has she shown any significant tendency to possessiveness, grievance, paranoia or mania. Whether such things are to be ascribed to a difference of 'level'
in neural organization, to her equable temper, or to strict
self-control, is not clear to me, but it is certain that Mrs Y.
– is almost alone of our extremely severely affected post-
encephalitic patients – preserves her 'upper storey' (her per-

_____
ently. This produced a very curious effect upon the eye (or 'ear') of
the observer – an effect of grotesquerie or surrealism, akin to that
produced by L. W.'s crises (see footnote to p. 82).

sonality, relationships, view-of-the-world, etc.) serene and free from the turbulent urges and affects which go on 'beneath' it. She experiences violent drives, but she herself is 'above' them. Her affects are never neuroticized, as her tics are never mannerized.

5. *Organization, 'level' and non-use of tics.* It is clear that Mrs Y.'s tics are far more complex in form than mere Parkinsonian jerks, jactitations or precipitations, and also more complex than the desultory, 'quasi-purposeless' choreic and hyperkinetic movements seen in most patients with ordinary Parkinson's disease with long administration of L-DOPA. Mrs Y.'s tics *look* like actions or deeds – and not mere jerks or spasms or movements. One sees, for example, gasps, pants, sniffs, finger-snappings, throat-clearing, pinching movements, scratching movements, touching movements, etc., etc., which could all be part of a normal gestural repertoire, and whose abnormality lies in their incessant, compulsive and 'inappropriate' repetition. One *also* sees bizarre grimaces, gesticulations and peculiar 'pseudo-actions', which cannot by any stretch of the word be called 'normal'. These pseudo-actions, sometimes comic, sometimes grotesque, convey a deeply paradoxical feeling, in that they *seem* at first to have a definite (if mysterious) organization and purpose and then one realizes that in fact they do not (like chorea). It is this odd simulacrum of action and meaning, this parody of sense which baffles the mind. (See footnote on L. W.'s crises, p. 82.) On the other hand, Mrs Y. has shown little or no tendency to utilize, rationalize, mannerize or ritualize her tics – and, in this way, stands in the sharpest contrast to Miron V., Miriam H., etc. The non-use of tics means that Mrs Y. herself can sit quietly (so to speak) 'in the middle' of her tics, paying remarkably little attention to them. It protects her from being 'possessed' or 'dispossessed' or

'taken over' by tics which become mannerisms, affectations or impostures – as happened, for example, with Maria G.[26] A special form of 'conflation' and 'cleavage' can be observed in Mrs Y.'s alternation of '*macro-tics*' (sudden, incredibly violent and massive movements, or fulgurations, which may bodily throw her off a chair or onto the ground) and '*micro-tics*' (multiple, minor tics, a twinkling or scintillation of innumerable tics). In general, Mrs Y.'s 'style' favours micro-*tics*' (multiple, minor tics, a twinkling or scintillation of violent startling macro-tics.[27]

6. *Relationships of tics and behavioural disorder*. It is possible that I am using the term 'tics' too widely, to denote the total physical-mental states which Mrs Y. shows. With continuing use of L-DOPA, she has shown a greater and greater tendency to 'split' into behavioural *fragments* – discrete, differentiated, behavioural forms. Thus she may, in the course of a minute, jump from a peculiar speech-pattern to a peculiar breathing-pattern, to a peculiar respiratory pattern, etc. – each such total-stage affecting different aspects of behaviour. One can easily see that these seemingly senseless 'unphysiological' jumps have a clear behavioural or dramatic unity; they are all reminiscent of or allusions to each other: one could say that they bear to one another a metaphorical relation, and to her total self or behaviour a metonymical relation. They thus follow one another like sequences of 'free association', and – like these – demonstrate, beneath their superficial 'randomness' or senselessness, the referential and epiphanic nature of even such 'primitive' behaviour.

26. I have similarly observed in youthful patients with multiple-tic (Tourette's) disease that *some* of these patients ignore their tics, and deny them any use or symbolic 'meaning', while others mannerize them, which leads the way to a schizophrenic fission of the entire personality.

27. One sees similar styles in Tourette's disease.

7. *Stationary states and kinematic states*. In addition to the above-mentioned disturbances, Mrs Y. *also* has periods when her movements, speech and thoughts seem virtually normal: her 'attacks' of normality, indeed, have something of the same paroxysmal and unpredictable quality as her behavioural disorders. When she is normal and undriven and unfettered, one can see what a charming and intelligent person she is, and how 'unspoilt' her original, pre-morbid personality. But these normal, free-flowing periods may themselves be interrupted – with great suddenness, and no warning – by sudden cessations of movement/speech/ thought, so that Mrs Y. will suddenly be arrested like a film in a 'freeze-frame'. These still-states may last a second or an hour, and *cannot* be broken by any voluntary action from Mrs Y. herself (indeed such action is impossible and unthinkable at such times). They may cease spontaneously, or with the merest touch or noise from outside, and then Mrs Y. moves immediately again into free-flowing motion/ speech/thought.[28] These states have no subjective duration

28. The fact that the *smallest possible* stimulus – a single photon of light or quantum of energy – suffices to dissipate these still-states shows us that they are totally *inertia-less*; this is further borne out by the fact that there is an *instantaneous* leap from absolute stillness to normal fluent motion. This absolute stillness of these extraordinary states, coupled with their proneness to sudden phasic transformations, suggest an analogy with the 'stationary states' and quantal 'jumps' postulated of atoms and electronic orbits; they suggest, indeed, that we may be dealing with a large-scale model of such micro-phenomena – 'macro-quantal states', if the term be allowed. Such inertia-less states stand in absolute contrast (and complementary) to the positive disorders of Parkinsonism (analysed in detail in the footnote to p. 85), with their intense inertia and resistance to change, their violent warpings of space and field; for *these* suggest miniature models of galactic phenomena, and so might be termed 'micro-relativistic states'.

It was such considerations which led me to write two years ago that 'our data not only show us the inadequacy of classical neurology, but give us the shape of a new neurophysiology of quantum-

whatever: they are identical with the *standstills* which started her illness. It is evident, from questioning Mrs Y., that her
perceptions of herself and the world have a very 'weird'
quality in these standstills. Thus everything seems sharp-
edged, flat, and geometric, with a quality like a mosaic or a
stained-glass window; there is no sense of space or time at
such times. Sometimes these 'stills' form a flickering vision,
like a movie-film which is running too slow.[29] When they

---

relativistic type ... in accordance with the concepts of contemporary
physics' (*Listener*, 26 October 1972). I will go further. It may be said
that even if such analogies are permissible or fruitful, the phenomena we are considering are extremely remote from 'ordinary' life,
as remote, in their way, as atoms and galaxies. But this, to my mind,
is neither interesting nor true. I think that a vast range of familiar
biological phenomena – from the forces and forms of our passions,
to the alternations of standstills and jumps in insects – lend themselves equally to analyses of a relativistic and quantal sort; so much
so, indeed, that I feel a certain astonishment that relativity and
quantality were not 'discovered' by biologists long before their discovery in physics.

29. Mrs. Y. and other patients who have experienced 'kinematic
vision' have occasionally told me of an extraordinary (and seemingly
impossible) phenomenon which may occur during such periods,
viz. the displacement of a 'still' either backwards or forwards, so
that a given 'moment' may occur *too soon* or *too late*. Thus, on one
occasion, when Hester was being visited by her brother, she happened
to be having kinematic vision at about three or four frames a second,
i.e. a rate so slow that there was a clearly perceptible difference between each frame. While watching her brother lighting his pipe, she
was greatly startled by witnessing the following sequence: first, the
striking of a match; second, her brother's hand holding the lighted
match, having 'jumped' a few inches from the matchbox; third, the
match flaring up in the bowl of the pipe; and fourth, fifth, sixth, etc.
the 'intermediate' stages by which her brother's hand, holding the
match, jerkily approached the pipe to be lit. Thus – incredibly –
Hester saw the pipe actually being lit several frames too soon; she
saw 'the future', so to speak, somewhat before she was *due* to see
it ... If we accept Hester's word in the matter (and if we do not
listen to our patients we will never learn anything), we are compelled
to make a novel hypothesis (or several such) about the perception of

achieve a certain critical rate, her sense of vision and of the world suddenly becomes 'normal', with the movement, space, time, perspective, curvatures and continuities expected of it. At times of great excitement, Mrs Y. may experience a kinematic 'delirium', in which a variety of perceptions or hallucinations or hallucinatory patterns may succeed one another with vertiginous speed, several a second; she is quite distressed and disabled while such deliria last, but they are, fortunately, quite rare.[30]

---

time and the nature of 'moments'. The simplest of these I think, is to take 'moments' as ontological events (i.e. as *our* 'world-moments') and assume that we 'take in' several at a time (as a moving whale continually swallows a swarm of shrimps), or that we keep a small hoard of them 'in stock' at any given time, and in either case 'feed them' into some internal projector, where they become activated and 'real', one at a time in their proper sequence. Normally, this proceeds correctly and easily; but in certain conditions, it would seem, our ontological moments may be fed to us in the wrong order, so that moments which are chronologically 'past' or 'future' get ectopically displaced, and presented to us as utterly convincing (but inappropriate) 'nows'. Somewhat allied hypotheses (of defective or mistaken 'time-labelling' in the nervous system) have been presented by Efron with regard to the commoner but still uncanny experiences of *déjà vu, jamais vu, presque vu*, etc. These are not associated with kinematic vision, but are apt to occur in states of intense and unusual nervous excitement (as in the singular cases of Martha N. and Gertie C.). All these states of *anachronism*, in company with other time-strangenesses described in this book, indicate how vast is the gulf between abstract and actual, chronological and ontological, in our conceptions and perceptions of time.

30. Shortly after completing this case history, and the other histories in this book, I had occasion to draw on what I had learned from Mrs Y., and from several other patients, in order to present as detailed and generalized a description of 'still states' as I could do; this description appeared in the course of an article published in the *Listener* ('The Great Awakening', 26 October 1972), and the following extract is taken from this:

'These states . . . may be described in purely visual terms, while understanding that they may affect *all* thought and behaviour. The

Summer 1972

Mrs Y. has become entirely accustomed to all of these strange states, and admits and discusses them freely with me, or with others. Although she lacks the investigative passion and capacities of another patient (Leonard L.), she accepts all of these singular, and potentially terrifying states, with a quite extraordinary equanimity, detachment and humour. She never feels persecuted or victimized by them, but seems to see them simply *as things which are there*, like her nose, or her name, or New York, or the world. Thus, she is never 'phased out' or 'flipped out' any more – as she was, for a day, when

---

still picture has not true or continuous perspective, but is seen as a perfectly flat dovetailing of shapes, or as a series of wafer-thin planes. Curves are differentiated into discrete, discontinuous steps: a circle is seen as a polygon. There is no sense of space, or solidity or extension, no sense of objects except as facets geometrically apposed. There is no sense of movement, or the possibility of movement, and no sense of process or forces or field. There is no emotion or cathexis in this crystalline world. There is no sense of absorption or attention whatever. The state is *there*, and it cannot be changed. From gross still vision, patients may proceed to an astonishing sort of microscopic vision or Lilliputian hallucination in which they may see a dust-particle on the counterpane filling their entire visual field, and presented as a mosaic of sharp-faceted faces. From here the patient may proceed to seeing lattices and networks which are no longer identifiable as familiar forms, until finally his entire sensorium may experience only a single point in one of these lattices, which is seen as an infinite concentricity of haloes, dense in the centre and fading at the edge ...'

I noted that the critical point at which a sequence of such stills ('kinematic vision') was replaced by normal, continuous, 'dynamic vision' occurred at about twenty stills or frames a second, i.e. the usual rate of 'flicker fusion frequency' at which a series of discrete visual, auditory, or tactile stimuli are fused into an illusion of continuity. It was pointed out by several readers of the *Listener* article that these observations supported the notion that existential 'time' and 'space' are *constructs* of a metaphysical sort, corresponding to Kant's 'synthetic *a priori*'.

such things first began. She is absolutely 'together' and will stay together, unlike less stable patients (Maria G., Margaret A., etc.) who became fragmented and schizophrenic under the strain of L-DOPA.

A second factor which has allowed Mrs Y. much greater freedom of action than would have seemed possible with her responses has been her skill and ingenuity in preventing, circumventing or utilizing her 'side-effects' – a skill which she shares with Frances D. particularly. Both of these ladies, with their sharp wits and their bizarre illnesses, have achieved a knowledge and a control of their nervous systems and reactions which not a neurologist anywhere in the world could approach. I scarcely know, here, who teaches whom: I have learned an immense amount from Mrs Y., and she, perhaps, learns something from me.[31] Moreover, Mrs Y. is always active in and out of the hospital – playing Bingo, seeing movies, visiting other patients, undertaking half a dozen projects at any time in occupational therapy or workshop, going to concerts, poetry-readings, philosophy classes, and – her favourite – excursions. She has as full a life as one can have at Mount Carmel.

The final source of Mrs Y.'s strength – as with so many patients – seems to have come from personal relations: in her case the 'discovery' of the son and daughter whom she had not seen in fifteen years or more, a discovery which she expressed a great longing for in her diary, in the dramatic days

31. A number of such strategies for 'pacing' and controlling postencephalitic patients are illustrated by Dr Purdon Martin in his excellent book *The Basal Ganglia and Posture*. A detailed theoretical and practical treatment is given in the last chapter ('The Control of Behaviour') of A. R. Luria's remarkable first book *The Nature of Human Conflicts*; he writes there that '... the healthy cortex enables [the Parkinsonian patient] to use external stimuli and to construct a compensatory activity for the subcortical automatisms ... That which was impossible to accomplish by direct will-force becomes attainable when the action is included in another complex system.'

of May 1969, and which was finally brought about by our untiring social worker. Her daughter, who had spent two decades in and out of mental hospitals since Mrs Y. became ill, is now a frequent and much-loved visitor at Mount Carmel – a reunion which has given deep pleasure and stability to both Mrs Y. *and* her daughter (the latter has steered clear of psychoses since the time of reunion). Equally affecting has been Mrs Y.'s reunion with her son, who after many years of a quasi-psychopathic life 'out West', has established home and roots in New York once again. Seeing Mrs Y. with her son and her daughter, one realizes the strength of her character and love; one sees what a remarkable person she is, and how solid and real she must have been as a mother. One sees why her children went mad with her illness, and why they are visibly healing as they return to her now.

Thus, despite the innumerable odds against her – the severity and length and strangeness of her illness, her preposterous responses to L-DOPA, and the grim institution which has housed her for years – Mrs Y. has emphatically awoken and returned to reality, in a manner which would have been unthinkable four years ago.

6. ROLANDO P.

Rolando P. was born in New York in 1917, the youngest son of a newly immigrated and very musical Italian family. He showed unusual vivacity and precocity as a child, acquiring speech and motor skills at an exceptionally early age. He was an active, inquisitive, affectionate and talkative child, until at thirty months of age his life was suddenly cut across by a virulent attack of *encephalitis lethargica*, which presented itself as an intense drowsiness lasting eighteen weeks, initially accompanied by high fever and influenzal symptoms.

As he awoke from the sleeping-sickness, it became evident that a profound change had occurred, for he now showed a completely masked and expressionless face, and had great difficulty in moving or talking. He would sit for hours completely motionless in his chair, seemingly inanimate except for sudden, impulsive movements of his eyes. If he was set on his feet, he would walk 'like a little wooden doll', with both arms hanging stiffly at his side; more commonly he would break into a run which would get faster and faster till he crashed into an obstacle and fell like a statue to the ground. He was generally taken to be mentally defective, except by his very observant and understanding mother, who would say: 'My Rolando is no fool – he is as sharp and bright as he ever used to be. He has just come to a stop inside.'

Between the ages of six and ten, he attended ungraded classes at a school for the mentally defective. He had become virtually unable to move or speak by this time, but conveyed to at least one teacher the impression of an intact but imprisoned intelligence: 'Rolando is not stupid,' said a report in 1925. 'He absorbs everything, but nothing can come out.' This impression of him as purely absorptive, as a sort of unfathomable, black and hungry *hole* was to be echoed over the next forty years by all who observed him closely; it was only superficial observers who thought him vacuous, stupid or inattentive. But schooling, such as it was, became increasingly difficult, with each passing year, due to an increasing loss of balance, and increasing salivation. In his last year at school, he had to be propped upright with cushions to each side; otherwise he would fall over as helplessly as an upset statue.

From his eleventh to his nineteenth year, he remained at home, propped before the speaker of a large Victrola gramophone, for music (as his father observed) seemed to be the only thing he enjoyed, and the only thing which 'brought

him to life'. Animated music would give the boy its animation, and allow him to nod, sing or gesture in time with
it; but as soon as the music came to a stop, he too would
come to a stop, and return at once to his stony immobility.
He was admitted to Mount Carmel in 1935.

The next third of a century, in a back ward of the hospital, was completely eventless in the most literal sense of
this word. Mr P. – who despite his disabilities had grown
into a well-proportioned young man – sat in his chair all day
like a statue. Every evening, however, between seven and
nine, his rigidity and frigidity would thaw out a little,
allowing some movement of the arms, some speech and some
emotional expression. At such times he might sing a snatch
of opera or embrace his favourite nurses, but – more commonly – he would inveigh against his fate: 'It's a hell of a
life,' he would shout; 'I wish I was dead.' Curiously enough,
his evening activity would continue during the first portion
of his sleep, when he would toss and turn, talk and verbiger-
ate, and show impulsions to walk in his sleep. After midnight these activities would die down, and he would lie like
a statue for the rest of the night.

He was submitted to an operation (a left-sided chemopal-
lidectomy) in 1958, which produced some loosening of the
rigidity on the right side of his body, but no alteration of his
akinesia, or his overall motionless, speechless state.

I examined Mr P. and talked to him several times between
1966 and 1969. He was a powerfully built man at this time,
who appeared far younger than his fifty-odd years; he could
easily have passed for half his actual age. He would always
be tied in his wheelchair, to prevent an otherwise irresistible
tendency to fall forwards. He showed great oiliness of the
skin, and continual sweating, lacrimation and salivation.

His voice was so soft as to be inaudible: sudden effort and
excitement, however, rendered exclamatory speech possible
for a few seconds. Thus, when I asked him whether his sali-

vation disturbed him much, he exclaimed loudly: 'You bet it does! It's one hell of a problem!' immediately afterwards relapsing into virtual aphonia. There was almost no spontaneous blinking of normal type, which contrasted with the frequency of spontaneous lid-clonus and forced closure of the eyes: a touch on the face, or indeed any sudden movement in the field of vision, elicited forced clonus or closure of the eyelids. Mr P.'s mouth tended to remain open unless deliberately closed.

He would sit in his chair, with his head bowed forwards and very little spontaneous movement, for hours on end. He showed intense rigidity of the neck and trunk muscles, and moderate rigidity of the limbs, the right side (which was more rigid before operation) now being slightly less rigid than the left. Cogwheeling was readily elicited at all major joints. The right hand was cool, the left cold, and both showed trophic changes of the skin and nails. There was no fixed deformity, and no tremor. There was very severe akinesia: asked to clench and unclench his hands, Mr P. could make only a slight finger-flexion, the movement decaying to zero after three or four repetitions. Asked to clap, Mr P. could make only three to five claps, the movement subsequently accelerating, becoming minimal in force, and finally tremulous, before its complete arrest. A sudden violent effort would enable Mr P. to rise to a standing position, but he was unable to stand unaided because of an irresistible tendency to fall backwards. Given much support, he could walk a few feet with very small, shuffling steps. On resuming his seat he would fall back rigidly, and statuesquely, without any segmental movements or reflexes. Mr P. was illiterate, but was able, using the left hand, to reproduce simple geometrical diagrams: these were much smaller than the originals which he had been requested to copy, and were produced only with great effort; there was too much akinesia in the right hand to allow even an attempt at such copying.

He was one of the most profoundly disabled post-encephalitic patients I had ever seen. I had no doubt that he would react to L-DOPA, but many doubts as to what would be his reactions, or his reactions to his reactions – for he had been out of the world, in effect, since the onset of his illness before he was three. But I started him on L-DOPA on 14 May 1969.

Course on L-DOPA

On 20 May, Mr P. said that he had an unusual feeling of 'energy', and an urge to move his legs: this urge was assuaged by 'dancing', which he did when supported by an orderly. The following day, Mr P. presented quite dramatic changes in his motor status, being able to walk the entire length of the ward (about 80 feet) and back, with only a finger on his back to support him.

By 24 May (the dose of L-DOPA had now reached 3 gm. daily), Mr P. was showing a variety of responses to the drug. His voice, previously almost inaudible, was now clearly audible at ten feet away, and could be maintained at this intensity without apparent effort. His drooling had ceased entirely. He was able to make fists, and to clap and tap his hands with a good deal of force. He was now able to *stride* around the ward, but still required assistance in view of his overwhelming tendency to fall backwards. The rigidity in his arms and legs was much reduced; so much so, indeed, that their tone felt somewhat *less* than normal. His neck and trunk muscles, formerly immovable, were now less rigid, although they did not display the amazing looseness of his arms. His face seemed flushed on this day, and his eyes were abnormally bright and somewhat protuberant. Lid-clonus and lid-closure had ceased to occur. He was also playful, giggly, and somewhat euphoric, and asked me whether he might improve so much as to be released for a day from the hospital. In particular, he showed a surge of sexual excitement, and a sudden development (or 'release') of libidinous phantasies, his desire to go out being partly the wish to have a sexual experience – his first. Motor activity, mood, and general arousal continued to increase over the weekend, Mr P. being loud in his demands for 'a woman – for Chrissake I *deserve* one after all these years!' On 27 May I found him very flushed, boisterous, insomniac, somewhat manic, and frenzied; his movements, previously so meagre and with so little dynamic background, were now violently forceful, and involved as background the whole of his body; he was intensely vigilant and over-alert. His eye-movements (which had been infrequent and unaccompanied by any head-movement) now had an incessant *darting* quality, and were accompanied by equally quick head-movements. His attention was constantly attracted hither and thither, and seemed to be intensified but also short-lived and distractible. Unexpected noises would startle him, and make him jump. Finally, I observed the onset of some akathisia – in particular, a restless shuffling of the legs, and a tendency to pound his bedside table if impatient. In view of this excessive arousal, I reduced his daily dose of L-DOPA from 3 gm. to 2 gm.

This permitted sleep, but he continued to show inordinate arousal. On 29 May, I was struck by the watchful, predatory expression on his face. Movements were now not only forceful but uncontrollable, and would tend to continual acceleration and perseveration, Mr P. being quite unable to halt them, once started.

On the positive side, Mr P. – who had been saddened and ashamed of his illiteracy since his earliest years – expressed a desire to learn reading and writing. He showed remarkable persistence in his efforts, and they were, initially, crowned with success. Unfortunately, his physiological disturbances made this increasingly difficult : he would either read too fast to take in what he read, or get stuck or transfixed on a single letter or word; his handwriting, similarly, would tend either to 'stickiness' and micrographia, or, more commonly, to be broken up into a multitude of impulsive jabbing strokes, which once he had started he could not control.

His akathisia, previously generalized and non-specific, now showed a differentiation into specific impulsions – a restless 'pawing' movement of the right leg (suggestive of a high-spirited, impatient horse), and a tendency to forced chewing and masticatory movements. Sexual and libidinous arousal was still more marked, and the transit of any female personnel across Mr P.'s field of vision would immediately evoke an indescribably lascivious expression, forced lip-licking and lip-smacking movements, dilation of the nostrils and pupils, and uncontrollable watching; he seemed – visually – to grab and grasp the object of his gaze, and to be unable to relinquish it till it passed from his field of vision.

On the evening of the 29th, I happened to see Mr P. asleep, and observed during his sleep an astounding exaltation of motor activities. In particular he showed incessant masticatory movements, waving and saluting movements of the arms, rhythmic ('salaam') flexions of the head on the chest, kicking movements of the legs, muttering, talking and singing in his sleep. He showed striking echolalia during sleep, immediately repeating my question when I spoke to him. After filming these movements, and taping his speech, I woke Mr P., and as he awoke there was an immediate cessation of all these activities. He himself had the impression of having slept soundly, and had no recollection of his speech or his movements. When he fell asleep once more, Mr P.'s motor activity resumed, and continued until about 1 a.m., at which time it stopped, not to reappear during the night. *Thus, his activities were an accentuation of phenomena already present before L-DOPA was given*. This was also apparent in Mr P.'s daytime cycles, with inordinate activation occurring each evening – a cycle which persisted however the doses of L-DOPA were shifted or timed. Thus, chewing and masticatory movements would start at 6 or 7 o'clock each evening, and persist, even during his sleep, till midnight, at which time they stopped.

Around 10 June, a new symptom appeared, which could be described as a voracity, an oral mania, or a devouring-urge. The taking of a first mouthful at any meal seemed to let loose an irresistible desire to grab, bite, and devour food, as fast as possible. Mr P. found himself impelled to stuff food into his mouth, masticate it violently (the mastications persisting after swallowing each mouthful), and when his plate was finished, to stuff his fingers or a napkin into his still violently and perseveratingly chewing mouth.

In the third week of June (his dose of L-DOPA remaining unchanged), symptoms of a more disquieting nature appeared, with agitation, perseveration, and stereotypy as their hallmarks. Mr P. would spend the greater part of each day rocking to and fro in his chair and chanting rhythmically: 'I'm crazy, I'm crazy, I'm crazy ... if I don't get out of this fucking place, I'll go crazy, crazy, crazy!' At other times he would hum or sing in a monotonous, perseverative, verbigerative fashion, for hours on end. With each passing day, the perseveration and stereotypy became greater, and by 21 June Mr P.'s conversation was made difficult by continual palilalic repetitions of words. His affect, which was intense at this time, alternated between anxiety (with fears of madness and chaos), hostility and intense irritability. Whenever he saw another patient look out of a window, he would yell: 'He's going to jump, going to jump, to jump, to jump, t'jump, t'jump, tchump, tchump ...' His attitudes, previously somewhat passive and dependent and abject, had now switched to goading, truculence, and bellicosity, although these were moderated, and made acceptable, by smiling and joking. Powerful sexual urges continued throughout this time, manifest as repeated erotic dreams and nightmares, as frequent and somewhat compulsive masturbation, and (combined with aggressiveness and perseveration) as a tendency to curse, to excited coprolalia, and verbigerative sing-song pornoloquies with obscene refrains.[32]

On 21 June, Mr P. complained that his eyes were being 'caught' by all moving objects, and that he could only 'release' his gaze by holding a hand in front of his eyes. This remarkable phenomenon could easily be observed by others: on one occasion, a fly entered the room and was impinged upon his visual attention; his gaze was then 'locked' onto the fly, and was drawn after it, irresistibly, wherever it flew. As the symptom grew more pronounced, Mr P. would find that his entire attention had to be concentrated upon whatever object compelled his gaze: and this phenomenon he called 'fascination', 'being spellbound' or 'witchcraft'. During this period, Mr P.'s 'grasp-reflexes' (which had been present, but mild and asymptomatic, before receiving L-DOPA) also became exaggerated, and caused forced grasping and groping of the hands, and a strong tendency for them to 'stick' to whatever they happened to touch.

Yet another symptom which became prominent during June was respiratory instability, which took the form of frequent, sudden, tic-like inspirations, occasional snuffling, and perseverative coughing – all of which, like his masticatory movements, pawing movements, etc., would come on in the evenings, clearly related to an innate rhythmicity, and not to the timing of his L-DOPA doses.

In view of Mr P.'s extreme emotional and motor excitement, and his distressing perseverations and 'stimulus-slavery', I reduced the dosage of L-DOPA to 1·5 gm. daily: his excitomotor syndrome continued, unabated, and it was therefore decided to try the effects of Haloperidol (a total of 1·5 mg. daily) added to the L-DOPA. Agitation and akathisia

---

32. This complex of motor, appetitive and moral disorder is reminiscent of that seen in severer cases of Gilles de la Tourette syndrome (who combine coprolalia, obscene obsessions, increased libido, orexia, excessive motor impetus and multiple tics).

still persisting, the dose of L-DOPA was reduced still further. I was astonished to find that so small a dose as 1 gm. of L-DOPA daily could still procure a useful activation of speech and movement, although at the expense of increased salivation. A return to the larger dosage at once caused excessive activation. By mid-July, we could predict the responses to L-DOPA with considerable precision, as tabulated below:

1·5 gm. daily	1 gm. daily
Great vocal and motor force	Moderate vocal and motor force
Excited, akathisic, insomniac	No excitement, akathisia, insomnia
Very little drooling	Profuse drooling
Prominent tics and perseverations	No tics or perseverations

It was evident that Haloperidol had an effect antagonistic in toto to that of L-DOPA, and not distinguishable from the effects of reducing L-DOPA dosage, and even on so minimal a dose as 1 gm. daily, paroxysmal and rhythmical activations were still prone to occur. Particularly striking, even on 1 gm. a day, was the sudden 'awakening' which occurred every evening – to flushed, bright-eyed, quick-glancing, loud-voiced, forceful, lascivious, expansive, manic-catatonic akathisia – a transformation which often occurred in a minute or less; equally acute (and equally difficult to ascribe to any simple, dose-related effect of the drug) was the reverse change – to compacted, contracted, aphonic akinesia. Thus, by mid-July, we came face-to-face with the essential problem in treating any case of very severe post-encephalitic Parkinsonism: how best to achieve a therapeutic compromise in a patient with an exceedingly unstable nervous system, a patient in whom all behaviour tended to have an oscillatory, bi-polar, all-or-none quality.

1969–72

In the past three years Mr P. has continued to take 1·0 gm. of L-DOPA daily: if he misses a dose he becomes deeply disabled, and if he misses a day he goes into stupor or coma. In autumn 1969, his days were almost equally divided between excited-explosive states and obstructive-imploded states, and he swung like a yo-yo from one to the other, making each passage within thirty seconds. In his excited states, Mr P. showed an intense desire to talk and move, and an equally intense hunger for all stimulation. Amongst these hungers was the hunger to read, and during these three months he made remarkable strides in this direction, considering he had been Parkinsonian since the age of three; he became able to read headlines and captions in the papers.

Since the beginning of 1970 Mr P.'s reactions to L-DOPA have become less auspicious, in that his Parkinsonian or 'down' periods have come to overshadow his excited-expansive states, and these latter are the only times in which he is really accessible. Very occasionally he shows a 'normal' or *middle* state, but these are only seen once or twice a month and then only last a few seconds or minutes.

A further problem has been the increasing incidence of stuporous or sleep-like states, accompanied by gesticulating and ticcing, gibbering and echolalia. Such states become more severe whether we increase or decrease the L-DOPA. On several occasions, we have tried the effects of amantadine – which, in some patients, reduces pathological responses to L-DOPA, and retrieves (if temporarily) its therapeutic effects. In Mr P., unfortunately, amantadine *exacerbates* pathological and stuporous responses.

His best moods and functioning are brought out by his family, when they take him home for occasional weekends or holidays. In particular Mr P. likes the Hi-Fi and swimming pool at his brother's country home. Very remarkably,

Mr P. can swim the length of the pool, and shows a great diminution of his Parkinsonism in the water; he apparently swims with an ease and fluency which he can never achieve when he moves on dry land. Effortless movement is also called forth by music on the Hi-Fi, especially *opera buffa* to which he is addicted; the music calls for singing, 'conducting' and occasional dancing, and at this time also, his symptoms are minimal. But Mr P.'s favourite occupation is to sit on the porch, watching the wild life which teems in the garden, or gazing at the wide prospects of up-state New York. Mr P. is always intensely depressed when he returns from the country, and the sentiments he expresses are always the same: 'What a goddamn relief to get out of this place!... I've been shut up in places since the day I was born ... I've been shut up in illness since the day I was born ... That's a hell of a life for someone to have ... Why the hell couldn't I have died as a kid? ... What's the sense, what's the use, of my fucking life here? ... Hey, Doc! I'm sick of L-DOPA – what about a *real* pill from the cupboard the nurses lock up? ... The *euthanazy* pill or whatever it's called ... I've needed that pill since the day I was born.'

Epilogue

In the American edition of *Awakenings* I added a short postscript to Rolando P.'s history, as follows: 'Early in 1973 Rolando P. pined away and died. As with Frank G. and others, no cause of death could be found at *post mortem*. I cannot avoid the suspicion that such patients died of hopelessness and despair, and that the *ostensible* cause of death (cardiac arrest, or whatever) was merely the means by which a sought-for *quietus* was finally achieved.' This cryptic postscript has given rise to many questions, and I feel it necessary and proper, therefore, to trace the course of Rolando's final decline, and its probable or possible determinants, in a fuller and more explicit way.

Rolando P.'s mother was exceptionally understanding and deeply devoted: thus it was she who would always defend him in his earliest years, when he was usually taken to be mentally defective or mad (see p. 147). Despite progressive age and arthritis she would visit Rolando every Sunday without fail (or else join him when he was invited to his brother's country home). By the summer of 1972, however, Mrs P. had become so disabled by arthritis that she was no longer able to come to the hospital. The cessation of her visits was followed by a severe emotional crisis in her son – two months of grief, pining, depression and rage, and during this period he lost twenty pounds. Mercifully, however, his loss was mitigated by a physiotherapist we had on the staff, a woman who combined the skills of her craft with an exceptionally warm and loving nature. By September of 1972 Rolando P. had developed a very intimate 'anaclitic' relation with her, leaning on her as he had previously leant on his mother; and the warmth and wisdom of this good woman's heart allowed her to play this motherly role with genuine, unsimulated, unconditional love, and without ever striking any false notes; indeed, her devotion was such that she would often come in on weekends or evenings, giving him the time and love he so needed. Under this benign and healing influence, Rolando's wound began to heal over – he became calmer and better-humoured, gained weight and slept well.

Unfortunately, at the start of February, his beloved physiotherapist was dismissed from her job (along with almost a third of the hospital staff) as a result of economies dictated by the recent Federal Budget. Rolando's first reaction was one of stunned shock, associated with denial and unbelief: he would have repeated dreams at this time that everyone had been dismissed *except* his new 'mother', that she had been enabled to stay by some special means – and he would wake from these sweet-cruel dreams with a smile on his face, followed by a cry of realization and anguish. But if these were his dreams, his conscious reactions were different – they were exceedingly 'sensible', exceedingly 'rational'. 'These things happen,' he would say with a nod. 'They are very unfortunate, but they can't be helped ... No use crying over spilt milk, you know ... One has to *carry on* – life goes on regardless ...' At this level, then, of consciousness and reason, Rolando seemed determined to bear with his loss and live on 'regardless'; but at a deeper level, so it seemed to me, he had sustained a wound from which he would not recover. He had once been saved by a surrogate mother, but now *she* had gone, and there was no prospect of another; Rolando had been deeply ill and dependent since his third year of life – he had the mind of a man, but the needs of an infant. I kept thinking of Spitz's famous studies, and I felt that the chances were against his survival.[33]

By the middle of February, Rolando was showing severe mental breakdown, compounded of grief, depression, terror and rage. He continually *pined* for his lost love-object; he continually *searched* for her (and kept 'mistaking' others for her); he had repeated *pangs of grief* (and psychic pain), in which he would turn pale, clutch his chest, cry aloud or groan. Admixed with his grief and pining and searching, he had a bewildered and furious sense of *betrayal*, and would

33. Spitz had provided unforgettable descriptions of the effects of human deprivation on orphaned children. These orphans (in an orphanage in Mexico) were given excellent mechanical and 'hygienic' care, but virtually no *human* attention, warmth or care. Almost all of them had died by the age of three. Such studies and similar observations upon the very young, the very old, the very ill, and the regressed, indicate that *human care is literally vital*, and that if it is deficient or absent we perish, the more quickly and surely the more vulnerable we are; and that death, in such contexts, is first and foremost an existential death, a dying-away of the will-to-live – and that this paves the way for physical death. This subject – 'dying of grief' – is discussed with great penetration in Chapter 2 ('The Broken Heart') of C. M. Parkes's book *Bereavement*.

rail wildly at Fate, at the hospital, and at her: sometimes he would revile her as 'a faithless fucking bitch', and at other times the hospital for 'taking her away'; he lived in a torment of bewailing and reviling.

Towards the end of February his state changed again, and he moved into a settled and almost inaccessible corpse-like apathy; he became profoundly Parkinsonian once again, but beneath the physiological Parkinsonian mask one could see a worse mask, of hopelessness and despair; he lost his appetite and ceased to eat; he ceased to express any hopes or regrets; he lay awake at nights, with wide-open, dull eyes. It was evident that he was dying, and had lost the will to live ...

A single episode (in early March) sticks in my mind: the medical staff, extremely alert for 'organic disease' (but seemingly blind to despairs of the soul), arranged for Rolando to have a battery of 'tests', and I was on the ward, that morning, when the diagnostic trolley came up, laden with syringes and tubes for blood, and accompanied by a brisk, white-coated technician. At first, passively, apathetically, Rolando let his arm be taken for blood, but then he suddenly burst out in an unforgettable, white-hot passion of outrage. He pushed the trolley and the technician violently away, and yelled: 'Can't you fuckers leave me alone? Where's the sense in all your fucking tests? Don't you have eyes and ears in your head? Can't you see I'm dying of grief? For Chrissake let me die in peace!' These were the last words which Rolando ever spoke. He died in his sleep, or his stupor, just four days later.

Newspaper headlines from the 1920s indicating the magnitude of the epidemic, and public alarm and horror in response to it.

SLEEPY SICKNE... SPREADING.

FATAL CASES.

HUNT FOR ELUSIVE GERM.

Sleepy sickness continues to spread New cases now reported as having oc-rred last week include :

BIRMINGHAM.—13; 5 deaths.
EFFIELD.—22; 1 death. Total cases
March 10, 217; deaths 26.
d Walters Sinclair, 58, an engin-Greenock, died yesterday from use after a week's illness, and are reported at Donaghmore, far the only cases reported in reland outside Belfast, where 10 deaths have occurred in cases were reported during and one death.
of Mr. C. Bower Ismay, nd sportsman, of Hazel-orthamptonshire, con-grave anxiety. Mr. ll 14 weeks ago while , and was found un-

PERIL OF THE SLEEPY MICROBE.

EPIDEMIC WORST IN BRITAIN AND ITALY.

RECORD DEATH-ROLL

CHILDREN AMONG THE VICTIMS.

TRAGEDIES OF SLEEPY SICKNESS.

WARPED MINDS AND BROKEN BODIES.

PLEAS FROM VICTIMS

Since The Daily Mail published t letter of Mr. E. W. Hore, of Manchest concerning the pathetic case of daughter, who is a sufferer from after-effects of sleepy sickness, we received a number of letters descri the tragic consequences of this dis Relatives write heart-broken

THE MYSTERY MALADY.

Alarming Spread of Sleepy Sickness.

WAR ON SLEEPY SICKNESS.

20,000 CASES LAST YEAR.

DEADLY AFTER-EFFECTS.

Sleepy sickness is without doubt the most devastating infective disease of modern times. The dreadful nature of this new disease is due not only to its high mortality but also to the very high percentage of victims who, even a year or two after the first attack, are visited with the most distressing after-effects. A form of paralysis agitans known as "Parkinsonism" [Parkinson in 1817 first described paralysis agitans] is a common sequel, even in children as young as 10 years of age.

This disease is characterised by a rigidity of the musculature of the body, so that all voluntary movements can only be carried out slowly. The face becomes devoid of expression, and in severe cases even speech is affected. As the condition advances, the unfortunate person, owing to the muscular stiffness, is unable to feed or dress himself, and finally may become bedridden, unable to turn himself without assistance.

Neurasthenia, in its various forms, intractable insomnia, and disturbances in the respiratory mechanism are some of the other sequelæ of the disease, often incapacitating the patient for months or years.

MORAL DEGENERATION.

But even more tragic are the changes in moral character which often follow the disease.

Docile and well-behaved children undergo a mysterious transformation. They become spiteful, untruthful, and unmanageable. They often steal, or make themselves objectionable in a score of wanton and mischievous ways. Unresponsive to any appeal, they sometimes find themselves in court, and unless the nature of their trouble is recognised, may be set on the road to becoming life-long criminals.

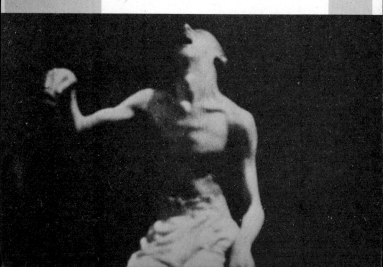

Asleep For Three Years

IN THE WORLD AND YET OUT

From Our Own Correspondent

OBAN, Tuesday.

THE tragic case of a man being in the world and yet out of it was described to me yesterday.

This man, workless and homeless, more than three years ago walked into the West Highland Rest Home. He complained of being terribly tired, and it was obvious that his complaint was genuine. He simply could not keep awake.

When the doctor examined him he found the man was suffering from sleepy sickness, and he was put to bed right away. He is still sleeping.

Spoken to no one

"He has spoken to no one during the time," stated Mr. Peter MacDonald, the governor of the home, yesterday, "though in a subconscious way he has managed to take his food.

"In these brief intervals his hand just seems to drift from the bedclothes, as if being guided by some mystic form of propulsion.

"He does not recognise anyone, and after each meal he literally returns to the state of a living corpse. It is truly pitiful. There is no form of bodily decay about him. He is, in fact, putting on flesh.

"No one can tell," added Mr. MacDonald, **"when, if ever, he will return to normal life. He is a problem and a vitally interesting one.**

"I cannot, for sentimental reasons," said Mr. MacDonald, "allow the patient's name to be published, but the facts concerning him are accurate."

I was subsequently allowed to visit the ward where this strangely silent man is accommodated.

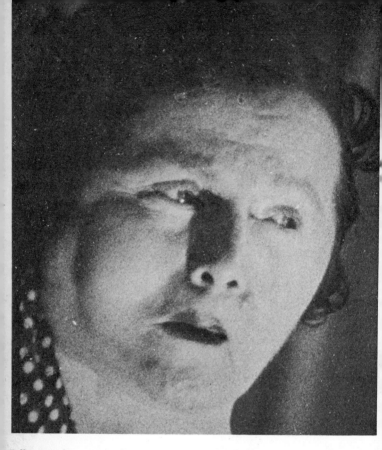

Following the great epidemic, numbers of patients passed into a strange, frozen 'sleep', in which they were transfixed in the endlessly prolonged first moment of their illness . . . This patient (*above*) had been transfixed in such a timeless entrancement since 1926; when 'awoken' briefly, in 1969, she felt that she was still in 1926 (see Rose R.).

(*Right*) This patient (Frances M.), shown here, motionless, in a state of frozen expectation, was also 'asleep', although she was sometimes able to walk and talk in a bemused, 'sleep-walking' way. Her expression – unlike Rose R.'s – looked towards the future, in perpetual expectation of a possible awakening. Whereas Rose R. could not bear the modern world suddenly thrust on her by L-DOPA, Frances M. greeted her awakening with gratitude and delight, accepting with good humour the forty years that she had 'lost'.

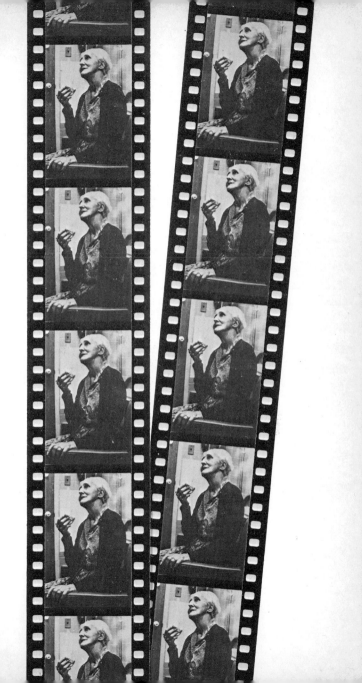

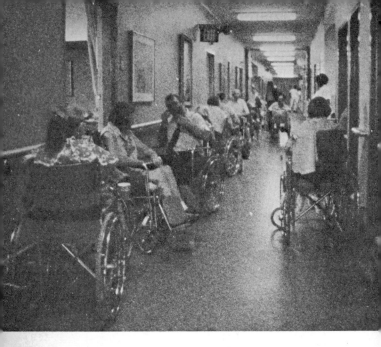

Unhappily, most large institutions are deficient in spaciousness and cosiness: their inmates tend to suffer from confinement and crowdedness, and from emptiness and loneliness.

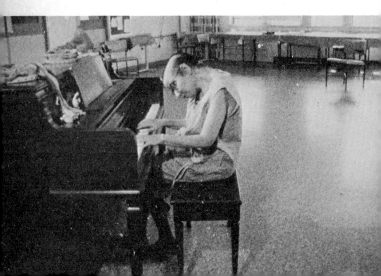

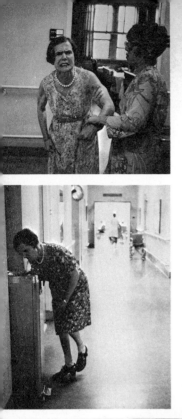

Institutions, insofar as they are *coercive*, aggravate the sickness of their inmates. Here we see one such patient driven, by the combined effects of disease, L-DOPA and institutionalization, into a state of panic and rage, and into perpetual, compulsive water-drinking. In contrast, both her Parkinsonism and her neuroses all but disappear in more human conditions – for example, in the hospital garden and, above all, when visited by her much-loved sister.

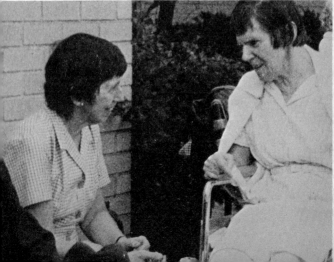

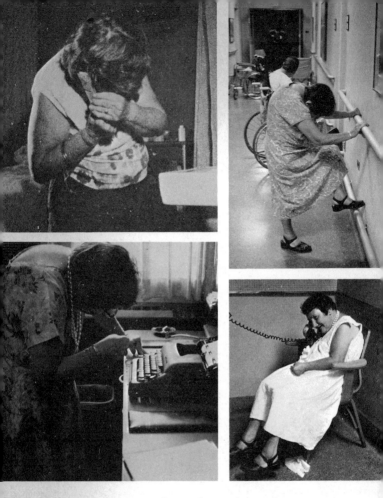

Some patients, however, despite disease, drug and
institutionalization manage to survive as vivid, individual,
idiosyncratic people. Here we see one such patient, who had
been in a state of virtual standstill for more than twenty
years, 'awakened' by L-DOPA: now, alive to her appearance,
she is seen doing her hair, despite the recurrence
of a partial standstill (after many minutes entirely
motionless, she is using her left hand to unlock her
'transfixed' right hand); we see her assiduously exercising
her long-frozen limbs, typing her journal, and laughing as
she speaks to her daughter on the phone . . .

7. MIRIAM H.

Miss H. was born in New York in 1914, the second child of a deeply religious Jewish family. Both of her parents died within six months of her birth – the first of many blows which life was to deal her. She was separated, as an infant, from her older sister, and sent to the old orphanage in Queens, where like Oliver Twist she was fed on thin gruel and threats. She showed considerable precocity from her earliest years, and was 'buried' in books from the age of ten. At the age of eleven she was pushed off a bridge, and sustained fractures of both legs, her pelvis and back. And at the age of twelve she developed a severe attack of *encephalitis lethargica* – the only one thus attacked in an orphanage-population exceeding two hundred. For six months she was so torpid that she would sleep night and day unless roused for food and other necessities, and for a further two years suffered from striking and frequent narcolepses, sleep-paralyses, nightmares, 'day-mares', and sleep-talking. Upon the heels of these sleep-disorders Parkinsonism followed, so that by the age of sixteen Miss H. had developed left-sided rigidity and a shrunken left hand, postural abnormalities, and an excessive rapidity and impetuosity of speech and thought. Her excellent intelligence was unimpaired by illness, and she was able to resume and finish high school. By the age of eighteen she was so disabled that she was transferred to Mount Carmel Hospital. Thus she had no chance to experience the 'outside' world, and could only learn of it from hearsay and books.

Her course, over the next thirty-seven years, was slowly but progressively downhill. In addition to a hemi-Parkinsonian rigidity and akinesia, she developed some spasticity and weakness of the left leg, and a shortening and deformity of the right leg, consequent upon her childhood accident. Des-

pite these difficulties, and superadded difficulties of balance
and marked festination, Miss H. was able to walk, with the
aid of two sticks, until 1966. In addition to great vocal hurry
and speed, she showed chewing and masticatory movements
of pronounced degree. Very distressing to her, and destructive to her self-esteem, were a variety of hypothalamic disorders which gradually overwhelmed her – extreme hirsutism
and obesity, a buffalohump and plethora, acne, diabetes and
repeated peptic ulcerations. She was painfully aware, in these
years, of her unattractiveness and grotesqueness, and this
reinforced her solitariness and seclusiveness, so that she buried herself, more and more, in what she could read. In the
early years of her illness, Miss H. used to suffer from sudden
paroxysms of left-sided pain, associated with anguish and
terror, of sudden onset and offset, and lasting some hours;
when I asked her about these, many years later, she answered
(as she was fond of doing) by a Dickensian example: 'You
keep asking me', she said, 'about the *location* of the pain,
and the only answer I can give is that which Mrs Gradgrind
gave: "I used to feel there was a pain *somewhere in the room*,
but I couldn't positively say that I had got it."' Following
the subsidence of these attacks, around 1940, Miss H. continued to suffer from an extreme sensitivity to pain on this
side of the body.

Until 1945, or thereabouts, Miss H. was prone to stormy
depressions and violent furies, but these gradually gave way
to a settled and somewhat apathetic depression. Miss H. remarked of this transition: 'I developed a violent temper after
the sleepy-sickness, quite uncontrollable, but it got *tamed*
with my disease.' There had also been a tendency to impatience and impulsiveness following her encephalitis, with
sudden violent screaming when frustrated, but this too had
subsided over the years. Miss H. referred with some embarrassment to these screaming attacks: 'It was as if something
built up and suddenly burst out of me. Sometimes I didn't

feel that I myself was screaming; I used to feel that it was something apart from me, something not controlled by me, which was doing the screaming. And I would feel awful afterwards, and hate myself.'

Apart from these occasional furies and screaming attacks, most of Miss H.'s hating and blaming was inflected inwards upon herself – or upon God. 'At first,' she said, 'I hated everybody, I longed for vengeance. I felt that people round me were somehow responsible for my disease. Then I became resigned to it, and realized that it was a punishment from God.' When I inquired whether she felt she had done anything to deserve the encephalitis, and why she felt she had been stricken in this way, she answered: 'No, I did not feel that I had done anything specially wrong. I am not a bad person. But I have been singled out – I don't know why. God is inscrutable.'

These feelings of inward blame and depression became greatly exacerbated and almost unbearable during the oculogyric crises from which Miss H. suffered. These crises, which started in 1928, would come with great regularity, every Wednesday; so much so that I could always arrange for my students to come on Wednesdays if they wished to witness such a crisis. Nevertheless, the times of these crises were modifiable to some extent: on one occasion I informed Miss H. that my students could not come on Wednesday, but would be coming on Thursday. 'OK,' said Miss H., 'I will put off the crisis to Thursday,' and she did. During her crises, which would last 8–10 hours, Miss H. would be 'compelled to look up at the ceiling', although there was no associated opisthotonos. She would be unable to wheel her chair, and only able to speak in a whisper. Throughout the crises she would be 'morose . . . sad . . . disgusted with life'. She would be forced to ruminate obsessively upon her miserable position, in hospital for thirty-seven years, without friends or family, ugly, disabled, etc. She would say to herself again and again: 'Why me? What did I do? Why am I being punished? Why have I been cheated of life? What is the use of going on? Why don't I kill myself?' These thoughts, which would repeat themselves in a sort of inner litany, could not be banished from her mind during the crises: they were reiterative, peremptory, overwhelming, and would exclude all other thoughts from her mind. When the crises were over, Miss H. would feel 'relatively cheerful', that she was herself again, and that perhaps, after all, things were not too bad. In addition to these crises, though sometimes combined with them, Miss H. – an extraordinary calculator – suffered from counting crises. These attacks, which occurred especially at night, consisted of compulsions to count to a particular number (like 95,000), or to raise 7 to the fifteenth power, before she would be allowed to stop thinking and sleep. In particular, like one of Jelliffe's patients, she was sometimes compelled to count in her oculogyric crises, and the crisis would/could not finish till she had reached her goal; if interrupted in her counting, at such times, she would have to return to 1 and start again; as soon as she reached her predetermined goal, her crisis would instantly cease at this moment.

Despite her many neurological and neuro-endocrinological problems, and despite the feelings of hopelessness which so often oppressed her, Miss H. fought bravely against her disabilities until 1967, being active in ward and synagogue affairs, an active debater in philosophy and other classes held at the hospital, an omnivorous reader and a close observer of current affairs. Following the exceedingly hot summer of 1967 – during which her anti-Parkinsonian medication was stopped for fear of the hyperpyrexia and heat-stroke which devastated our post-encephalitic patients that year – Miss H. regressed neurologically and emotionally, becoming intensely rigid in the left arm, chair-ridden, withdrawn and apathetic: she seemed to have lost all her former motivations, and would sit motionless in her chair all day, staring dully at the wall in front of her. Anti-depressants made very little difference to this state, and resumption of her previous so-lenaceous medicines diminished her salivation, but were of no use to her in other respects. She was considered to be ir-reparably damaged, a hopeless 'backward' patient at the time L-DOPA was first administered.

Before L-DOPA

When examined in May 1969 – just before the administration of L-DOPA – Miss H. was a grossly obese, heavily bearded, acromegalic and Cushingoid woman sitting motionless, slumped and apathetic in her wheelchair. Her face was greatly masked and devoid of any play of emotional expression, while the dullness and hopelessness of her appearance and attitudes was shown by the almost opaque spectacles – clearly uncleaned for many months – which she wore over her protuberant and myopic eyes. When these were removed, the eyes seemed to stare dully at nothing, showing nothing of the alert, attentive movements which are some-times the only sign of animation in severely akinetic patients. The pupils were small and unequal in size (the left being somewhat larger), but gaze was normal in all directions save for a moderate deficit of convergence. There was no spontaneous blinking, but glabellar tap or visual approach would elicit a protracted forced closure of the eyelids. Her skin was greasy, showed extensive acne and sebarrhoeic dermatitis, and sweated profusely, especially on the left side of the body.

Miss H.'s voice was clear and intelligible, although it alternated between vocal blockings and extreme vocal hurry, every clause being jetted out suddenly, and rapidly decaying into aphonia. In addition to this irregularity of speech-force and rhythm, there were occasional expiratory and phonatory tics (grunting) which further interrupted coherent speech. Her breathing was scarcely perceptible, but she showed occasional, impulsive deep inspirations. Salivation was increased, although there was no actual drooling. She was unable to protrude her tongue, and could only move it slowly and tremulously from side to side, writhing her mouth when requested to wag it quickly. She showed intermittent chewing movements when her attention was not actively engaged, and these (I later had occasion to observe) persisted during sleep in the early part of the night. Miss H. showed a striking unilaterality of rigidity and akinesia, the left side of her body being much more severely affected. The left arm was intensely rigid, with dystonic deformity and contracture of the hand, and had almost no capacity for independent movement. The right arm had only slightly increased rigidity, and the right hand was able to make six to seven clenching movements before akinesia set in. There was intense axial rigidity with almost no available movement of the trunk or neck muscles. The entire left side of the body showed a combination of hypalgesia with intense hyperpathia and over-reaction to painful stimuli. The legs showed some spasticity and weakness of upper motor neurone type: all tendon-reflexes were pathologically increased, and plantar responses were extensor on both sides. Miss H. was quite unable to rise from her chair, and even when supported was unable to stand or walk.

It was astonishing to observe, in a patient of such unprepossessing and regressed appearance, the sudden outcroppings of high intelligence, wit, and charm, for these lay buried, most of the time, by extreme withdrawal compounded by 'block'; so much so, indeed, that those who did not know Miss H. well generally took her to be mentally defective.

Course on L-DOPA

The administration of L-DOPA was started on 18 June 1969. No changes were observed in the first week of L-DOPA medication, while the dosage was being slowly increased, and Miss H. made no complaints of nausea, dizziness, or other symptoms commonly experienced in the first days of receiving the drug. The following are extracts from my diary.

27 *June*. Now on a dose of 2 gm. L-DOPA daily, Miss H. appears more alert, more cheerful, and more interested in her surroundings.

1 *July*. Miss H. continues to be alert and cheerful, and now, for the first time in many years, takes an interest in her appearance, requesting that she be shaved three times a week, that her skin-problems be attended to, and if she might wear a dress each day, rather than a shapeless hospital-gown. She has arranged to borrow a novel from the library – she had had no wish to read for more than two years – and has started to keep a diary in a minute, but daily enlarging, handwriting. There is now a quite remarkable dissolution of rigidity in the left arm, and Miss H. has planned a series of exercises to 'limber up' this previously petrified limb. She has become able to open and close the left hand freely, although separate finger-movements still remain impossible. In view of this auspicious therapeutic response, and the absence of any adverse effects, I am raising the dosage of L-DOPA from 3 gm. to 4 gm. daily.

9 *July*. Miss H. has shown further improvement on an increased dose of L-DOPA, although there are now a number of adverse effects also, none of them, fortunately, too serious. Her left arm, aided by physiotherapy, has become more skilful, and discrete finger-movements are now possible: this allows Miss H., amongst other things, to handle a knife and fork in a normal fashion, and to take the paper off sweets and chocolates (to which, despite her obesity and diabetes, she is somewhat addicted).

Miss H. has also become more demanding and impatient; she is now able to make her needs known in a loud voice, if need be, and if this is not heeded screams shrilly. These

occasional screamings are felt as ego-alien, and are followed
at once by contrition and apologies. She continues to show
vocal hurry, but her speech-pattern is altogether more even
and coherent, and has entirely ceased to have any delay after
each clause or sentence. Indeed, I have never seen a human
being who can speak like Miss H.: she could easily beat any
news-announcer, because she can talk at 500 words a minute
without missing a syllable. Her rapidity of speech, combined
with her rapidity of thought and calculation, makes her
more than a match for any of my medical students: When I
ask her, for example, to take 17s away from 1,012, she per-
forms these serial subtractions as fast as she can speak. [Mas-
ticatory movements had become more marked, and were especially gross in the evenings, continuing after Miss H. had
fallen asleep, but they neither annoyed nor inconvenienced
her. An entirely novel symptom which had developed on the
increased dose of L-DOPA was a *tic*, a lightning-quick movement of the right hand to the face, occurring about twenty
times an hour. When I questioned Miss H. about this symptom, shortly after its inauguration, she replied that it was
'a nonsense-movement', which had no purpose that she was
aware of, and which she did not wish to make: 'I feel a tension building up in my hand,' she said, 'and after a time it
gets too much, and then I *have* to move it.' Within three
days of its appearance, however, this tic had become associated with an intention and a use: it had become a mannerism,
and was now used by Miss H. to adjust the position of her
spectacles. Her spectacles were indeed loose, and prone to
slip down over the bridge of her nose: 'You better not get
them fixed,' Miss H. remarked, with insight and humour,
'otherwise I will have to find a new use for this hand-move-
ment of mine.' There was no doubt of the relief when this tic
became mannerized, when a 'nonsensical' dynamism became an action with reference. Miss H. was always prone

to give a rationalization and a referential form to her 'involuntary' movements; she could not stand mere impulses, like Mrs Y. for example.]

21 *July*. Miss H. has continued to show an even and satisfactory therapeutic response – alertness without insomnia, good humour without excitement, excellent function in her left arm, and now, with the aid of physiotherapy, a capacity to stand with assistance for a few seconds, although the spastic weakness in her legs is unchanged.

1 *August*. 'It has been the best month I have had in years,' says Miss H., summarizing the events of July. Amongst the other desirable effects of L-DOPA has been the cessation of oculogyric crises, which had tormented her regularly for more than forty years.[34] Although equable under normal circumstances, Miss H. now shows the quick temper which characterized her reactions in the early post-encephalitic years.

Throughout August Miss H. maintained her stable and satisfactory improvement, and, with the aid of physiotherapy, became able to stand on her feet and walk a few steps once more. As striking as the neurological and functional improvement, and most obvious to a stranger's eye, was the transformation which had occurred in Miss H.'s cosmetic appearance and behaviour. Two months previously, she had been a pitiful, motionless, apathetic, backward patient, misshapen and unwholesome in appearance, bundled into an anonymous white hospital gown. Now she was neatly dressed, with a style of her own, shaven, powdered, made-up and permed. Her obesity, her acromegaly, and her slightly masked face could easily be overlooked now with her new

---

34. One of the most welcome effects of L-DOPA in post-encephalitic patients generally was to rid them, for a while, of their disabling and hellish oculogyric crises; see 'Oculogyric Crises and L-DOPA' by Sacks *et al.*, *Lancet*, July 1970.

poise and smartness, and especially when one was listening to her admirably witty and fluent conversation. The Ugly Duckling was nearly a swan.

1969-72

In her fourth month on L-DOPA (September–October 1969) Miss H. started to show respiratory 'side-effects' to L-DOPA (her dose having been maintained at 4·0 gm. a day). The first such effect was hiccup, which would come in hour-long attacks, starting at 6.30 every morning, a little after Miss H. had awoken and *before* her first dose of L-DOPA for the day. Three weeks later a 'nervous' cough and throat-clearing started, associated with a recurrent tic-like feeling of something blocking or scratching her throat; the hiccup disappeared with the onset of throat-clearing and coughing, as if it had been 'replaced' by these symptoms. In late November Miss H. started to develop a tendency to gasping and breath-holding, which in turn 'replaced' the throat-clearing and coughing. From here she proceeded to increasingly severe 'respiratory crises' which had some similarity to those of Miss D.[35] Towards the end of the year Miss H.'s crises grew intolerably severe, and were accompanied not only by a marked increase of pulse and blood pressure, but by intense emotional excitement, blocking of speech and recrudescence of Parkinsonism and oculogyria.

She further experienced forced and quasi-hallucinatory 'reminiscences' and phantasies during her crises which were responsible for her peculiar facial expression during these and her 'block'. Thus Miss H. would suddenly 'remember' (in her crises) that she had been sexually assaulted by 'a beast' of an elevator-attendant in 1952, and that in consequence of this she now had syphilis; she 'realized' (in her

35. Miss H. and Miss D. were 'pet enemies' at this time, were unhappy if apart, and spent most of each day sitting opposite one another having crises at one another.

crises) that this horrible story was known to everyone round her, and that the entire ward was whispering about her 'looseness' and its pathological outcome. It was two weeks before Miss H. could bring herself to divulge these thoughts to me; when I asked if the assault had actually happened, etc., she replied: 'Of course not. That's a lot of nonsense. But I'm *forced* to think it when I have one of my crises.' By the end of December her crises had become virtually continuous one with another, and it was therefore necessary to stop her L-DOPA.

A month went past, during which Miss H. recovered from her crises, but showed a degree of Parkinsonism considerably in excess of her pre-DOPA state. In February 1970, Miss H. said to me, 'I think I'm ready for L-DOPA again. I've done a lot of thinking in the last month and I've worked my way through that sexual nonsense. I will lay you 20–1 I have no more crises again.' I started her back on L-DOPA again, and worked up once more to 4·0 gm. a day.

Miss H. again had good therapeutic efforts, though not as marked as the first time she had taken it. She continued in fair shape until the summer of 1970, when she again started to have 'side-effects' of various kinds. These did not take the form of hiccups, coughs, gasps or other respiratory symptoms – as Miss H. herself had predicted and wagered; but they took the form of multiple tics. These had a most bizarre form, 'punching' each arm alternatively into the air, as if swatting mosquitoes which buzzed over her head. By July her rate of ticcing was 300 per minute, her arms moving up and down like streaks of lightning, almost too quickly for the eye to follow. Other activities became impossible at this time and Miss H. herself asked us to re-stop her L-DOPA.

In September 1970, Miss H. said to me, 'Third time lucky! If you give me L-DOPA once again, I promise you no complications this time.' I did so, and Miss H. proved correct. In the last two years she has continued to take 4·0 gm. a day with a clear-cut if unspectacular therapeutic response. She does have an occasional tantrum or crisis, but not too often and never severe. She *has* continued to maintain her 'spectacles-adjusting' mannerism, which seems to absorb or discharge or express her ticcish propensities, or an undue building-up of psychomotor excitement: 'It's my conduit,' Miss H. says. 'You leave it alone.'

In general Miss H. lives as much of a life as is possible with the disabilities she has, and in the situation she is: she makes a point of going to excursions and movies, whenever she can; she is a terror at Bingo, at which she invariably wins, because there is no one in the hospital who can match her shrewdness or her lightning-quick thought; and she is warmly devoted to her one remaining sister. For most of the day however, Miss H. is absorbed in reading and writing: she reads with great speed and intentness and devours what she reads – it is always something 'old-fashioned' (usually Dickens) and never contemporary; she thinks a great deal and keeps her thoughts to herself, confiding them to volume after volume of her extensive diaries. Thus, all in all, Miss H. has done well – amazingly so, considering the existence she has led. Against all odds, Miss H. has always managed to be a real *person* and to face reality without denial or madness. She draws on a strength unfathomable to me, a health which is deeper than the depth of her illness.

8. LUCY K.

Born in New York, in 1924, an only child, Miss K. apparently had no childhood illnesses of note, and in particular no febrile illnesses characterized by lethargy or restlessness. At the age of two, however, she developed a paralysis and divergence of the left eye: this was ascribed to a 'congenital strabismus', despite its suddeness of onset (over the course of six weeks), and the normality of gaze before its occurrence. Miss K. is described by her mother as having been eager and quick to learn as a child, as having been very 'good' and obedient in early childhood, although developing a 'nasty disposition' (stubbornness, naughtiness, stealing, lying, tantrums, etc.) at about the age of six. She was greatly attached to her father, and it was shortly after his death (when she was eleven) that Parkinsonian symptoms became plainly manifest.

The first physical abnormalities were observed in her walking, which became by degrees stiff and wooden, and particularly unstable when she faced a downwards flight of stairs, which she would be impelled to descend with uncontrollable speed, usually falling to the bottom. Her face had become 'expressionless and shiny – like a doll's face' by the age of fifteen. Concurrently with these motor symptoms, Miss K. developed increasing emotional disorder, becoming inattentive and quarrelsome at school – which she had to leave at the age of fourteen – and more and more parasitically attached to her mother at home. By degrees, she became more withdrawn, losing interest in her friends, her books, and her hobbies, increasingly disinclined to leave the house, and gradually drawn into a closer and more hostile intimacy with her mother – an intimacy uninterrupted by the presence of a father, of other children, of school, of friends, or of any other interests or emotional attachments. She never dated, despite her mother's 'encouragement', variously maintaining that she despised, hated, or feared the other sex, and that she was 'perfectly happy' at home with her mother. It is evident, from close questioning of the mother, that this domestic bliss was broken by frequent violent quarrels, apparently started either by Lucy or her mother.

Rigidity, first of the left side, then of the right, set in during her early twenties, and by the age of twenty-seven

Miss K. could no longer walk and was confined to a wheel-chair. Despite mounting and seemingly impossible difficulties, she remained at home, totally dependent upon her mother, who devoted every hour of the day to caring for her. On one occasion, Miss K. was taken to a neurology outpatient clinic where she was given some pills, and where continued outpatient care and possible surgery were advised. Miss K.'s mother threw away the pills, was shocked by the suggestion of surgery, and never took her daughter back to the clinic.

Eventually, in 1964, when total nursing care had become necessary, Miss K. was brought to Mount Carmel Hospital by her mother. At the time of her admission, the picture was one of severe rigidity, akinesia, ophthalmoplegia, and auto-nomic disturbances, but with a relatively well-preserved and audible voice. Her admission precipitated a month of violent rages and belligerence, which was followed by a marked and sudden withdrawal and deterioration of her neurological status: in particular, Miss K. ceased to speak, to feed herself, to move in bed, or to show any signs of independent func-tioning.

About six months after Miss K.'s admission, she became greatly attached to a male orderly on the ward who showed her some human concern and kindliness. During the two months that this orderly was on the ward, Miss K.'s voice returned, and she recovered the ability to feed herself, to turn in bed, etc. When he left the ward her state suddenly and profoundly declined once again; and she remained in a severely regressed and incapacitated state after this time.

Between 1965 and 1968 Miss K. presented a picture of ex-treme uniformity, of an almost inhuman monotony, except on certain occasions of violent 'release'. She remained un-cannily motionless, with a tense, an *intense* motionlessness somewhat different from Parkinsonism; and totally speech-less, again in a forced, constrained manner different from the aphonia of Parkinsonism.

Sometimes, when watching a movie, she would be swept by an access of terror or pleasure, and this would suddenly 'break' her clenched silence and immobility, and lead to a loud high scream ('Eeehhh!' accompanied by a child-like clapping of the hands, or a sudden raising of them to the face (as in an infant's startle-reflex). She was also notorious for her rages, which would come on extremely suddenly, with scarcely a moment's warning: during these she would curse with great violence and fluency in a particularly sarcastic and wounding way, which showed how closely and clever-ly she had watched all those around her (when she was im-mobile and seemingly dead to the world), and how gifted she was in mockery and caricature; at such times she would glare balefully, wave her clenched fists, and occasionally hit out with a good deal of force. The unmistakably murderous qual-ity of these rages, combined with their total unexpectedness, had a peculiarly unnerving effect. These paroxysms of terror or pleasure, of laughter or rage, would rarely last more than a minute or so; they would vanish as abruptly as they had come, and Miss K. would suddenly revert, without any in-termediate stages, to the violent fixity of her 'normal' state.

Her general appearance, during these years, was pathetic – and grotesque. She was heavily and powerfully built, giv-ing the impression of great physical strength clenched in restraint. She looked (like most post-encephalitics) much younger than her age – one could easily have supposed she was in her twenties, not her forties. Her bizarre 'baby-doll' appearance was accentuated by the immense pains her moth-er took to 'prepare' her every day. Miss K., when 'prepared', would sit in the hall rigid and motionless in her over-size chair, invested in an embroidered and ambiguous child's or bride's nightgown. Her jet-black hair would be heavily brai-ded, and her face chalky-white from its coating of powder (she suffered from constant sweatings and sebarrhoea). Her dystonic, crippled hands (with fingers immovably flexed at the knuckles) were heavily ringed, and had long scarlet nails. Her inverted feet were daintily slippered. She looked like – I could never decide: like a clown, or a geisha, or Miss Haversham, or a robot. But most of all like a baby-doll, in the most absolute and literal sense of the words: a living reflection of her mother's mad whim.

And, indeed, as I progressively came to realize, not only Miss K.'s appearance, but a great deal of her pathology, was inseparably associated with her mother's behaviour, and could not be considered as a thing-in-itself.

Thus her mutism was in part a *refusal* to speak (a block or veto or interdict on speech), which mirrored the warnings of her paranoid mother. 'Don't speak, Lucy,' she would say every day. 'Ssshhh! Not a word! They're against you round here. Give nothing away – not a move, not a word ... There's nobody here you can trust in the least.' These dire warnings would alternate with hours of crooning, maudlin baby-talk: 'Lucy, my baby, my little living *doll* ... There's nobody who loves you like me ... Nobody in the world *could* love you like me ... For you, little Lucy, I have given my life ...'

Miss K.'s mother would arrive at hospital very early in the morning, seven days a week, undertake the feeding and total care of the patient (despite the efforts of the nursing staff and others to dislodge her from this despotic position), and leave late at night, when the patient was finally and safely asleep. She avowed, truthfully, that she was complete-ly devoted to her daughter, and that she had 'sacrificed' the last twenty-five years to looking after her, and 'protect-ing' her. It was evident, however, that her attitude was deeply contradictory, and involved hatred, sadism, and destruc-tiveness no less than an inordinate love and devotion. This was particularly manifest if I chanced to walk through the ward with my students: Miss K.'s mother, on spotting our group, would suddenly seize her daughter and jerk her into a sitting position, straightening her neck with a vicious crack; she would then beckon us to approach, and would start a cruel goading of the patient: 'Lucy,' she would say, 'which is the best-looking one? That one there? Wouldn't you like to kiss him, wouldn't you like to marry him?' At this stage, a tear would roll down Lucy's face, or she would utter a hoarse roar of fury.

Early in 1969, I suggested L-DOPA, thinking at this time that there was nothing to lose. For Miss K. was not only mute and motionless from 'wilfulness', refused, 'block' and negativism, etc., but deeply and distressingly Parkinsonian as well. She showed – insofar as could be detected 'beneath' catatonic rigidity – a severe plastic rigidity of Parkinsonian type, more on the left, and easily elicited cogwheeling at all major joints. Her crippling dystonic contractures ('bilateral hemiplegic dystonia') have already been noted, and were associated with coldness, waxiness and some atrophy of hands and feet.

She showed paroxysms of 'flapping' tremor on both sides, and occasional massive myoclonic jerks. Particularly severe was her endless salivation, a constant stream of viscid saliva; which not only necessitated the use of a bib and constant mopping – in itself a humiliation – but by its quantity (approaching a gallon each day) continually threatened her with dehydration. Continual tremor of the lips was present, and – when excited – a rhythmical grimace (her mother called it 'snarling') which bared all her teeth.

She showed an alternating exotropia, with widely skewed eyes, which seemed to shine, when open, with anguish and spite (they were concealed, for much of the day, by tonus/clonus of the eyelids, or anablepic rotation – which exposed only sclera). Her eyes, and these alone, were freely mobile, and were painfully eloquent in expressing her feelings. These were extreme, contradictory, and wholly irresoluble. When Miss K. was hostile and negativistic (as she seemed to be, most of the time), all requests elicited 'refusal': a request to look at one caused looking-away; a request to show her tongue caused clenching of the jaws; a request to let herself 'go loose' made her rigid with spasm. At other times, more rarely, she would have a tender, submissive and melting expression, and 'gave herself' unreservedly, catatonically, to those who examined her; at such times, the merest intimation elicited *compliance*, or as much as was possible in her disabled state. Even her Parkinsonian rigidity seemed to 'melt' at such times, and her usually rigid limbs could be moved with some ease. Thus Miss K.'s Parkinsonism, catatonia and psychotic ambivalence formed a continuous spectrum, all interlocked in inseparable relation.

Early in 1969, then, I suggested L-DOPA. I suggested it once and many times subsequently. (My enthusiasm at that time was scarcely qualified, and I tended to simplify the most complex situations.) 'Lucy is helpless,' I said. 'She needs to be cured. L-DOPA, nothing else, can come to the rescue.' Her mother, however, was implacably opposed, and expressed her opinion in front of the patient: 'Lucy is best as she is,' she asserted. 'She'll get stirred up, she'll *blow up* if you give her L-DOPA.' And she added, piously: 'If it is God's will that Lucy should die, then she must die.' Miss K., of course, heard this without speaking, but expressed in her eyes a tortured ambivalance – wish-fear, 'yes–no' – of unlimited degree.

1969–72

In 1969, I started to revise my own opinion: I *saw* several 'blow-ups' in other patients on L-DOPA. I became far less eager to press it on Miss K. I ceased to mention it when I saw her or her mother. But as my enthusiasm waned, Miss K.'s increased. She became more stubborn and defiant in relation to her mother, and stiffened herself in board-like rigidity. Their contact became a wrestling together, with Miss K. 'winning' by sheer catatonia.

Late in 1970, her mother came to me. 'I'm exhausted,' she said. 'I can't cope any more. Lucy's killing me with her hate and her badness ... Why did you ever mention that *cursed* L-DOPA? It's come like a curse between Lucy and me ... Give her the drug, and we'll see what we'll see!'

I started L-DOPA with a very small dose, and gradually built it up to 3 gm. daily. Miss K. was mildly nauseated; her Parkinsonism and catatonia, if anything, became more severe. But there was nothing else – only a sense of *something* impending. In her fourth week on L-DOPA, she did react, and – as her mother predicted – she 'blew up' completely. It happened very suddenly one morning without warning. The staff-nurse, usually staid, came running to my office: 'Quick!' she said. 'You must come along quickly. Miss Lucy's moving and talking a mile to the minute ... It suddenly happened a few minutes ago!' Miss K. was sitting up alone in bed (something normally impossible for her), was flushed and animated and waving her arms. I smiled, rather dazedly, and quickly examined her: not a trace of rigidity in her arms or her legs; akinesia quite vanished; free movement except where contractured.

Her voice was loud and clear, and immensely excited: 'Look at me, look at me! I can fly like a bird!' All the nurses were standing around, exclaiming, congratulating and hugging Miss K. And her mother was also there, saying nothing at all, with an unfathomable expression contorting her features. That evening, when I visited her alone (her mother had gone, and the nurses had cooled down), I went over the examination again. In the course of this I said, 'Will you give me your hand?', and Miss K. said, 'Yes, yes, I'll give you my hand.'

She continued excited, elated, and very active the next day. When I did rounds in the evening, she took the initiative: 'Dr Sacks!' she said, her words tumbling over themselves in her excitement. 'You asked for my hand. It's yours!

... I want you to marry me and take me away. Take me
away from this horrible place ... And, promise – you'll never
let *her* come near me again !'

I calmed her down as best I could, explained I was her doctor, not anything else; that I liked her and would do my best
for her, but – Miss K. gave me a long, anguished, and
furious glare: 'OK,' she said. 'That's *it*. I hate you, you
louse, you rat-fink, you ...' She sank back exhausted, and
said nothing more.

The next morning, Miss K. was totally mute and blocked
and rigid, salivating grossly, and shaking with tremor.
'What happened?' asked the nurses. 'She was doing so well.
The L-DOPA can't fade as quickly as that.' Her mother,
when she came in, broke into a smile: 'I knew it would happen,' she said. 'You pushed Lucy too far.'

We continued the L-DOPA, for another three weeks, even
raising the dose to 5·0 gm. a day, but it could have been
chalk for the effect it had. Miss K. *had* exploded – and imploded again, contracted herself to an intransigent point,
infinitely withdrawn, Parkinsonian and rigid. She had been
exposed and extended – and totally rebuffed; and that was
it – she was having no more; we could fill her with L-DOPA,
but react *she would not*. This, at least, was my guess about
her feelings and reactions; I could learn nothing directly,
because her silence (including her 'motor silence') became
absolute. When I stopped the L-DOPA, she showed no further reaction of any type.

In the months that followed, Miss K.'s Parkinsonism continued profound, and she perhaps came to terms, a little,
with what had happened on L-DOPA. She never spoke again
to me, but occasionally she smiled.

She seemed, from this time on, to be less tense, less em-
phatic, less rigid in her posture. Some of the *violence* of her
feelings seemed to abate. But she grew sadder and more withdrawn, as far as I could judge. I had the feeling of something

broken, irremediably, inside her. There were no more curses or outbursts at others, and she now sat at films without attending or reacting. Her eyes lay closed for most of the day – not clenched, just closed. Her behaviour was that of a ghost or a corpse – of someone who'd *had it*, and had done with the world.

She died, quietly and suddenly, in July 1972.

9. MARGARET A.

Margaret A. was born in New York, in 1908, the youngest daughter of a poor Irish immigrant couple who were intermittently employed. There was nothing in her early years to suggest retardation, major emotional disturbances, or any significant physical illnesses. She was a student of at least average competence, who graduated from High School at the age of fifteen, a good athlete, and apparently easy-going and equable in her emotional life.

In 1925, at the age of seventeen, she developed an acute illness with overwhelming sleepiness and depression. She did indeed sleep almost continuously for ten weeks, although she could be roused from her sopor to be fed, and was exceedingly lethargic, fearful, and depressed for a year after this. This illness was at first ascribed to 'shock' (her father, to whom she was closely attached, had died shortly before the onset of her symptoms), but subsequently recognized as *encephalitis lethargica*.

Following a year of lethargy and depression, she apparently made a complete recovery, working as a secretary and book-keeper, playing tennis, and being sociable and popular among a large group of friends. In 1928–9, however, she developed the first symptoms of a very complex post-encephalitic syndrome.

Among her first symptoms were a tendency to gross tremor of both hands, some slowness of gait and impaired balance, a tendency to drowse during the day and be wakeful at night, a 'monstrous' appetite (which caused her to gain 100 lb. in two years), insatiable thirst and need to drink, and a tendency to sudden brief elations and depressions which seemed to bear little relation to the actual circumstances of day-to-day living. Two other paroxysmal symptoms developed in the early thirties: severe oculogyric crises which would last ten to twelve hours, and come on, characteristically, on Wednesdays, and frequent short staring spells ('crises of fixed regard') which would suddenly arrest her, and hold her 'in a sort of trance state' for a few minutes. Her bulimia and inversion of sleep-rhythm became less marked after 1932–3, but her other symptoms have gradually worsened over the past forty years.

Miss A. was able to continue working in a clerical capacity until 1935, and subsequently lived at home with her mother – apart from a number of brief hospital admissions – until she entered Mount Carmel Hospital in 1958. Miss A. is reluctant to speak of these other brief periods of hospital care: it is evident, from summaries we have received, that the presenting symptoms in each case were those of depression, hypochondriasis and suicidal rumination. Treatment was made difficult by the fact that these periods of depression, for all their severity, would last only a few days, being succeeded by elations and denial of all problems. It was never necessary, apparently, to administer shock-treatment or anti-depressant medication. She would be discharged with the somewhat vague diagnosis of 'Parkinsonism with psychosis', or 'Parkinsonism with a typical schizophrenia'.

During her ten years at Mount Carmel, Miss A.'s state has very slowly worsened, although she has continued to be able to walk without assistance (despite a strong tendency to festination, and a number of falls), to feed herself, to dress herself with some assistance, and at her 'good times' to type. Her thirst and urge to drink have continued to be very prominent: her daily input of water varies between 10 and 15 pints, and there is a commensurate output of very dilute urine. She has shown strongly marked cycles and paroxysmal alterations of alertness, motor activity, and mood. Thus every day, between 5 and 6.30 p.m., she becomes overwhelmingly sleepy, and may fall asleep, quite suddenly, while eating or washing, etc. The drowsiness is accompanied by greatly increased blepharoclonus, uncontrollable drooping of the eyelids and repeated forced closures of the eyes. This drowsiness can be resisted for a few minutes, but will invariably lead to short sleep. There tend to be somewhat milder attacks of drowsiness in the early afternoon, shortly after 1 p.m.; these may occasionally be of almost narcoleptic abruptness. Her motor activity is at its height between 2 and 4.30 p.m., at which time her voice, normally low-pitched and monotonous, is loud and expressive, and her small-stepped shuffling gait is replaced by striding with exaggerated swinging of the arms, and synkinetic involvement of the trunk-muscles. Her motor capacities are at their lowest ebb in the early morning hours (5–8 a.m.), when she is fully alert but barely able to speak audibly or rise to her feet. She displays both wakefulness and increased motor activity after seven in the evenings, and has great difficulty going to sleep at 9 p.m., the usual time at which our patients retire. Even after she has fallen asleep around 10 p.m., she displays unusual motor activity during sleep, in particular turning-and-tossing in bed, sleep-talking, and on occasion sleep-walking. This motor activity ceases around 1 a.m., and for the remainder of the night her sleep is tranquil. She has no feeling of tiredness in the mornings, and no recollection of talking or other activities during her sleep.

Her depressions and elations both have a rather stereotyped quality. During the former, she feels that she is 'bad,

repulsive . . .' etc., she hates herself and feels that she is hated
by the other patients, she feels they despise her for her woe-
begone expression and for drinking at the water-fountain
fifty times a day, that her life is worthless, pitiful, and not
worth going on with, and above all she is tormented by the
conviction that she is going blind. Her hypochondriacal fears
of blindness have an obsessive, reiterative quality: she re-
peats to herself innumerable times, 'I am going blind, I know
it, I'm really going blind,' etc., and at such times she *cannot*
be reassured.

On the other hand, when she is in one of her elated moods,
she feels 'gay as a skylark' (a favourite and much-repeated
phrase), care-free, pain-free ('I haven't an ache or pain in
my whole body – I feel so good, there's nothing, nothing at
all the matter with me,' etc.), full of energy, very active,
very sociable and inclined to gossip. These changes of mood
and attitude, which are very abrupt and extreme, are rarely
connected with any realistic change in her circumstances:
she herself says, 'I'm often depressed when there's nothing to
worry about, and gay as a skylark when there are all sorts of
problems.' Sometimes, however, one of her hypochondriacal
depressions may come on during the course of an oculogyric
crisis (when indeed she cannot see, because of extreme upward deviation of the eyes), and outlast it; and on several
occasions a depression has switched to elation during a crisis.

In terms of her *general physical and neurological condition* (understanding that this tends to fluctuate a good deal
during the course of each day, and according to mood, etc.)
Miss A. was a rather thin woman, appearing considerably
younger than her sixty-one years, with a rather greasy and
notably hirsute skin, but without clear signs of acromegaly,
thyroid or other endocrine disturbance. She experienced considerable salivation, having to wipe her mouth clear of saliva
every few minutes. Her face appeared rigid and masked, with
some tendency (especially during inattention and sleep) to

an open-mouthed posture. There was a resting tremor of the lips, and a gross rotary and intromittent tremor of the tongue. Spontaneous blinking was rare, but forced blinking, blepharoclonus and protracted forced closure of the eyes were readily elicited by glabellar tap, or sudden stimuli in the visual field. When sleepy, she showed incessant attacks of blepharoclonus, and a tendency to 'micro-crises' with forced lid-closure and upward deviation of the globes for several seconds. Her voice was monotonous and uninflected, low in pitch and volume (occasionally decaying into inaudibility), with some tendency to hurry (vocal festination), but no palilalia. The pupils were small (2 mm.), equal, and reactive, the eyes moist from excess lacrimation, and the gaze full in all directions save for a mild convergence-deficit.

She showed extreme rigidity of the axial musculature, with almost no available neck-motion, and mild-moderate rigidity of the limbs. She showed a very gross ('flapping') tremor of the arms when anxious, excited, or standing, but not at other times. Asked to clench her hands repeatedly, the movement would decay in volume after 2–3 repetitions, then accelerate, and after 6–8 repetitions automatize, decompose rhythmically, and be replaced by uncontrollable flapping tremor. Miss A. tended, when sitting or standing, to assume a strongly flexed posture of the trunk, and could only straighten herself for a few seconds. She would usually arise slowly and with difficulty, and shuffle slowly forwards with her arms held flexed, rigid, and motionless by her sides. Propulsion, laterpulsion, and retropulsion could be elicited with extreme ease, and she showed a considerable tendency to pitch forwards, especially if caught in uncontrollable festination. Although very rigid and bradykinetic at the start of an examination, Miss A. showed a remarkable ability to 'activate' and loosen herself by exercise (her functional state before and after physiotherapy were strikingly different), and she could also be activated for a few minutes, even in her most akinetic early-morning period, if she chanced to sneeze. Her mood, if depressed, would show dramatic improvement *pari passu* with her motor activation. Before being placed on L-DOPA, she had had no full-blown oculogyric crises for over a year. She had received a great number of solenaceous and similar drugs, which controlled her salivation and tremor to some extent, but had made little difference to her flexed posture, bradykinesia, instability of gait, hypophonia, crises, or mood-changes. She was started on L-DOPA on 7 May.

Course on L-DOPA

No effects of any kind were experienced or observed until the dosage had been raised to 2 gm. daily. At this dosage (12 May), Miss A. experienced mild nausea and dizziness, and started to show frequent opening of the mouth – the mouth-posture of yawning, although there was no actual yawning; this alternated with occasional clenching of the teeth. Miss A. described both movements as 'automatic' and involuntary.

By 15 May (the dose had now been raised to 3 gm. L-DOPA daily), Miss A. showed striking changes in many ways. Her expression had become alert and keen, and her features more mobile; she had ceased to have drowsy periods or sopors in the course of the day. Her posture was maintained upright without effort. Her rigidity was distinctly reduced. The abnormal mouth-movements had declined in frequency. She described a state of unprecedented energy and well-being.

On 17 May (with raising of the dosage to 4 gm. L-DOPA daily), there was further reduction in rigidity and akinesia – a variety of daily skills were now within her reach, e.g. dressing and undressing, which had been impossible previously without considerable assistance. She could rise to her feet without hesitation, and stride the length of the corridor swinging her arms. Her face was mobile, and she smiled readily. Her eyes were now very wide open all day, and appeared very 'bright'. Forced opening and clenching of the jaws again became prominent with the raising of dosage-level.

On 19 May (still on 4 gm. L-DOPA daily), Miss A. started to show some disconcerting effects from the drug. She felt extremely wakeful and had found it impossible to sleep for two nights running. Her pupils were dilated (5 mm.), though normally reactive. Her legs felt restless, and she had an urge to cross and uncross them, to tap either foot, and generally to move about. She felt a need, even in bed, to perform her physiotherapy exercises over and over again. Her mouth-movements had become exceedingly conspicuous, and had formed the focus of some paranoid anxiety – that other patients, and nursing staff, were 'watching' her, laughing at her, etc. In view of this excessive arousal – akathisia, agitation, agrypnia – the dosage was reduced to 3 gm. daily.

For several days (18–25 May), on a dosage of 3 gm. daily, Miss A. maintained a steady improvement of posture, gait, and voice, and virtual disappearance of her rigidity and akinesia, without any manifestation of the inordinate arousal seen on the larger dose. We entertained hopes that a stable plateau of improvement had been reached.

On 26 May, however, renewed and novel manifestations of arousal were exhibited. Miss A. felt constant thirst and ravenous hunger – she felt impelled to drink at the water-fountain almost incessantly, and her appetite and voracity reminded her of what she had experienced in the early thirties. Her mood became exalted: she felt 'a wonderful flying and floating feeling inside', became intensely sociable, talked continually, found reasons to run up and down the stairways ('doing errands'), and wished to dance with the nurses. She beamed at me and said she was sure she must be my 'star patient'. Between other activities, she filled twelve pages of her diary with happy, excited, and partly erotic reminiscences. Her sleep was again diminished and disturbed, with a tendency to toss and turn all night after the action of her night-sedative had worn off. On this date we observed the appearance of a new symptom – a rather sudden 'let-down', with feelings of weakness and drowsiness – coming on between $2\frac{1}{2}$ and 3 hours after each dose of L-DOPA.

The following day (27 May), she showed still greater activity, and felt driven to perform her physiotherapy exercises by the hundred: 'I had such a *storm* of activity', she complained, 'that it frightened me. I *could not* keep still.' An additional feature seen on this day were sudden *tic-like movements* – lightning-quick impulsions to touch either ear, to scratch her nose, etc.

Two days later (despite reduction of her dosage to 2 gm. L-DOPA daily), her akathisia was still more marked: Miss A. felt 'forced' (her word) to move her arms and legs continually, shuffling her feet, drumming her fingers, picking up objects and immediately putting them down, 'scratching' (despite the feeling that there was nothing to scratch), and making sudden darting movements with her hands to her nose and ears. She said of these sudden tic-like actions: 'I don't know why I make them, there's no reason for it, I just suddenly *have* to make them.' Palilalic repetition of phrases and sentences was also observed for the first time on 29 May, although this occurred only occasionally: her speech in general was pressured and hurried (tachyphemic). Her insomnia continued to be severe, and barely responsive to chloral or barbiturates; her dreams were extremely vivid, with a tendency to nightmares; and her mood, though consistently excited, was labile in affect, with sudden veerings from stormy hypomania to fearfulness and agitated depression. Her intermittent mouth-openings had been replaced by a strong drive to clench her teeth. Thirst and hunger continued to be inordinate, and Miss A. – normally delicate and restrained in her table-manners – felt the urge to tear her food and stuff it into her mouth. Her water-intake increased to

5–6 gallons a day; tests for *diabetes insipidus* were invariably negative, and her drinking seemed rather to be a compulsion or mania.

With further reduction of dosage (down to 1·5 gm. daily), Miss A. remained comparatively stable for a further week: euphoric but not exalted, able to sleep (but only with sedation), very active, sociable and talkative. At this period akathisia was only seen if she was constrained to sit still, as at mealtimes: at such times, in her own words, her 'muscles would feel impatient', and she would be forced to shuffle and kick her feet under the table.

During the second week of June, her tendency to festinate became more marked. Her walking would be quite stable, although it had a hurried, urgent quality about it, until she encountered an obstacle, or the necessity for negotiating a corner. This would elicit sudden festination and forward-impetus, so that she started to suffer the first of many falls. Her mood continued to be elevated, but her attitudes were now marked by increasing impatience and demand, and sometimes by stamping if her demands were not met instantly. Her 'let-downs' in the third hour after medication became more sudden and severe: she would seem to pass within two or three minutes from forceful, noisy bustling into a near-speechless akinesia with intense drowsiness. In view of this, it was decided to give her a smaller dose of L-DOPA spaced at shorter intervals.

On 13 June (an exceedingly hot and sultry day) Miss A.'s emotional excitement became manic in quality. She had an uncontrollable urge to dance and sing, and did so continuously while I was trying to examine her. Her thoughts and speech were very pressured and exalted: 'Oh Dr Sacks!' she exclaimed breathlessly, 'I am so happy, so very very happy. I feel so good, so full of energy. So tingly, like my blood is champagne. I am bubbling and bubbling and bubbling inside. Dance with me!... No? Well I'll sing to you then –'

(sings 'O what a beautiful morning, O what a beautiful day,' with occasional palilalic repetitions).

Added to the manic pressure there appears to be a considerable element of motor, bulimic, and other drives: she cannot sit still, but constantly dances and prances across the room; she shuffles her feet, crosses and uncrosses her legs, suddenly belches, straightens her dress, pats her hair, belches again, claps her hands, touches her nose, and belches a third time, exuberantly and without apologies. She looks warm and flushed, has very dilated pupils, and a bounding tachycardia of 120. Her feeding shows insatiable voracity and hurry: she tears at her food in an animal-like way, grunting with excitement, and stuffing it into her mouth, and when finished gnaws her fingers in an uncontrollable perseveration of greed. I observed too that when she ate, her tongue would shoot out of her mouth as she brought the morsel to her lips: I had the feeling that her tongue was *enticed* out by the food, and that eating evoked voluptuous pleasure.

Other oral automatisms and urges were also in evidence during this peak of excitement: a tendency to tonic protrusion of the lips ('*schnauzkrampf*'), to make sucking noises, and – most astonishingly of all – to *lap* milk from a saucer: the tongue-movement during lapping was amazingly quick and expert, clearly not under voluntary control, and was called by Miss A. 'automatic . . . it just seems to come naturally to me' (compare Maria G.).

On the afternoon of the 13th her excitement and tachycardia became more extreme, and she exclaimed: 'I feel jam-packed with energy like a rocket. I'm going to take off, take off, take off . . .' It was therefore decided to tranquillize her, and to our surprise a minute (10 mg.) dose of parenteral thorazine brought her 'down' in an hour, to an exhausted, drowsy, almost akinetic state. Her dose of L-DOPA was then further reduced, to 1 gm. daily.

The day following this reduction of dose found Miss A.

torpid, sad, somewhat rigid and akinetic. Moreover, she had an oculogyric crisis lasting several hours, her first for more than a year. During her oculogyric crisis, Miss A. sat absolutely motionless. Describing it afterwards she said: 'I had no impulse to move, I don't think I could have moved ... I had to concentrate on the bit of ceiling I was forced to look at – it filled my mind, I could think of nothing else. And I was afraid, deathly afraid, as I always am in these spells, although I knew there was nothing to be afraid of.'

Following the crisis, L-DOPA was discontinued for two days. Through these two days, Miss A. showed an *exacerbation* of her pre-DOPA state, being intensely rigid, scarcely able to speak or move, and deeply depressed: 'trombone-tremor' of the tongue also recurred at this time, with extreme intensity. A short trial of Haloperidol ('Haldol': 0·5 mg. b.i.d.) only served to aggravate these symptoms. On 18 June, therefore, Miss A. was put back on a very modest dose of L-DOPA (750 mg. daily).

In the ensuing week, there was a satisfactory return of speech and motor force, but this was now combined with some disquieting new symptoms. Miss A.'s expression became somewhat blank and confused, although she was at no time disoriented or unaware of her surroundings. She would have to make a notable effort to speak, but the effort notwithstanding she would speak in a whisper quite different in quality from the hypophonia she had shown in her pre-DOPA days. She conveyed to us, in a whisper, that she had the feeling of 'some force, some sort of obstruction' which stopped her speaking loudly, although she was able to whisper to us without impediment. During this period, a different set of abnormal mouth-movements made their appearance: forced protrusions of the lips, propulsion of the tongue, and occasional choreic dartings of the tongue. Most alarming of all, the tendency to festination and hurry, which had come on ten days beforehand and become slowly worse (despite the fluctuations of drug-dosage, and of her other symptoms), now took a frightening paroxysmal form. Where previously she would festinate only on encountering an obstacle in her path, she would now have a sudden, spontaneous urge to run, and would be impelled forward in a frenzy of little, stamping steps, which were accompanied by shrill screams, tic-like movements of the arms, and a terrified expression. This stampede was followed, after a few steps, by an inability to lift her feet, and inevitably she would fall forwards on her face. Sometimes these paroxsyms would take an even more acute form, in which she would be impelled to lunge forwards while remaining (in her own words) 'rooted to the spot'. It became necessary, therefore, to have someone accompany her in order to moderate her walking and save her from falling. It at once became apparent that provided Miss A. could be walked (or persuaded to walk) slowly and gently, no problems would arise, but that as soon as she hurried (or was pushed or pulled beyond a given pace), a sudden resistance would develop which 'rooted' her to the spot. This phenomenon appeared analogous to her speech-problems at this time, where an attempted exclamation immediately evoked resistance and 'block', but a gentle whisper could 'get through' without impediment.

It was clear that these paroxysms, whatever their nature, were terrifying and indeed dangerous, and that some functional instability (or series of instabilities) had arisen, and was perpetuating itself, despite the very nominal dose of L-DOPA which she was receiving. With regret, but feeling that it was necessary, we therefore replaced the drug-capsules by placebo. The speech-block and stampeding attacks persisted, with lessening intensity, for a further forty-four days, and then ceased. Her rigidity, bradykinesia and other symptoms reverted to their pre-DOPA level. Towards the end of July, therefore, a small dose of L-DOPA was again started (750 mg. daily), and Miss A. now appears (three weeks later) to be enjoying a substantial stable, though limited, improvement (in terms of speech, walking, balance, etc.), without any return of the adverse and paroxysmal effect encountered earlier.

1969–72

In May of 1969 Miss A. reached her high point, her zenith, her 'stardom'; the last three years have seen her decline and fall. In June 1969, Miss A., at the acme of her excitement, started to come apart like the sky-rocket she compared herself to; the last three years have seen a continual increase of her schism or fission. If these problems are to be ascribed to L-DOPA (i.e. to the particular reactivity of this so-excitable, so-fissionable person to L-DOPA), why did we not stop the drug? *We could not:* like Maria G., Hester Y., and other such patients, Miss A. became critically dependent on the continuance of L-DOPA, and by 1970 would move not merely into exacerbated Parkinsonism and depression but into immediate stupor or coma, if it was stopped for a day; thus we were forced to continue the drug. Miss A. herself was well aware of the dilemma: 'It's driving me mad,' she would say; 'but I'll die if you stop it.'

She has indeed lost almost all possibility of a modulated 'middle' state, and has almost nothing in between coma and hyper-vigilance, Parkinsonism and frenzy, depression and mania, etc.; her responses have become extreme, abrupt and all-or-none, reflected and rebounding from one behavioural pole to another. *Both* poles, indeed, may simultaneously occur, and Miss A. will declare – within two or three minutes – that she feels wonderful, terrible, can see perfectly, is blind, cannot move, cannot stop moving, etc. Her will is continually vacillating or paralysed; she wants what she fears, and fears what she wants; she loves what she hates, and hates what she loves. She is driven this way and that by intense contradictions, impossible decisions between impossible choices.

In the presence of excitement and perpetual contradiction, Miss A. has split into a dozen Miss A.'s – the drinker, the ticcer, the stamper, the yeller, the swinger, the gazer, the sleeper, the wisher, the fearer, the lover, the hater, etc. – all struggling with each other to 'possess' her behaviour. Her real interests and activities have practically vanished, and have been replaced by absurd stereotypies, continually ground smaller in the mill of her being. She is completely reduced, for most of the time, to a 'repertoire' of a few dozen thoughts and impulsions, increasingly fixed in phrase and form, and repeated, compulsively, again and again. The *original* Miss A. – so engaging and bright – has been *dispossessed* by a host of crude, degenerate sub-selves – a schizophrenic fission of her once-unified self.

But there are still a few things which bring her together, or which recall her former un-broken self. Music calms her, relieves her distraction, and gives her – if briefly – its coherence and concord; and so too does Nature, when she sits in the garden. But, above all, she is recalled by a single relation, the only one which still preserves for her undivided meaning and feeling. She has a favourite younger sister who lives out-of-state, but who comes to New York once a month to visit her. This sister always takes Miss A. out for the day – to an opera, or a play, or a good meal in the city. Miss A. is radiant when she returns from these excursions, and describes them in detail, with feeling and wit; at such times there is nothing 'schizophrenic' in her thought or her manner, but a return of wholeness and the sense of the world. 'I can't understand', her sister once said to me, 'why Margaret is called crazy or broken or strange. We had a wonderful day "on the town" together. She was eager and interested in everything and everyone – chock-full of life, and full of enjoyment … She was easy and relaxed – none of

the pushing and the drinking you all make so much of ...
She talked and laughed the way she used to in the old days,
back in the twenties before she got ill ... She goes mad in
your madhouse because she is shut off from life.'

10. MIRON V.

Miron V. was born in New York in 1908 and had the flu
severely in 1918, although he showed no symptoms which
were recognized as encephalitic at this time. After High
School he started work as a cobbler, and by the age of thirty
owned his own shoe-shop, had married, and had fathered a
son.

In 1947 Mr V. showed the first signs of a Parkinsonian
syndrome associated with restlessness and impulsiveness, tics
and mannerisms, and a tendency to periods of staring and
'trance' – an unmistakable post-encephalitic syndrome.[36] He
was able to continue work as a cobbler until 1952, and to
stay at home until 1955, at which time increasing disability
necessitated his admission to hospital. Immediately following
his admission to Mount Carmel, Mr V. developed an 'admission psychosis' – an intense paranoia, with hallucinatory
images of castration, degradation, abandonment, vengeance,
spite and impotent rage.[37] With the fading of his acute

36. Miron V. thus showed a period of almost thirty years between
what must be presumed to have been a sub-clinical attack of *encephalitis lethargica* in 1918 and the development of an indubitable
post-encephalitic syndrome. Even longer 'incubation periods' may
occur: thus another patient (Hyman H.) had severe manifest sleeping-sickness in 1917, recovered from this completely, but developed
an unmistakable post-encephalitic syndrome in 1962.

37. Such 'admission psychoses' are not uncommon when patients
are unwillingly consigned to what is, in effect, a terminal institution
like Mount Carmel. I have seen such psychoses in dozens of patients.

psychosis, ten days later, he passed into a state of intensely exacerbated Parkinsonism and catatonia – a state so intense as to render him virtually speechless and motionless. This state continued unchanged till he was given L-DOPA.

This Parkinsonian-catatonic state was accompanied by a mixture of intense aloofness, negativism and withdrawal. In the words of his wife, 'Something happened to Miron when he stopped working, and then when he left home and went into hospital. He used to be such a warm man ... He loved his work more than anything in the world ... And then he changed ... He came to hate us and to hate everyone and everything. And maybe he hated himself.' Mr V.'s iciness and hostility were deeply disturbing to his family, who 'responded' by refusing to visit him soon after he had been institutionalized, thus completing and compounding a vicious circle of neurotic reaction.

Over the ensuing fourteen years Mr V.'s state remained essentially the same, although he developed extremely profuse sebarrhoea and sialorrhoea. I frequently saw him between 1966 and 1969, and was always impressed by his almost absolute immobility, which was such that he might sit fifteen hours in a chair without the least hint of spontaneous movement. He did, however, show occasional tics and impulsions – sudden 'saluting' tics with either hand, or sudden throat-clearing or 'giggling' noises – in startling contrast to his overall background of complete immobility and silence. Although exceedingly disinclined to speak, Mr V. could say a few words in a very staccato, exclamatory fashion – sufficient to indicate his intelligence, his bitterness, his hopelessness, and his indifferent awareness of everything round him. He could neither rise to his feet nor walk without aid. When I asked him whether he wished to try L-DOPA, he said, 'I don't care ... It's up to you.'

Mr V.'s response to L-DOPA, in July 1969, had the same sudden and almost magical quality seen in so many other severely affected post-encephalitic patients. Within the course of a single day he regained an almost normal power and pattern of movement and speech. He also showed feelings of amazement and joy, although these were still overcast by his habitual suspicion, coldness and constraint. Within two weeks of this initial reaction, Mr V.'s state had swung to the opposite extreme: he became exceedingly impulsive and hyperactive, hypomanic, provocative, impudent and amorous – everything was velocity, audacity, salacity. His previously rare tics now became much commoner, so that he would find occasion to 'adjust' his spectacles, or clear his throat, two or three hundred times an hour.

Mr V.'s reactions, over the next nine months, were all extreme, erratic and contradictory. He showed abrupt alternations between totally immobile states and dangerously hyperactive impulsive states. He sustained innumerable falls and no less than three hip fractures due to his impetuosity and folly in his hyperactive states.[38] But his attitudes were mixed, and he also showed, during these difficult months, an increasing interest in people about him, a diminution of hostility and withdrawal, and some affection for his wife and son, who – after a twelve-year gap – started to visit him again. He also became very handy about the ward – he was extraordinarily adept in the use of his hands – and expressed a longing for work of some kind.

The real change came when we set up a last and a cobbler's bench for Mr. V. in our Sheltered Workshop, in May 1970. When he was taken to see these he showed an amazement

38. If the commonest *secondary* problems stemming from the activation procured by L-DOPA were mouth-movements and mouth-damage (see the footnote to p. 77), the most serious, by far, were falls and fractures. Thus of some eighty patients (about half post-encephalitic, and half with common Parkinson's Disease) put on L-DOPA in Mount Carmel in 1969, *more than a third sustained serious (and sometimes multiple) fractures* (similar figures are reported from elsewhere in similar situations).

and joy without the least admixture of suspicion or constraint. His old skills returned to him with amazing speed, and so did his admiration and his love for his work. He started to do cobbling and repairs-jobs for more and more of the patients in hospital, and to show a craftsman's skill and love in making new shoes. With this return to his work, and his *relation* with his work, Mr V.'s reactions to L-DOPA became better and stabler: he ceased to have dangerously impulsive 'ups' and ceased to have depressive-Parkinsonian-catatonic 'downs' with anything like the severity with which they had initially occurred. He became far more affable and accessible, and recovered a good deal of his lost self-esteem: 'I feel like a man again,' he once said to me. 'I feel I've got some use and a place in the world ... A man can't live without that.'

Since the summer of 1970, Mr V. has done extraordinarily well – miraculously well considering the severity and hopelessness of his original state, and the extreme and erratic reactions he first showed on L-DOPA. It cannot be said that his speech and motor patterns are in any sense 'normal' – they still show a good deal of abruptness and freezing – but they are adequate and controllable, and they allow him to do a full day's work at his last every day, to walk round the hospital, to converse fairly freely, and to go home for occasional weekends with his wife. Of the forty or so post-encephalitic patients at Mount Carmel who showed extremely severe Parkinsonian-catatonic syndromes before L-DOPA, Mr V. – finally – has done by far the best; he has been the *only* one among them able to tolerate the continuous administration of L-DOPA without interruption, and to develop such stability after so unstable a start.

11. GERTIE C.

Mrs C. was born in New Hampshire in 1908, the youngest daughter of a harmonious and close-knit family. She had a happy childhood without neurotic distresses or difficulties of significance, made friends easily, did well at school, and worked as a typist-stenographer until the age of twenty-five when she married. She continued in seemingly perfect health, enjoying a full social life and bringing up a family of three children, between her marriage and her thirty-eighth birthday. Shortly after this, however, she developed a violent shaking of both hands, which was first ascribed to the rigours of a New York winter, but recognized a few weeks later as Parkinsonian in nature. In the next six years her illness proceeded relentlessly and rapidly, combining tremor, rigidity, akinesia, pulsions and extremely profuse sweating, salivation and sebarrhoea. By the age of forty-four Mrs C. had been rendered totally immobile and virtually speechless. Her tremor and rigidity could be diminished somewhat by atropine-like drugs, but her disabling akinesia and aphonia showed no response to these. Despite great difficulties and the necessity for nursing assistance round the clock, Mrs C.'s devoted family kept her at home for another ten years (i.e. until 1962).

When I first saw Mrs C. in 1966, I found that she had developed dystonic contractures of all her extremities and showed the most intense rigidity of all her musculature. It was just possible for her to whisper with very great effort. It was clear, however, that she followed everything that was said to her perfectly. She did not in the least seem inert, indifferent and unreactive (like Mrs B.) but conveyed the impression of an intense inner activity which was motionless and enclosed in itself. Her eyes seemed to shine with intense peacefulness, as if she were contemplating a beautiful picture or a landscape. She gave the impression of being *rapt* not inert.

I started Mrs C. on L-DOPA in the middle of June 1969. She showed remarkable sensitivity to this, and on a dose of no more than 1 gm. a day started to show a striking restoration of her voice and of all movement, and an equally striking reduction of rigidity and salivation. With a further increase of dosage to 1·5 gm. daily Mrs C.'s voice became virtually normal in strength and timbre, and revealed a full and subtle range of intonation and modulation. Her strength had now become such that she could feed herself and turn the pages of a book, although these activities were difficult because of irreversible contractures in the hands. Her mood was calm, happy and equable, with no hint of anxiety or emotional extravagance. During this halcyon period Mrs C. was able to talk freely for the first time in almost twenty years, and spoke to me at length about the state she had been in for much of this time.

It had been, she explained, a state of 'great inner stillness' and of 'acquiescence'; her attention would dwell for hours on whatever object or thought entered its field; she would feel herself completely 'absorbed' and 'engrossed' by all of her postures, perceptions and thoughts; she said, 'My mind was like a still pool reflecting itself.' She would spend hours and days and even weeks reliving peaceful scenes from her own childhood – lying in the sun, drowsing in a meadow, or floating in a creek near her home as a child; these Arcadian moments could apparently be extended indefinitely by the still and intent quality of her thought. Mrs C. added that she had always had a vivid imagination and had been able to picture things clearly, but that its vividness was increased by the motionless concentration which accompanied her Parkinsonism. She stressed that her sense of time and duration had become profoundly altered during the previous two decades;

that although she was aware of what was happening and what the date was, she herself had *no feeling of happening*, but rather the feeling that time itself had come to a stop, and that every moment of her existence was a repetition of itself.

Four weeks after starting L-DOPA her responses became less favourable and she experienced impulses to gasp and swallow, and reversions to Parkinsonism and aphonia, after each dose. Feeling that Mrs C. was moving along into a pathological reaction, I decided to stop the L-DOPA for a few days. With its cessation, Mrs C. at once reverted to severe Parkinsonism, and to this was added a rather deep depression and somnolence which had not been part of the original picture.

Re-starting her on L-DOPA towards the end of July we found it impossible to regain the beautiful response seen in the previous month. In an effort to try and retrieve the original response we added a small dose of amantadine (100 mg. b.i.d.) to the gram of L-DOPA per day she was receiving – a measure we had found useful in a number of other patients. The effect of this addition was absolutely catastrophic. Within three hours of receiving her first amantadine capsule, Mrs C. became intensely excited and deliriously hallucinated. She would cry out, 'Cars bearing down on me, they're crowding me! They're crowding me!' Her voice would rise to a scream of terror, and she would suddenly clutch my arm; at this time she also saw faces 'like masks popping in and out' – which would snap and mock and grin and yelp at her. Occasionally she would smile rapturously and exclaim: 'Look what a beautiful tree, so beautiful!' and tears of pleasure would enter her eyes. But in general this state was one of a disorganized and terrifying hallucinatory paranoia with multiple Lilliputian hallucinations of sight and sound. It was accompanied by a violent rhythmic thrashing of her head from side to side, and by rhythmic tongue-protrusion, screaming and tic-like movements of the eyes. These hallucinations and movements were at their worst if Mrs C. was left alone or if the room was darkened; a familiar and friendly presence, or speaking to her, or holding her hand could deliver her from apparitions and movements, and restore her to herself for a few seconds or minutes. Although the L-DOPA and amantadine were immediately stopped with the onset of this state, it continued of its own momentum for more than three weeks, during which time only the heaviest doses of sedation or tranquillization could reduce her excitement. In September her delirium suddenly ceased, leaving her exhausted and torpid, although perfectly rational. It was clear from talking to her, and from observing her, that she retained no conscious memory whatever of the extraordinary state which had possessed or dispossessed her in the preceding three weeks.[39]

At the beginning of October we very cautiously tried Mrs C. on L-DOPA again, this time giving her a total dose of only one quarter of a gram daily. This immediately induced a considerable restoration of her voice and strength, but also evoked a new disorder – a tendency to sudden, tic-like jabbings and swattings in the air, as if she were fending off flies or mosquitoes. After ten days of this combination, Mrs C. abruptly returned to her hallucinatory delirium; the onset of this precisely coincided with the cessation of her tics, which suggested that the latter might have served as 'lightning-conductors', discharging her excitement in a relatively

39. It may be asked whether Gertie C. perhaps retained *unconscious* memories of this time, memories *repressed* from consciousness because of their deeply frightening and traumatic nature (such pseudo-amnesias, or inhibitions of memory, are not uncommon after frightful events – which include, of course, frightful psychoses). It is possible that there was some element of this, but it seems altogether more probable to me that Mrs C. – who was given neither to psychoses nor to crypto-amnesia – retained *no memory whatever* of the preceding three weeks, because these were filled with *delirium*, not psychosis.

harmless way. The L-DOPA was immediately stopped again, but this did not diminish her excitement in the least. It became necessary to put side-rails on her bed and to have a nurse in constant attendance lest she injure herself in her extremity. On the night of 10 October, while her nurse had left the room for a minute, Mrs C. uttered a scream of terror, climbed over the side-rails, and fell heavily to the ground breaking both hips and her pelvis.

The following months were months of great physical and mental torture for Mrs C.: she was in great pain from the injuries she had received; she developed a bedsore over the sacrum which had to be probed and washed several times a day; she lost 40 lb. in weight; her dystonic rigidity and contractures grew more severe; and finally she was tormented by evil hallucinations which persisted without the least diminution for more than *five months* after the discontinuance of L-DOPA. By the summer of 1970 Mrs C. had come through the worst: her bedsore was healing, her rigidity and dystonia had become less extreme, and most important, her hallucinatory delirium was beginning to fade out.

As her periods of delirium diminished, and her intervals of lucidity increased, Mrs C. voiced a certain wistfulness: 'They're all disappearing now,' she said, 'the little people and *things* which have been keeping me company. Then I'll be my old plain self again.' But this was not to be. The day *after* delirium finally ceased, she had a strange experience while lying in bed. It started as an *uncanny* feeling – the sense that something extraordinary was about to happen; she felt herself compelled to look out of the window, and there to her amazement she saw a masked man climbing the fire-escape; when he drew level with her he brandished a stick and poked it in her direction, which filled her with terror; he then gave a 'devilish grin' and retreated down the fire-escape – *taking the fire-escape along with him.* It was this which indicated to Mrs C. that she had had 'a

vision', and that she had not only hallucinated a man but a
fire-escape into the bargain. When Mrs C. described this to
me the next day she shuddered all over, but also evinced, in
her manner and choice of words, an unmistakable relish.
The next evening the masked man on the fire-escape again
appeared and this time came closer and flourished his stick
in a fashion not only threatening but brazenly suggestive.
On the third day Mrs C. decided to 'have it out' with me:
'You can't blame me,' she said. 'I haven't had anything for
the last twenty years, and I'm not about to get anything
now, you know ... You surely wouldn't forbid a friendly
hallucination to a frustrated old lady like me!' I replied that
if her hallucinations had a pleasant and controllable character, they seemed rather a good idea under the circumstances.
After this, the paranoid quality entirely dropped away, and
her hallucinatory encounters became purely amicable and
amorous. She developed a humour and tact and control –
never allowing herself an hallucination before eight in the
evening and keeping its duration to thirty or forty minutes
at most. If her relatives stayed too late, she would explain
firmly but pleasantly that she was expecting 'a gentleman
visitor from out of town' in a few minutes' time and she felt
he might take it amiss if he was kept waiting outside.

Mrs C. is alive and as well as she can be considering the
severity of her illness. The deep peaceful look has returned to
her eyes, and she seems to have regained her power for timeless contemplation of childhood scenes and moments. The
only change in her from pre-DOPA days is that she now
receives love, attention and invisible presents from a hallucinatory gentleman who faithfully visits each evening.

12. MARTHA N.

Miss N. was born in New York in 1908, the only daughter of devout Irish Catholic parents. She almost died from the flu in 1918, but did not suffer any clear-cut encephalitic symptoms then. After finishing High School, she started work with a telephone company; she was a thrice-elected 'Beauty Queen' at this time, and a valued companion at functions and dates. Parkinsonism presented itself when she was twenty-one years old, and caused such tremor that she ceased work that year. Concurrently she developed sleep-talking and sleep-walking. After this initial outburst of symptoms, her illness remained static for twenty-two years, during which time she lived at home with her parents, was able to walk, visit friends, play golf and attend to all household and shopping duties.

With the death of her parents in 1951, Miss N.'s illness abruptly became worse, and in particular rigidity and dystonia developed, and overtook her, so that within two years she had become deeply disabled, losing the ability to walk or stand, and her voice and swallowing were also impaired. This precipitous deterioration in her status led to her institutionalization in 1954. Once admitted to hospital, her illness again seemed to come to a standstill, although the dystonia had led on to dystonic deformities.

I often saw Miss N. between 1966 and 1969 and found her intelligent and charming and pleasant to talk to. She showed at this time an immovable dystonic rigidity of both legs, a severe torticollis, a very soft voice, and extremely voluminous salivation. She was conspicuously sociable and affable in comparison with many other post-encephalitic patients. For fifty-one weeks in the year Miss N. was conspicuously 'to-together' and sane, but in the fifty-second week she had an

'Easter Psychosis'. This took the form of increasing rigidity, lessened ability to move or speak or swallow, depression, masking of the voice and sometimes oculogyria. On Good Friday she would feel herself dying, and in a scarcely audible whisper request that we bring a priest to administer Last Rites. This done she would sink into a motionless, speechless 'swoon', remaining this way till Easter Sunday, when she would rather suddenly 'come to' with a feeling of rebirth. Her voice, her movement and all her abilities would be strikingly better than 'normal' for two or three weeks following this annual rebirth, and the diminution in her Parkinsonism and other problems was very remarkable during these weeks.

Miss N. was started on L-DOPA in June 1972. Her initial response to this was a retropulsion or insucking of the tongue, so severe that speech was impossible, and she was in continual danger of swallowing her tongue. In view of this her L-DOPA (2 gm. a day) was stopped. She was restarted on L-DOPA later, in the middle of July, and this time the tongue-pulsions and gaggings were not evoked at all, but, on the contrary, a striking improvement occurred. Her voice became much louder, her salivation virtually ceased and her arms lost almost all their rigidity and akinesia; in effect Miss N. was 'normalized' except, of course, for the irreversible contractures of her feet and her neck. This superb therapeutic action showed itself with remarkable suddenness – in the course of an hour – and was induced by a mere 750 mg. of L-DOPA a day.

Her excellent state was maintained until 4 August – the day following my own departure for London. On this day Miss N. became extremely agitated, frightened, and depressed, showed intense tremor and rigidity alternating in her limbs, presented a fixed and corpse-like expression, and demanded Last Rites for her impending death. Her L-DOPA was stopped once again, and after a day she returned to her pre-DOPA self. On my return she asked me once more to try her on L-DOPA. 'It wasn't the drug which upset me,' she said. 'It was your going away. I couldn't be sure you would ever come back. I felt so afraid, I thought I would die.'

In September for the third time I gave her L-DOPA and her responses were *now* quite different from either of the first two times. She complained of rapid breathing and difficulty in catching her breath, and she had the beginnings of respiratory crises. She developed very rapid 'saluting' tics in both of her arms, her hands flying from her lap to her face three or four times every minute. She also developed palilalia, repeating her words innumerable times. Her reaction at this time was remarkably similar to that of her room-mate Miss D., so much so that I wondered if either was automatically 'imitating' the other. By the middle of September, Miss N. was ticcing 60 times to the minute, 60 minutes to the hour, and saying an incessant palilalic repetition of the following verse she had learned years before:

> I thought it said in every tick,
> I am so sick, so sick, so sick.
> Oh death, come quick, come quick, come quick!
> Come quick, come quick, come quick, come quick!

Since she was exhausting herself and maddening her fellow patients, I again found it necessary to stop L-DOPA.

Following this excited state Miss N. showed a severe 'rebound' when L-DOPA was stopped, becoming so rigid, tremulous, akinetic and voiceless, and having so much difficulty in swallowing, that we had to tube-feed her. This 'withdrawal-reaction' continued for the remainder of September without any lessening in severity whatever.

In October I started Miss N. on L-DOPA for the fourth time and this time she again did well for some weeks, although she was more easily excited than usual, and when excited showed recurrence of her tics and palilalia. It was noted by the nursing staff, at this time, that she particularly showed tics when I was around. Miss N. knew that I was fascinated by tics, and that they would always attract my attention and interest.

In December, during a period of particularly grim weather, Miss N. again passed into a death-like stupor similar to that which she had shown on L-DOPA in August (and before L-DOPA, in her 'Easter Psychoses'). This time neither my presence nor anything I could do could alter her state: she lay motionless and frigid as if already a corpse. After three days of this state I stopped her L-DOPA, but this did not seem to make any difference. She continued in stupor for another ten days and during this time required total nursing care and tube-feeding once more. On Christmas day the sun came out and shone brilliantly for the first time in more than two weeks. Miss N. was taken in her chair onto the porch outside. Five minutes later she suddenly 'came to', and within a few seconds was restored to herself. Her description of this was impressive and moving: 'I saw the sun,' she said. 'I saw the people all around me living and moving. I realized I was neither dead nor in Hell. I felt life stirring inside me. I felt something like a shell breaking inside me. And suddenly I could move and speak again.'

We gave Miss N. three months to recover from these experiences and to restore her physiological and psychological equilibrium. In March 1970, at her request, we started L-DOPA for the fifth time. Here, as before, there was a gratifying reduction of Parkinsonism and other symptoms for about three weeks. Then she started to develop singular hallucinations every evening, which always took essentially the same form. They would start with a feeling of *uncanniness*, a feeling that something unimaginably strange was about to happen, and the feeling that it had happened once before, in a dream or a past life, and that her coming experience would be a revisiting of the past. In this strange state, Miss

N. would suddenly see two bearded men enter the room. They would walk to the window with an unhurried gait, and there light an old-fashioned lantern which they swung to and fro ('like a censer'). Miss N. would feel this swinging light was designed to capture her attention or 'bewitch' her, and she would feel intensely tempted to gaze at the light. At this point she would turn her head violently away and say, 'Get behind me, get behind me, you devils, you devils!' It was this sudden violent turning of the head and exclamation which drew the attention of Miss N.'s room-mate to the fact that she was having 'queer experiences' of some kind. Her equivocal visitors would then come to the head of her bed, would take pieces of shimmering gauze from their pockets and wave these in circles in front of her eyes; she felt herself both shrinking and swooning as they did this before her, not knowing whether their activities were a curse or a blessing. Both men would bend over her face and kiss her, brushing her cheeks with the bristles of their beards. They would then walk gravely out of the room. With their departure Miss N. had an immense sense of regret and relief inseparably mixed. The feeling of 'strangeness' would disappear, and Miss N. would feel herself once again. These episodes would last ten or twelve minutes and would start on the stroke of eight every evening. When I asked Miss N. whether she thought her 'visitors' were real, she said: 'Yes and no. Not real like you, Dr Sacks, or the nurses, or this place. A different sort of reality, as if they had come from another world.' She later said, 'First I thought they were ghosts of patients who had died in this room, and then I realized they were supernatural. I could never decide whether they came from Heaven or Hell ... it's funny – I am not usually superstitious, I don't normally believe in ghosts or spooks, but when the mood comes on me I *have* to believe.'

Since for two weeks the *status quo* was preserved, her apparitions coming at 8.00 and leaving sharp at 8.10, we continued Miss N. on her dose of L-DOPA; it was apparent, moreover, that she had started to derive a good deal of pleasure from the regular visits, for she would make herself up carefully 'in readiness' each evening. In her sixth week on L-DOPA, the visions assumed a more severe and ominous quality; the two bearded men were joined by a third and fourth and fifth and sixth, until the entire room was crowded with bearded men making supernatural gestures; moreover they would stay past their time, and continue their silent, sinister milling-around till 9.00 or 10.00 or 11.00 at night. At this stage Miss N. agreed that perhaps L-DOPA might be stopped. Her hallucinations continued for three weeks after the withdrawal of L-DOPA and then suddenly stopped: it was remarkably abrupt – one evening Miss N. failed to make herself up after supper and, when we asked why, said: 'There'll be no company this evening.' And, indeed, her 'company' never returned.

We gave Miss N. the remainder of the spring and the entire summer to recover her balance, and in October 1970 we started her on amantadine (an L-DOPA-like drug). And here, as with L-DOPA, there was an initial improvement in voice and movement and rigidity, etc. But after three weeks Miss N. complained of *pruritus vulvae*. We sent her to a gynaecologist, but he could find nothing the matter. Her pruritus then became a formication – a feeling that ants were crawling inside her; Miss N. would shudder all over as she described these symptoms, but would also exhibit unmistakable relish. Finally, the ants became tiny ant-sized men, crawling up her vagina, trying to get inside her. At this point Miss N. became violently agitated, and begged us to stop both the assault and the drug. We stopped the amantadine, but the hallucinatory assault persisted for more than six weeks before it disappeared, quite suddenly, without any warning or slow 'fading-out'.

Thus Miss N. – in her five trials on L-DOPA and her addi-

tional trial on an L-DOPA-like drug – showed remarkably
different reactions on all six occasions. It was clear that the
action of the drug was, in a sense, unpredictable, in that it
might call forth a variety of behaviour: given the initial
form of behaviour – whether therapeutic, catatonic, ticcy-
palilalic, formicatory, or hallucinatory – the rest of the reaction would follow this form. Miss N. showed strikingly little
physiological constancy in her reactions to L-DOPA, but a
striking dramatic unity in them once they were started. In
view of her six so-strangely-mixed but ultimately uncontrollable reactions, we have not given Miss N. L-DOPA or amantadine again. She has returned to her pleasant, easy-going,
good-humoured and prosaic self. She even 'skipped' her
'Easter Psychosis' in 1971 and 1972 – her first such omission
in at least twenty years. She says, 'I have had enough visions
and what-not to last me a lifetime.'

13. IDA T.

Mrs T. was born in a village in Poland in 1901, had an un-
eventful childhood, and became a bride at sixteen and a
mother at seventeen. In her twentieth year her life was cut
across by a double tragedy: the death of her young husband,
and the sudden onset of impatience, irritability, impetuosity,
increased appetite and a violent temper – a monstrous transformation of her previous character. The increasing violence
and appetite of their bulky daughter was a source of great
alarm to her peace-loving and penurious family, who found
themselves wondering if a devil had possessed her. In her
twenty-first year – when she had trebled her weight and ter-
rorized the entire village – symptoms of a new kind appeared: increasing stiffness and slowness of movement, and
other signs of a Parkinsonism which *held in* without dimin-

ishing her impulses to violence. At this juncture, her family took medical advice, and decided to ship off their now bomb-like daughter to the fabled doctors in the New World, who would doubtless know how to treat her.

By the end of her four-month transatlantic voyage 'Big Bertha' (as her shipmates had come to call her) had become completely motionless and speechless and stiff as a board, and on her arrival in the New World was at once moved into the newly opened 'Home for the Crippled and Dying'. For the next forty-eight years Mrs T. (or 'Big Bertha', as the hospital staff too now called her) continued to lie in Parkin-sonian state, rigid, mute, motionless and glaring, upon her specially reinforced catafalque of a bed, attended by relays of diminutive nurses. She received no communication whatever from her family, who had evidently decided to 'dump' her and to retain possession of her effectively orphaned, infant daughter. On rare occasions, if in pain or frustrated, Mrs T. would explode and chatter in fury like a maddened machine-gun. She continued to display a voracious appetite, which was soon joined by a voracious anality, her only demands being for enemas or food. She was, however, sensible of at-tention and kindness, and would occasionally smile to her nurses, or smackingly kiss them in a manner as explosive as her greeds and rages. Indeed, all the nurses who came and went were fond of 'Big Bertha' and devotedly looked after her physical needs; she would never have survived the 1920s without their devoted and sedulous attentions.

When I first saw Mrs T. in 1966, she was a seal-shaped woman weighing 400lb., entirely bald and covered with sebum. The back of her head was totally flat, having been moulded from a half-century of lying supine upon it. Her entire body was immovably rigid, and there were crippling dystonic-dystrophic, flipper-like deformities of her hands and her feet. (These flipper-like extremities, combined with her gigantic, greasy, streamlined bulk, often gave one the curious impression of an enormous Channel-swimmer 'frozen' miraculously, stroboscopically, in mid-stroke.) Her eyes were as unblinking and hard and glowering as a basilisk's. She was virtually without movement of any kind, and even her breath was hardly perceptible. She greatly resented my presence and questions, answering them with grunts, expectorations, or spat-out monosyllables. Along with Miss K., she was at once the most formidable and the most pathetic human being I had ever seen.

This continued to be her state for the next three years, until I brought her to our post-encephalitic 'community' and started her on L-DOPA. I must confess that she refused the L-DOPA when I asked her about it, and that I had it administered, at first, by stealth, in her food. I did this after much inner conflict, in which I was finally swayed by the nurses who had so long attended her, who felt that there was 'a lovely person' beneath the formidable exterior of 'Big Bertha', confined and longing to get out. She had no family or friends to say 'Yea' or 'Nay' for her.

The effects of L-DOPA were remarkably striking and sudden, and came on at a dose-level of 4 gm. a day. The frozen rigidity of her body suddenly 'cracked' and melted to a liquid, free-flowing motion, and her voice became much louder and more fluent, losing much of its explosive-obstructive sputtering-stuttering quality. I was summoned to the ward by an amazed and excited staff-nurse, and when I arrived I found Mrs T. smiling and gesturing and talking to the nurses nineteen-to-the-dozen; to me she said, 'Wonderful, wonderful! I'm moving inside – that dopey's a *Mitzphah* ... Thank God you had sense to get it inside me!' To celebrate her 'awakening', Mrs T. announced in a stentorian voice that she wanted a quart of chocolate ice-cream with each meal every day, and 'a big olive-oil enema – but Big!' morning and evening. In the next three weeks, she talked a great deal to herself in Yiddish, or in guttural English with a strong Yiddish-Polish accent, chuckling and gurgling as she did so : all her talk was of the village where she had grown up as a child. At this time she also took to singing old Yiddish folk-songs and ballads in a sea-captain's rollicking bass – to the fury and amusement of everyone near her. The Sleeping Beauty had assuredly awoken, but as yet in a manner completely regressive and nostalgic; her mouth, her colon and her past were the only things which mattered to her at the moment. She had yet to allow a *current* relationship.

At this stage I gave Mrs T. a small present, a token, a succulent cactus with a hideous yet beautiful spiny bulbosity. She was charmed with this plant and became immediately devoted to it, tending it and watching it for hours on end. I had the impression that it represented not only her first possession but her first *relation* in her forty-eight years 'underground' at Mount Carmel Hospital.

In the autumn of 1969, Mrs T. started to recognize and appreciate *as a person* a physiotherapist who was with us, who bathed and massaged her hands every day, and who designed special implements for them which she could hold in a pinch-grasp. Before this time, I think, Mrs. T. had not clearly distinguished or differentiated between the nurses who served her, but had regarded and treated them as identical – somewhat as a Queen Termite treats her tiny Workers. When not with her beloved plant or physiotherapist, she was still implacably hostile, greedy, suspicious, stubborn, negativistic, belligerent, querulous, and accusing. But the plant and the physiotherapist brought out the best in her.

The most moving event took place at the end of 1970 when our social worker – after almost three years of persistent inquiry – was able to locate her long-lost daughter; her daughter had, in fact, come to America in the 1930s, but had never attempted to seek out her mother because the rest of the family had said she was dead. The reunion was not a simple one – it was a speechless weighing-up and gazing on

both sides, but it was a start; there were months of disagree-
ments, rages, silences and quarrels, but – somehow – by the
middle of 1971, a deep mutual relation had been forged,
and each would greet the other with unmixed pleasure. One
could see, in these intervening months, how Mrs T. became
humanized from week to week, as she emerged from her pit
of regression, desolation, and unreality. This one good relation was the thread which led the way from the maze of
madness, which drew her forth from the depths of Unbeing.

In the last year there have been some complications from
the continued use of L-DOPA – some return of her rigidity
and stuttering, etc. But, all considered, she is still doing incredibly well considering she was dead for forty-eight years.

14. FRANK G.

Mr G. was born in 1910, did reasonably at school and seemed
normal in all respects until the age of thirteen when he contracted the sleeping-sickness, and spent nine weeks in a state
of deep stupor during which he was totally helpless and had
to be tube-fed. When he recovered from this he showed a
gross skewing of the right eye outwards and other signs of a
third nerve palsy. He also seemed 'queer in the head', 'sorta
strange', 'not myself any more'. He was unable to continue
school, was considered mentally defective, and sent to work
in a corrugated-box factory. For the next twenty years Mr
G.'s life was monotonous and exemplary. He arrived at the
factory on the dot each morning, worked at a steady unvarying rate, left the factory at five each evening, had supper and
sat with his parents, went to bed at ten and got up at six.
His behaviour during these twenty years was conventional to the point of stereotypy : he would always greet the
same people in the same words each day, make a comment

about the weather and subside into silence; he would read the headlines and a few sub-headings in the papers each day; he had no hobbies, no interests, no friends, and no social or sexual relations at all. He moved like a robot on his dull, undeviating, lifeless course – like a million 'chronic ambulatory schizophrenics' in the streets of America. Two or three times a year he would suddenly fly into a violent rage and attack someone, always an older man, whom he would allege to have been staring at him and trying to seduce him.

In his thirty-fifth year Mr G. found himself unable to maintain his rate of work, having developed a certain slowness of movement and speech. In his thirty-seventh year he was discharged from his job – to join the half-million population of out-of-work Parkinsonians. With the loss of his job Mr G. 'went to pieces', and became agitated, depressed and unable to sleep. The monotonous structure of his life had been shattered, and he walked the streets, unkempt and dirty, swearing and muttering to himself at intervals. In this state Mr G. was admitted to a state mental hospital where he gradually regained something of his former equability and monotony, and in 1950 was transferred to Mount Carmel Hospital.

During his twenty years at Mount Carmel Mr G. slowly 'deteriorated' in a number of ways: although he was physically quite able to look after himself, wander around the hospital, or go out in the streets, he became increasingly withdrawn and narrowed-down in the range of his activities with each passing year. He developed a multitude of fixed rituals and routines, but no real relationships with anyone or anything. He became prone to stare and hallucinate for several hours each day, but he kept his hallucinatory experiences to himself and kept them apart from his behaviour and actions. His attacks of panic and rage became somewhat commoner and would usually occur two or three times a month:

they were always connected with the feeling of being slighted or seductively pressured.

In 1969, before he received L-DOPA, Mr G. showed 'flapping tremor' of both arms, some rigidity and flexion of the neck, profuse salivation and bilateral ptosis, his eyelids so drooping that his eyes were almost closed. His postural reflexes were considerably impaired. He showed mild akinesia, but no rigidity of the arms. Additionally – quite unusual among the post-encephalitic patients I have seen – Mr G. showed bilateral signs of upper motorneurone deficit and a mild mental dullness besides his 'queerness'. Finally Mr G. showed a 'humming tic' – a melodious sound (mmmm . . . mmmm . . . mmmm . . .) with each expiration.

Mr G. was placed on L-DOPA in May 1969, the dose being gradually increased to 2 gm. a day. In these first three weeks Mr G. showed exacerbation of his tremor and hurrying of gait as well as sudden myoclonic jerks and spasms at times. He also showed an increase of his expiratory humming tic and a tendency to toss, grunt and mutter during his sleep.

After a month these effects died away and Mr G. returned to his previous state. Although continuing on 2 gm. of L-DOPA he showed *no* reactions to this apparently for the ensuing three months. In October Mr G. developed violent out-thrustings ('propulsions') of the tongue, which was forced out to its roots 12 or 15 times a minute. When after two days of this we suggested stopping L-DOPA, Mr G. said, 'Don't – they'll stop by themselves.' An hour later the tongue pulsions *did* stop, and were never indeed to be seen again. For the ensuing six months Mr G. again reverted to his reactionless state, until in March 1970 he was carried away by a new wave of responses. He seemed to become irritable and touchy, and had a constant feeling that his right cheek was itching; he would scratch this impulsively and repeatedly in a tic-like way, and so violently that he continually caused it to bleed. He also showed an increased libido, spent many hours masturbating, and repeatedly exposed himself in the passage. During this distressed and agitated period Mr G.'s humming tic became a refrain ('*tic d'incantation*'), a palilalic verbigeration of the phrase 'keep cool'. During the course of the day Mr G. would murmur 'keep cool, keep cool, keep cool . . .' hundreds if not thousands of times a day.

By May 1970 Mr G.'s exposures and assaults on other patients had become so frequent that the hospital administration threatened to transfer him to a state hospital – a threat which filled him with terror and impotent rage. The day after this threat Mr G. developed an oculogyric crisis combined with catatonia – the first he had ever had in his life: his eyes stared upwards, his neck was retracted with extraordinary violence, and the rest of his body showed statuesque immobility and cataleptic flexibility; he became completely inaccessible to all contact, and also, apparently, unable to swallow. This crisis or stupor lasted for ten days without interruption, during which time Mr G. required tube-feeding and nursing. When he 'came to' at last, he seemed a different man – as if he recognized defeat, and was broken inside. His impulsions and itching and tics and erotic and hostile excitement had all disappeared, and he now moved like a sleep-walker or a man in a dream. He was polite and pleasant and perfectly oriented, but his whole being seemed to be immured in a sort of 'sleep' or swoon; he gave an uncanny impression of being absent-as-a-person, and no longer in the world. He seemed almost disembodied – like a wraith or a ghost.

In August 1971 he died in his sleep. No cause of death was visible at *post mortem*.

15. MARIA G.

Miss G. was born on a Sicilian farm in 1919, the younger daughter of strict and affectionate, if neurotic, Italian Catholic parents. She seemed intelligent as a child and did well at her school, although she had a reputation for being sprightly and 'fey'. In her eighth year she had a terrible nightmare which seemed to go on all night: she dreamt she had gone mad and been taken to Hell. This was the start of a month-long delirium with fever, hallucinations, and extraordinary movements; she scarcely slept at this time and could not be sedated. As the acute delirium faded away it became evident that a profound change had occurred in her character; for she was now intensely restless and violent and easily enraged, and lewd and impudent and always 'in trouble'. This behaviour was deeply shocking to her God-fearing parents and evoked from them hatred and threats and punishment. Indeed, her mother, speaking of all this to me more than forty years later, said: 'It was a punishment from Heaven because she was so evil. She was a naughty disobedient hateful child, and she deserved her sickness – she deserved all she got.'

By the age of twelve Miss G.'s behaviour had become constrained by a progressive stiffness and slowness of movement, and by the age of fifteen she was deeply Parkinsonian. For the next thirty years her parents – who in the meantime had moved to the United States – kept her in a back-room where no one could see her; here she would lie face down on the carpet, sometimes biting it or chewing it with rage; her food would be thrown in like scraps to an animal, although a priest would be brought to see her every Sunday without fail.

In 1967, in view of her parents' increasing age and a heart ailment which was disabling her mother, Miss G. was admitted

to Mount Carmel Hospital. At this time I found her profoundly Parkinsonian and catatonic : she showed a divergent
squint and an internuclear paresis; salivation, which was
exceedingly profuse and viscous; rigidity and akinesia of
severe degree; violent 'flapping' tremor of her right hand
at times; continual closing and clonus of the eyelids; and an
impairment of postural reflexes so profound, that she would
sit doubled over with her head on the ground. Her voice was
very soft, but impulsive, and scarcely intelligible. She seemed
quite intelligent and soon came to recognize everyone around
her. Twice a month, she would have an oculogyric crisis,
and on rare occasions a most violent rage; during her rages
she would be able to rise to her feet and walk and yell and
hit with great force; but for most of the time she was totally
motionless. This was her state until given L-DOPA.

I started L-DOPA on 18 June 1969. Her response, which
occurred at a dose-level of 1·2 gm. a day, was exceedingly
swift and dramatic, occurring within hours on one particular day. She experienced a sudden surge of energy and
strength, and a complete abolition of all her rigidity. She
became able to walk the length of a passage, battling her
stooping-tendency by the use of main force; her voice became
loud and clear, though hurried, with a tendency to speak in
short sentences or phrases; her salivation ceased almost completely; and her mood became joyous with a touch of elation.
Her parents were summoned and visited her at once – their
first such visit in her two years at hospital : her father em-
braced her with great gratitude and joy, and her mother
exclaimed: 'A miracle from Heaven ... a completely new
person.' There followed a single wonderful week in which
Miss G. was transformed in all possible ways. Her mother
had bought her a wardrobe of dresses to celebrate her 'rebirth'. Dressed up in her finery, poised and made-up, Miss
G. looked beautiful and much younger than her age : the
nurses now called her 'The Sicilian bombshell'.

In the first week of July various problems appeared. Miss G.'s high spirits turned to violence and mania, and she started to feel that she was being 'seduced' and 'teased'; she felt patients and staff were conspiring to 'get' her, and she was at once thrilled, terrified and infuriated by the feelings this aroused. The merest glance would call forth a yell or the sudden violent flinging of whatever was to hand. She continually asked me how children were born and whether sex was 'natural' or punished by death. She became intensely anxious about her mother's health and made continual phone calls to home; the question she asked was always the same: 'You feeling OK, mother? You ain't going to die?' and she would weep and shudder after each of these phone calls. By the middle of July her days had become an ontological switch-back of 'ups and downs' – five furies a day followed by exhaustion and contrition. She was exceedingly formidable in these outbursts of fury, and would howl with great force like a maddened gorilla; she would rush down the corridors striking everyone round her, and if there was no one she would hit at the walls. Towards the end of each outburst she would bang her head on the walls and yell: 'Kill me, kill me! I'm bad, I must die!' Tiny doses of thorazine (largactil) – a mere 5 mg. – would 'break' these furies within a few minutes, but threw Miss G. into a deeply Parkinsonian, catatonic and almost stuporous state.

On 16 July I reduced her L-DOPA from 1·2 gm. to 1·0 gm. a day. This immediately acted like a large dose of thorazine, bringing Miss G. to a Parkinsonian-stuporous standstill. She spent four days in a profoundly disabled and depressed state, far more severe than her pre-DOPA state, and begged me repeatedly to increase her L-DOPA. On 20 July I increased it, infinitesimally, by 0·1 gm. a day. This immediately re-awakened the worst rage we had seen. Miss G. exploded into a murderous-catatonic fury with snarling, screaming, growling and roaring, clawing, scratching, smashing and hurling; she scowled and glared in a bestial way, and looked like a great carnivore preparing to kill. In this state, she also showed violent out-thrustings of the tongue and a continual tonic protrusion of the lips ('*schnauzkrampf*'). Since she seemed unable to speak, I gave her a pencil and paper, but she thrust these into her mouth and chewed them to pieces. After twenty-five hours of continuous fury – unmitigated by stopping her L-DOPA or injections – she collapsed into an exhausted, motionless sleep, curled up like a baby, with her thumb in her mouth. Feeling that Miss G. needed some weeks to 'cool off', and since I myself was going away for a month, I did not re-start her L-DOPA till my return in September.

On my return, I found Miss G. was still intensely Parkinsonian-catatonic-depressed, immovably imploded in a physiological Black Hole – a state far worse than her pre-DOPA state, and one which necessitated near-total nursing care. She seemed scarcely alive now without her L-DOPA, but I feared she would become uncontrollably violent again if I re-started the drug. It seemed an impossible choice between impossible alternatives, but I could only try (and hope) for an intermediate state. I started Miss G. back on L-DOPA, therefore, using doses so small we had to make our own capsules. At 100 mg. a day, she showed no response; at 150 mg., 200 mg. and 250 mg. a day, she showed no response; at 300 mg. a day she suddenly '*exploded*', and went Super-Nova as she had done in the past.

This time her explosion went further than before, and caused her to shatter into behavioural fragments. In the ensuing two months her behaviour lost what unity it had shown before, and broke into innumerable 'sub-behaviours', each perfectly organized and profoundly regressive – like a schizophrenic process, but deeper and more acute than any I had seen. I felt we had opened a Pandora's Box, or disclosed a nest of ontological snakes. And yet it was impossible to stop the L-DOPA, or even to reduce it by the minutest fraction, for her response to this was immediate coma, with depressed respiration and signs of anoxia. I tried this twice, both times with results which could have been fatal. She had lost any state between death and madness; she had lost the *possibility* of any intermediate state once she started overreacting to L-DOPA.

In these two months, Miss G. became very sensitive, and would shield her food and her possessions with her hands, fearfully and angrily scowling at 'stealers'. She developed an insatiable hoarding urge, and surrounded herself with a miscellany of objects – torn papers, gnawed candies, and pencils and fruit, the contents of her handbag, bits of bread, and occasionally faeces – all gathered together in her chair and her bed. She showed lightning-quick tics and impulsions of gaze, her eyes darting around with extraordinary speed; frequently her gaze would be 'captured' or captivated by some object or other which had chanced to enter its field; flies, in particular, compelled her attention; when her gaze was caught she would have to make a violent effort of her entire body to 'release' it. She was continually 'bewitched' by objects around her, and forced to watch them, or touch them, or lick them, though at times she could countermand these enticements with 'block'. She showed insatiable appetite and uncontrollable voracity, and after eating would have an irresistible urge to lick her plate, and to stuff her fingers and the utensils into her still-chewing mouth. When drinking, her tongue would be violently extended, or she would *lap* with an incredibly cat-like celerity.

She repeatedly complained that she was filthy and shameful, and was continually picking and brushing her person, her hands moving separately as if independently controlled. Occasionally, she would pick at or brush the people around her. At times she felt the whole world like a goad, or a horde of pestering, picking impingements, and she would shrink

down in her chair and cover her face, or lie on the floor in a
foetal position. Increasingly she lived in a world of her own,
battling with or surrendering to her own apparitions. Each
day she became more narcissistic and regressive, and less
prone to react to anything round her. She developed innumerable strange habits and mannerisms, some of them so
strange as to defeat interpretation, and others which were
plain tokens of self-destruction – biting and kicking herself,
choking and scratching herself, putting her head in an invisible noose, or laying it flat on an invisible block, panto-
mimes and evocations of violence and death. Only in the
evenings would her torments diminish, and a calm would
descend on this distracted woman: at such times she would
go back to weaving a basket, which she had been engaged on
for several months, and which – alone – had been exempt
from her rabid destructions. I last saw Miss G. on the evening of 21 December, calmly weaving her basket in bed. She
was found dead and cold in her bed the next morning, her
rigid arms still clutching her favourite basket.

16. RACHEL I.

Following an attack of *encephalitis lethargica*, Mrs I. developed a progressive Parkinsonian disability which by 1964
had completely immobilized her with intense rigidity and
dystonia of her trunk and extremities. Her speech, curiously,
was an aspect of function scarcely touched by her otherwise
so-engulfing Parkinsonism, and showed that she retained her
intelligence, memory and humour despite having been so
long 'walled up' in her immobilizing syndrome. Twice a
month, usually on Sundays, her condition would be transformed by peculiar attacks in which she would feel herself
flooded by wave upon wave of unlocalizable pain and an-

guish which compelled her to scream out in a high perseverative voice. These attacks, which began and ended quite
suddenly, and had occurred for twenty or more years, had
never been demonstrably associated with any physical disease
and were therefore presumed to be *crises* or 'thalamic attacks'
of an unusual sort. They demonstrated a potential for affective and catatonic excitement which was inapparent or dis-
guised at all other times.

In the latter part of 1967 Mrs I. started to show a slight
senile deterioration of recent memory although her general
intellectual organization remained quite intact and above
normal in quality. I had several times approached her about
the use of L-DOPA, but she was very fearful regarding its
use and would say, 'No, I won't try it – it'll blow me to
pieces.' In September 1970, she changed her mind, saying,
'I suppose at this stage I have nothing to lose.'

Her reaction to L-DOPA was catastrophic from the start.
Ten days after beginning the drug and on a dose of 1 gm.
daily, without any therapeutic effect or warning signs whatever Mrs I. *did* 'blow up'. She became intensely excited, deliriously hallucinated, seeing tiny figures and faces all
around her, and hearing voices, which suddenly appeared
and disappeared in all parts of the room; she also became
uncontrollably echolalic, repeating anything one said to her
in a shrill screaming voice hundreds or thousands of times
in succession. Haunted by hallucinations and echoing indefinitely to external stimuli, Mrs I. gave the impression of a
hollow, untenanted, ghost-filled house, as if *she herself* had
been 'dispossessed' by echoes and ghosts. Despite stopping
L-DOPA immediately, and despite the heaviest possible use
of sedatives and tranquillizers, it proved impossible to stop
this monstrous excitement. It continued unabated for three
weeks, and almost twenty-four hours a day, during which
time she had no rest except for short-lived exhausted stupors.
During this period she showed a sharp decline in her intel-

lectual status, becoming visibly less able to recognize familiar figures, and less able to create complex hallucinations, with each passing day; it was impossible to avoid the impression that she was being combusted or 'burnt out' by the uninterrupted intensity of her cerebral excitement. In the fourth week the excitement suddenly came to an end and was replaced by a state of coma. This continued for a month, during which time she required total nursing care, tube-feeding, etc. When Mrs I. awoke from her coma she had lost the power to recognize anyone or anything, could make only non-verbal noises, and showed no recognizable signs of mental 'presence' at all. She seemed to have become a complete mental blank, wiped clean of all structure like a terminal dement. She lingered in this mindless and functionally decorticate state for seven weeks before expiring in an attack of pneumonia.

17. AARON E.

Mr E. was born in 1907, the elder of fraternal twins. His parents had immigrated to the States a few years before, and at the time of Mr E.'s birth had established a flourishing delicatessen in the right part of Brooklyn. Mr E.'s early life was one of work, seriousness, and laborious self-improvement, delivering newspapers and half a dozen other jobs as a boy and adolescent, and supplementing his education with night classes, public lectures and long hours spent in the Brooklyn public library. By the age of twenty-three Mr E. had established himself as an up-and-coming accountant, was able to marry and take out a mortgage.

Over the next thirty years Mr E. showed exceptional vigour and enterprise, and was able to expand into a six-man corporation. During these intervening years he enjoyed excellent health and never lost a day's work through illness or 'indisposition'. He was a freemason, a prominent member of the local synagogue, a vice-president of the local school board, and actively interested in civic affairs. He had a large circle of friends and business acquaintances, went to the theatre every Thursday, played golf every Sunday, and went on a camping trip with his wife and five children to the Adirondacks every summer. He was the epitome of the self-made man and the American success-story.

It is probable, in retrospect, that his first symptom of Parkinson's disease might have showed itself in his trips to the mountains in situations of unusual exertion or stress. At such times he would occasionally show a tendency to stutter, and an unusual impatience, restlessness and alacrity of movement; he would also get abnormally tired and find particular difficulty in 'getting going' once he had 'settled down' in his chair. But if these were Parkinsonian symptoms they were unrecognized at the time, and it was only in 1962, in his fifty-sixth year, that Mr. E. developed an unmistakably Parkinsonian tremor of the hands and an increasing rigidity of his arms and back. His symptoms were considerably helped by artane and similar drugs, and he fought them off with his usual vigour, continuing to do a full day's work, maintain his social life and play golf until 1965.

In 1965, Mr E. felt that everything was becoming too much for him; these feelings had been brewing for more than a year, and had been fought down by him again and again; when they finally broke through, they did so suddenly and explosively. With no warning, and with none of his usual deliberation, Mr E. precipitately announced his retirement from work, his resignation from the local school and synagogue boards, and a great reduction of all his other activities and commitments. He 'renounced' his life as an active man, and almost as a member of society. He now spent the greater part of his time at home, looking at the newspapers and television, and pottering in the garden at the back of the house. He continued to follow the market and keep in touch with his broker, but to a smaller and smaller degree with each passing month, ceasing altogether in 1966. Prematurely retired, and no longer the bread-winner, Mr E.'s status at home very sharply declined; he partly fell from, and partly resigned, his position as paterfamilias and master of the house, letting all major decisions be undertaken by his wife and his sons. He started to show signs of depression, anxiety, dependence, passivity, self-pity and querulousness – incredible to those who had known him as an active, driving, powerful and resourceful man only a few years before. His loss of status and general autonomy, and his Parkinsonian symptoms, seemed to play upon and reinforce one another; and by 1967 Mr E. had not only become a complete invalid, but had developed the personality and traits of one.

In view of his severe disability and depression and dependence, Mr E. was admitted to Mount Carmel Hospital as a private patient in the summer of 1967. This greatly increased all his symptoms, Parkinsonian and otherwise; he saw his hospitalization not as 'a new start' and 'a form of therapy' – as his family and the hospital brochures suggested – but as a 'putting-away' and a sign that 'everything was finished' as far as he was concerned. When I saw him at this time, he showed a picture of Parkinson's disease which was severe, but could not possibly be mistaken for a post-encephalitic picture. He exhibited very little spontaneous speech or movement, although when spoken to he would liven up and talk with a touch of his old animation. He was unable to rise without aid from his chair, to initiate gait or to walk stably once started, having strong tendencies to 'freezing', festination and pulsion. He was thin and haggard, and looked older than his age. His posture was listless and stooped, and his face had a hopeless look under its Parkinsonian mask. He showed moderately severe rigidity in all his limbs, and much shaking of the hands when tired or distressed. He presented the picture of a man who was both severely disabled and broken in spirit, and I could scarcely believe that he had been in full command of a vigorous and varied life only two years before. Mr E. continued in this disabled and defeated state, until he was given L-DOPA.

He was started on L-DOPA in March 1969. The dose was slowly raised to 4·0 gm. a day over a period of three weeks without *apparently* producing any effect. I first discovered that Mr E. was responding to L-DOPA by accident, chancing to go past his room at an unaccustomed time and hearing regular footsteps inside the room. I went in and found Mr E., who had been chairbound since 1966, walking up and down his room, swinging his arms with considerable vigour, and showing an erectness of posture and a brightness of expression completely new to him. When I asked him about these effects he said with some embarrassment : 'Yes ! I felt the L-DOPA beginning to work three days ago – it was like a wave of energy and strength sweeping through me. I found I could stand and walk by myself, and that I could do everything I needed for myself – but I was afraid that you would see how well I was and discharge me from hospital ... you see, I've gotten so used to depending on people and having them take care of my needs, I've lost all confidence in myself ... I've got to unlearn the habit of depending, I suppose ... you'll have to give me time for this, you know.' I reassured Mr E. that I understood his position, and would in no sense hurry him or force him beyond his wishes or capacities.

The requisite dose of L-DOPA (5·5 gm. a day) was achieved after another two weeks and brought about a virtual 'normalization' in every way. Mr E. now talked and walked with perfect facility, and could do everything he wanted : he was no longer detectably Parkinsonian in any way. But he remained very fearful of expanding his so-constricted life, and did much less than his capacities allowed. It took a

month before Mr E. plucked up courage to leave his room
and walk freely around the hospital; it took four months
before Mr E. ventured outside the hospital to walk round
the block and look at the world 'outside'; and it was nine
months before Mr E. said he felt sufficiently well and confident to return to his home and former style of life. During
those nine months he presented a picture of health; he had
filled out again, had a good colour and no longer looked older
than his age. Thus, to overcome Mr E.'s Parkinsonism was a
matter of days; but to overcome his invalidism and fear and
pessimism took all of nine months.

Mr E.'s leaving the hospital and return to his home had a
moving and triumphal quality about it; half the hospital
turned out to see him off, and the *New York Times* itself
published a picture; it was the first time in fifty years that a
Parkinsonian patient who had entered Mount Carmel had
ever left it to return to his home. There followed three pleasant and full months during which Mr E. – still taking 5.0
gm. of L-DOPA a day – resumed a fairly active domestic and
social life, seeing friends and neighbours he had turned
away from in 1965, gardening a little, playing golf on Sunday, and even discussing the market a bit with his broker.
He appeared increasingly confident and tranquil during
these first three months at home.

In his thirteenth month on L-DOPA, however, some problems arose, affecting his movements and emotional reactions.
He developed sudden flickering movements (chorea), especially
severe about the mouth and face, and tending to dance from
one muscle group to another;[40] his actions became rather

40. Chorea (literally 'a dance') was rather rare before the advent
of L-DOPA, usually being seen only in the hereditary Huntingdon's
chorea, and the chorea which sometimes occurred with rheumatic
fever ('St Vitus's Dance'). Now chorea is extremely common, since
virtually every patient with Parkinsonism placed on L-DOPA develops chorea sooner or later – so much so that some neurologists have
spoken of chorea as 'anti-Parkinsonism'. It is certainly very striking

abrupt and precipitate, and he now started to gesticulate
a great deal with his arms and body when he was speaking
(he was not formerly given to such gestural exuberance).
He became impatient and restless; he became somewhat irritable and inclined to quarrel; he developed a hectoring and
bullying manner, with apprehension and anxiety beneath.
In short, he was now showing a progressive psychomotor
excitement induced by L-DOPA. Mr E. tended at this time
to minimize all his symptoms: 'They're nothing,' he would
say, 'nothing to speak of ... I don't mind them, why should

---

and convincing to see, in such patients, the interconversions of the
two: the massive hardness and tension of Parkinsonian rigidity
transformed to the softness and fluttering of (anti-Parkinsonian)
chorea; particularly dramatic, in patients with *dystonia musculorum
deformans*, is to see a heavy, sluggish, rolling wave of dystonia
break into a fine, sparkling spray or spume of chorea ... Chorea is
a sort of physiological confetti, and gives the impression of being
weightless and forceless; choreic movements occur 'spontaneously',
requiring neither deliberate effort, nor the convulsive tension which
eventuates in tics; they 'happen', suddenly, without effort or warning, in a way which suggests a complete absence of resistance, indeed
a complete absence of inertia. One can treat chorea stochastically
or statistically, and say that such-and-such an amount is likely to
occur in such-and-such a time; but it is impossible to treat its movements *individually* – to say *when* or *where* the next movement will
occur. Nor is experience of any use here: one realizes, after a while,
that choreic movements are *inherently* unpredictable in individual
terms – one can no more say when and where they will occur than
one can predict this of bubbles in a boiling liquid, or of the disintegration of atoms in a radioactive substance ... or other *essentially
quantal phenomena* which can only be quantized in probabilistic
terms. We have spoken earlier of the need for relativistic and quantal
models in neurology, and we see that we do not have to go as 'far
out' as the peculiar standstills (considered on p. 141) to find biological
'macro-quantal' phenomena. Seeing chorea as a sparkling emission,
and Parkinsonism or dystonia as strongly constrained travelling
waves; seeing, above all, their interconversions, one enjoys a sort of
double vision, the contrast and complementarity of two basic modes
– the discrete and the continuous, the quantal and the relativistic.

anyone else mind? ...' And indeed, the choreic and urgent quality of Mr E.'s behaviour was not in itself a real disability; it prevented him from nothing that he wished to do; it was far more obvious to others than it was to himself; and it was obviously a state far preferable to his previous Parkinsonian-depressive state. These movements could be reduced only partially by reducing the L-DOPA: thus I found Mr E. best on 4·0 gm. a day; on 4·5 gm. he was far too choreic, and at 3·5 gm. a day he showed reversion to his Parkinsonism. At this stage, therefore, Mr E. had begun to walk a tight-rope of 'normality' with chasms of 'side-effects' to either side.

In the sixteenth month on L-DOPA Mr E. started to develop spontaneous reversions to Parkinsonism, tiredness and depression which were at first infrequent and brief. Within two weeks of their onset these fluctuations had become abrupt, severe and frequent, and Mr E. started swinging, several times a day, between states of driven excitable chorea and states of intense weariness and Parkinsonism. Finally, the excited choreic states ceased altogether, and Mr E. found himself clenched, without any intermission at all, in an intolerably severe Parkinsonian state – *much* more severe than his pre-DOPA state. Attempts to alter his state by increasing his L-DOPA – the recommended treatment – were entirely useless. Motionless, almost speechless, salivating, intensely rigid, Mr E. was brought back to Mount Carmel Hospital. His return in this state was not only intensely humiliating to himself, but caused a wave of apprehension among the seventy other Parkinsonian patients receiving L-DOPA. They had seen Mr E. leave in triumph, and now they saw his tragic return. I frequently overheard such comments as, 'He was the star patient – he did better than anybody. If *he* gets into such trouble, what'll happen to *us*?'

With Mr E.'s readmission to hospital I stopped his L-DOPA – a withdrawal which caused great weakness and lassitude and apathetic depression, as well as a violent resurgence of Parkinsonian tremor. This acute 'withdrawal syndrome' lessened after two weeks, and Mr E. seemed to return to his pre-DOPA status. With his state apparently stable once more, I restarted him on L-DOPA, hoping for a renewal of his original reaction. This, however, did not occur: Mr E. now showed himself to have become unusually and pathologically sensitive to L-DOPA, so that on a dose of no more than 1·5 gm. a day he immediately re-developed chorea and swung into the up-and-down cycle which he had shown before, culminating once again in an intense contracted Parkinsonian akinesia. It was therefore necessary to withdraw his L-DOPA again, and I decided to let two months elapse without L-DOPA in the hope of restoring his original reactivity. In October 1970 I started him on L-DOPA for the third time, using the smallest possible doses, and increasing these extremely slowly. This time Mr E. showed a still more inordinate sensitivity to the drug, becoming violently choreic on a dose no greater than 250 mg. a day – less than a twentieth of the dose that he had originally been taking – and for the third time L-DOPA had to be stopped. I therefore decided that six months had to elapse before we tried L-DOPA again.

During these six months Mr E. fell into a peculiar state, completely unlike anything he had ever shown before. He would sit motionless in his wheelchair in the corridor all day with his eyes open but curiously blank; he seemed wholly indifferent to everything around him, and also to his own fate as a person. When I asked him how he felt he would reply, 'Comme ci, comme ça,' or 'That's the way it goes,' without any expression. He showed no active attention to anything around him, although he registered its happening in a mechanical way. I tried hard to elicit some feeling from Mr E. and failed completely; and he himself said: 'I have no feelings – I've gone dead inside.' During these months Mr E. looked somehow dead, like a ghost or a ghoul or a zombie.

He had ceased to convey any feeling of living presence, and had become a mere absence seated in a wheelchair. During this time (March 1971) I tried L-DOPA for the fourth time, and now Mr E. showed no reaction whatever: where he had reacted so intensely six months before to 250 mg. a day, he now showed not a trace of any reaction to 5,000 mg. a day. He said: 'I knew this would happen – I'm burnt out inside. Nothing you can do will make any difference.' I could not help wondering whether he was right, and whether we had indeed in some way totally destroyed his potential for reacting to L-DOPA or to anything else.

In the summer of 1971 Mr E. – who had not been taking L-DOPA or other drugs since the spring – started to look and feel more *alive*, and to show a return of reactions and feelings which had been in abeyance for the previous nine months. In October 1971 I started him on L-DOPA for the fifth time, and his reactions to this have been substantially and moderately successful up to the present time (September 1972). Mr E. has shown nothing to match the marvellous effect seen in 1969; there is never a time when he could be mistaken for 'normal'; he has bouts of chorea and Parkinsonism and depression and occasional festination, and a new symptom – dystonic spasms affecting his neck; but, despite these problems, his overall mobility and mood are obviously much better than they were in the days before L-DOPA. He is able to get around the hospital and look after his own physical needs, for most of the time, and once a month or so he feels up to a weekend at home. He reads the papers and gossips, and takes a very real interest in everything about him. Although his life is constricted and monotonous – as is unfortunately true of so many patients in such institutions – he nevertheless seems to have achieved a real and useful equilibrium over the last ten months, and perhaps he will continue to hold this indefinitely in the future.

18. GEORGE W.

Mr W. was born in the Bronx in 1913, left school at fourteen and joined his father in the family laundry business. He married in his early twenties and combined his daily slogging in the laundry with a full family and social life.

In his fiftieth year Mr W. noticed a tendency for his right hand to tremble if he became over-excited or over-tired – a symptom which was initially dismissed by his doctor as a 'nervous tremor'. Two years later, he started to experience some difficulty with quick or fine movements in his hand and found that his handwriting was becoming smaller. Subsequently he developed an overall stiffness of the entire right side of his body.

These and other symptoms were so slowly progressive that when I first saw Mr W. as a private patient – eight years after the onset of his tremor – he was still able to do a full day's work in his sweltering laundry, to drive his car, to walk several blocks and to look after himself in every way. He did, it was true, show considerable rigidity and akinesia of his right side, and when he walked showed no swing of the right arm and a tendency to drag his right foot; his voice was virtually normal; his face was moderately masked. The only change which had been necessitated by his illness was that Mr W. had had to learn to write with his left hand – he had always, fortunately, been 'ambidextrous'. Although there was no sign of Parkinsonism on the left side of his body, I had the impression that his left arm was a trifle hyperactive, because he seemed to gesticulate a good deal with his arm and showed a tic-like or manneristic tendency to adjust his spectacles every two or three minutes.[41]

41. When I first saw Mr W., I was uncertain as to whether this over-activity of the left arm was pathological, or whether it was

Mr W. had found artane and similar drugs quite useful since 1965, and was in two minds about the use of L-DOPA when he first came to see me in 1970. 'I hear it's a wonderful drug,' he said. 'They keep calling it a "miracle drug" in the papers. I've often talked with Mrs W. about taking it, but we can't make up our minds. I can still do a full day's work, and almost everything else I want, but things are getting more difficult from one year to another. Maybe I could carry on for another few years ... Of course, it would be wonderful if I could get back the full use of my right side. But then there are all of these "side-effects" I keep hearing about.'

There was no urgency in the matter, and Mr W. and I postponed any decision about the use of L-DOPA until the summer of 1971. We finally decided to try it after he had shown an excellent reaction to amantadine during April and May of that year. Mr W.'s initial reaction to L-DOPA was rather strange, and consisted of the development of manifest Parkinsonism in his 'normal' left side. This negative reaction disappeared after a few days and was replaced by a remarkable loosening-up and mobilization of his right side – to such an extent, indeed, that Mr W. seemed and felt absolutely normal in all ways in his third week on the drug. In his fourth week on L-DOPA (he was taking at this time 3·5 gm. a day) he developed a distressing restlessness and alacrity which drove him to walk much too fast: 'I'm sort of scared by all this *drive*,' he said at the time. 'I hurry so much I'm practically running – I'm scared I'll get a heart-attack or something. I keep having to tell myself to walk more slowly.' At this time he also developed some chorea, grimacing, irregularity of breathing, stuttering, and periods of exhaustion and rigidity in the middle of each day. At this time we

---

simply a 'compensation' for the deficiency of activity on his right side: his subsequent reactions to L-DOPA showed that its activity was in fact pathological.

discussed stopping L-DOPA but Mr W. said, 'Let's wait a bit longer – maybe things will settle down and I'll adjust to the stuff.'

Things did settle down and Mr W. did adjust to his L-DOPA. His 'side-effects' disappeared within a month – his dose of L-DOPA remaining unchanged – and he returned once more to a state of complete or apparently complete 'normality'. He is still maintaining this now – more than a year later. But it is normality with a catch to it, as Mr W. and those who know him are fully aware. I have recently (September 1972) had a letter from Mr W. in which he says: '... I've been on L-DOPA for fifteen months now. It's amazing stuff but there is a "but" ... At best I feel completely normal and I can do everything I want. At these times nobody would know there was anything the matter with me ... but I've become very over-sensitive, and the moment I over-exert myself or over-excite myself, or if I am worried, or get tired, all the side-effects immediately come back. If anyone even talks about "side-effects", or if I think about them, they also come back. Before I took L-DOPA I had Parkinson's all the time. It was always there and never changed too much. Now I'm OK. I'm *perfect* when everything is going smoothly, but I feel like I'm on a tight-rope, or like a pin trying to balance on its point.[42] If you ask whether L-DOPA

42. Many other patients besides George W. use such images to express their sense of an extremely fined-down and precarious balance, an ever-diminishing fulcrum or base, an ever-increasing liability to upset ... Such patients, although they appear perfectly normal *when* they are normal, have lost the latitude, the broad base, of true health or stability, and have entered the knife-edged state of *meta-stability*: they have lost the 'give', the resilience, the *suppleness* of health, and are now in a state essentially *brittle* – a 'rigid-labile state', in Goldstein's term. One feels of such patients – and this too is an image frequently voiced by them – that they no longer dwell in a world of gentle slopes and gradients, a secure and familiar terrestrial landscape, but that they have been transported to a sort of nightmare world, a moonscape of fearful pinnacles and precipices, a (literally)

is good or bad for me, I'd say it was *both*. It has wonderful effects but there is a hell of a "but" . . .'

19. CECIL M.

Cecil M. was born in London in 1905, developed the sleeping-sickness during the great epidemic, but appeared to have made a complete recovery from this until the onset of Parkin-

---

horrid realm of points and edges . . . We have seen, again and again, how the morbid comes to resemble the mechanical in its lack of intrinsic stability and control. Thus the horrid, punctate, acicular state of metastable patients is extraordinarily evocative of the world which Newton devised, and precisely shares its character, its improbability, and its peculiar perils : '. . . To suppose that all the Particles in an infinite Space should be so accurate poised one among another', Newton writes, '. . .[were] as hard as to make not one Needle only, but an infinite number of them . . . stand accurately poised upon their Points . . . the Principle . . . is a precarious one' (Newton : second letter to Bentley).

Given this mountainous, precarious landscape, where there is no safe point of equilibrium and stability, it is inevitable that these DOPA-inflamed Parkinsonian patients should be liable to violent crashes and falls. Images of exciting heights and terrible falls (metaphorical perceptions of their precarious states) may haunt or obsess such endangered patients, and be vividly conveyed to all those around them. Thus Lucy K. (p. 179) : 'Look at me, look at me ! I can fly like a bird !' and Margaret A.'s 'wonderful flying floating feeling' (p. 187); but these elevated states are accompanied by indefinable yet intense anxieties – thus Rose R., her jubilation darkened by a shadow from the future, exclaims : 'Things can't last. Something awful is coming !' No patient depicted an Icarus-flight and an Icarus-fall more vividly and memorably than Frances D. : 'I'd done a vertical take-off,' she said (p. 76). 'I'd gone higher nad higher on L-DOPA – to an impossible height. I felt I was on a pinnacle a million miles high . . . And then . . . I *crashed* . . . I was buried a million miles deep in the ground.'

I see, equally, how my own feelings and images were half-conscious

sonian and other symptoms twenty years later (1940). His initial symptom was megaphonia – a tendency to bellow and raise his voice – which was followed by the development of grunting, and a tendency to clench and grind the teeth. Within a few months of their onset these presenting symptoms disappeared, and were replaced by a Parkinsonian syndrome with impairment of balance, a tendency to backwards-falling, festination, freezing, and predominantly left-sided rigidity and tremor. By 1942, the clinical picture had stabilized and was to show no significant changes for the next quarter of a century. Mr M., who was an intelligent and resourceful man, found that he could lead a full life despite his symptoms: he continued to drive to business each day, to lead an active family and social life, and to maintain his many interests, hobbies and physical activities – especially swimming, of which he was particularly fond, and which allowed a far more fluid and fluent motion than walking.

Mr M. was placed on L-DOPA in 1970. His initial responses

---

reflections of those of my patients. Thus, in the happy summer of 1969, I too had obscure presentiments of trouble; and in my notebooks, subsequently paraphrased here, I wondered whether my patients might not be facing 'enticing ascensions' or 'fraudulent heights' (p. 282 n.). I see how these faint premonitions or trouble-to-come were hideously realized in the time that followed, how these faint foreshadowings became 'the heights of exorbitance' and 'crashes . . . into subterranean depths' (p. 298).

I think that such images of proud and tempting inner heights, of climbs which are folly and must end in falls, have metaphorical relevance at a variety of levels. At an energetic–economic level, one sees that over-excitement, excess stimulation, *must* cause a sudden exhaustion of resources; at a metaphysical level, one sees that an ever-increasing tension and charge, a continual intensification of force and field, an ever-greater distortion of ontological 'space', *must* eventuate in a catastrophic event – a sudden, critical, inwards collapse (like the gravitational collapse which leads to 'Black Holes'); lastly, at an allegorical level, what amounts to an ever-increasing ontological *hubris* has to provoke and be followed inevitably by *nemesis*.

may be described in his own words: 'In the early stages it seemed to have given me a new lease of life. I felt exhilarated and rejuvenated. The stiffness went out of my left arm and leg. I could use my left arm to shave and also to type. I could bend down with ease to do my shoe up. And of course I could walk with complete freedom and enjoy moving about, which is something I dreaded doing before. And the tremor in my left arm almost disappeared.'

On the sixteenth day of taking L-DOPA, when Mr M. was enjoying his new-found mobility and feelings of energy, he started to suffer from a recrudescence of the 'lock-jaw' or *trismus* he had briefly experienced in 1940. Over the next week Mr M.'s trismus became intense and continual, so that he could no longer open his mouth to eat or speak. Concurrently with this he experienced a return and indeed an exacerbation of his Parkinsonian freezing, rigidity and tremor. At this point he indicated that he wished the L-DOPA to be stopped.

Mr M. has declined any subsequent trials of L-DOPA. He says: 'I have had this condition for more than thirty years and I have learnt to live with it. I know exactly where I am, what I can do, and what I can't do. Things don't change from day to day – or at least they didn't change till I was given L-DOPA. Its effect was very pleasant at first but then it turned out more trouble than it was worth. I can get along perfectly well without it – why should I try L-DOPA again?'

20. LEONARD L.

I first saw Leonard L. in the spring of 1966. At this time Mr L. was in his forty-sixth year, completely speechless and completely without voluntary motion except for minute movements of the right hand. With these he could spell out

messages on a small letter-board – this had been his only
mode of communication for fifteen years and continued to be
his only mode of communication until he was given L-DOPA
in the spring of 1969. Despite his almost incredible degree of
immobility and disability, Mr L. was an avid reader (the
pages had to be turned by someone else), the librarian at the
hospital, and the producer of a stream of brilliant book reviews which appeared in the hospital magazine every
month. It was obvious to me, from my first meeting with Mr
L. – and this impression was reinforced by all my subsequent
meetings with him – that this was a man of most unusual
intelligence, cultivation, and sophistication; a man who
seemed to have an almost total recall for whatever he had
read, thought, or experienced (he once called himself the
'Buchmendel' of Mount Carmel[43]); and, not least, a man
with an introspective and investigative passion which ex-
ceeded that of almost any patient I had ever seen. This
combination of the profoundest disease with the acutest investigative intelligence made Mr L. an 'ideal' patient, so to
speak, and in the six and a half years I have known him he
has taught me more about Parkinsonism, post-encephalitic illness, suffering, and human nature than all the rest of my
patients combined. Mr L. deserves a book to himself,[44] but I
must here confine myself to the barest and most inadequate
outline of his state, before, during and after the use of
L-DOPA.

   The picture which Mr L. presented in 1966 had not changed
since his admission to the hospital, and indeed he himself

43. 'Buchmendel' is a story by Stefan Zweig concerning an eccentric bibliophilic scholar who devotes every hour of his life to reading.
Zweig calls him 'a British Museum catalogue on two legs'.
44. My own notes on Leonard L. run to 100,000 words or more, and
Mr. L. himself wrote a remarkable autobiography at the height of his
therapeutic reaction to L-DOPA (see pp. 250–51 and n.). I hope that
I may be able to conflate his autobiography with my own biography
of him in a separate volume at some future date.

– like so many other 'mummified' post-encephalitic patients
– seemed a good deal younger than his chronological age: in
particular he had the unlined face of a man in his twenties.
He showed extreme rigidity of his neck, trunk and limbs and
marked dystrophic changes in his hands, which were no larger than those of a child; his face was profoundly masked,
but when it broke into a smile the smile remained for minutes or hours – like the smile of the Cheshire Cat; he was
totally voiceless except at times of unusual excitement when
he could yell or bellow with considerable force. He suffered
from frequent 'micro-crises' – upturnings of the eyeballs,
associated with transient inability to move or respond; these
lasted a few seconds only, and occurred dozens, and sometimes hundreds, of times a day. His eye movements, as he
read, or glanced about his surroundings, were rapid and sure,
and gave the only external clue to the alert and attentive
intelligence imprisoned within his motionless body.

At the end of my first meeting with Leonard L. I said to
him: 'What's it like being the way you are? What would
you compare it to?' He spelt out the following answer:
'Caged. Deprived. Like Rilke's "Panther".'[45] And then he
swept his eyes around the ward and spelt out: 'This is a
human zoo.' Again and again, with his penetrating descriptions, his imaginative metaphors, or his great stock of poetic
images, Mr L. would try to evoke the nature of his own being
and experience. 'There's an awful presence,' he once tapped
out, 'and an awful absence. The presence is a mixture of
nagging and pushing and pressure, with being held back
and constrained and stopped – I often call it "the goad and

45.   Sein Blick ist vom Vorübergehn der Stäbe
        So müd geworden, dass er nichts mehr hält.
        Ihm ist, als ob es tausend Stäbe gäbe
        Und hinter tausend Stäben keine Welt.
(His gaze from going through the bars has grown so weary that it can
take in nothing more. For him it is as though there were a thousand
bars, and behind the thousand bars no world.)

halter". The absence is a terrible isolation and coldness and shrinking – more than you can imagine, Dr Sacks, much more than anybody who isn't this way can possibly imagine – a bottomless darkness and unreality.' Mr L. was fond of tapping out, or voicelessly murmuring – in a sort of soliloquy – passages from Dante or T. S. Eliot, especially the lines:

> Descend lower, descend only
> Into the world of perpetual solitude,
> World not world, but that which is not world,
> Internal darkness, deprivation
> And destitution of all property,
> Desiccation of the world of sense,
> Inoperancy of the world of spirit ...

'At other times,' Mr L. would tap out, 'there's none of this sense of pushing or active taking-away, but a sort of total calmless, a nothingness, which is by no means unpleasant. It's a let-up from the torture. On the other hand, it's something like death. At these times I feel I've been castrated by my illness, and relieved from all the longings other people have.' And when he was in *these* moods Mr L. would think of Abelard, and would tap out or mumur:

> For thee the fates, severely kind, ordain
> A cool suspense from pleasure and from pain,
> Thy life a long, dead calm of fix'd repose;
> No pulse that riots, and no blood that glows.
> Still as the sea, 'ere winds were taught to blow,
> Or moving spirit bade the waters flow.

At other times, Mr L. would describe for me states of perception and being to which he was frequently prone, both in his waking and his dreaming states – states which I have elsewhere called dynamic vision, and kinematic-mosaic vision.[46] My knowledge of such states, as they occur in post-

---

46. Such states may also occur in other intoxications induced by belladonna, LSD, etc., in psychoses, and especially during migraine attacks: see Ch. 3 and figs. 5b and 5c in my book *Migraine*.

encephalitic patients, has been especially derived from Mr L., who is so articulate, and from other patients (particularly Hester Y. and Rose R. as well as other patients whose histories are not given here), who frequently experienced such states without having Mr L.'s passion and power to describe them.

It was only very gradually, over the following years, with Mr L.'s help and that of his devoted mother – who was continually with him – that I was able to form any adequate picture of his state of mind and being, and the way in which this had developed in the preceding years. Mr L. had shown precocity and withdrawal from his earliest years, and these had become much accentuated with the death of his father when he was six. By the age of ten he would often say: 'I want to spend my life reading and writing. I want to bury myself among books. One can't trust human beings in the least.' In his early adolescent years Leonard L. was indeed continually buried in books, and had few or no friends, and indulged in none of the sexual, social or other activities common to boys of his age. At the age of fifteen his right hand started to become stiff, weak, pale and shrunken : these symptoms – which were the first signs of his post-encephalitic disease – were interpreted by him as a punishment for masturbation and for blasphemous thoughts; he would often murmur to himself the words of the 137th psalm ('If I forget thee, O Jerusalem, let my right hand forget its cunning') and 'If thy right hand offend thee cut it off.' He was reinforced in these morbid phantasies by the attitude of his mother who also saw his illness as a punishment for sin (compare Maria G.). Despite the gradual spread and progression of his disability, Leonard L. was able to go to Harvard and to graduate with honours, and had almost finished a thesis for his Ph.D. – in his twenty-seventh year – when his disability become so severe as to bring his studies and activities to a total halt. After leaving Harvard, he spent three years at home; and at the age of thirty, almost totally petrified, he was admitted to Mount Carmel Hospital. On his admission he was at once given charge of the hospital library. He could do little but read, and he *did* nothing but read. He indeed became buried in books from this time on, and thus, in a sense, achieved a dreadful fulfilment of his childhood wish.

In the years before I gave him L-DOPA I had many conversations with Leonard L., conversations which were necessarily somewhat one-sided and cursory since he could only answer my questions by painfully tapping out answers on his spelling-board – and his answers tended to assume an abbreviated, telegraphic, and sometimes cryptic form. When I asked him how he felt he would usually tap out 'meek', but he would also intimate that he sometimes had a sense of intense violence and power which was 'locked up' inside him, and which he experienced only in dreams. 'I have no exit,' he would tap out. 'I am trapped in myself. This stupid body is a prison with windows but no doors.' Although for much of the time, and in many ways, Mr L. hated himself, his disease and the world, he also had a great and unusual capacity for love. This was especially apparent in his reading and his reviewing, which showed a vital, humorous, and at times Rabelaisian relish for the world. And it was sometimes evident in his reaction to himself when he would spell out : 'I am what I am. I am part of the world. My disease and deformity are part of the world. They are beautiful in a way like a dwarf or a toad. It's my destiny to be a sort of grotesque.'

There existed an intense and mutual dependence between Mr L. and his mother, who came to the hospital to look after him for ten hours a day – a looking-after which included attention to his most intimate physical needs. One could see, when his mother was changing his nappies or bib, a look of blissful baby-like contentment on Mr L.'s face, admixed with impotent resentment at his degraded, infantilized and dependent state. His mother, similarly, showed and expressed a mixture of pleasure with her life-giving, loving and mothering role, admixed with intense resentment at the way in which her life was being 'sacrified' to her grown-up but helpless 'parasite' of a son. (Compare the relationship of Lucy K. and her mother.) Both Mr L. and his mother expressed uncertainty and ambivalence about the use of L-DOPA; both of them had read about it, but neither had actually seen its effects. Mr L. was the first patient in Mount Carmel whom I put on L-DOPA.

Course on L-DOPA

L-DOPA was started in early March 1969 and raised by degrees to 5·0 gm. a day. Little effect was seen for two weeks, and then a sudden 'conversion' took place. The rigidity vanished from all his limbs, and he felt filled with an access of energy and power; he became able to write and type once again, to rise from his chair, to walk with some assistance and to speak in a loud and clear voice – none of which had been possible since his twenty-fifth year. In the latter part of March, Mr L. enjoyed a mobility, a health and a happiness which he had not known in thirty years. Everything about him filled him with delight: he was like a man who had awoken from a nightmare or a serious illness, or a man released from entombment or prison, who is suddenly intoxicated with the sense and beauty of everything round him. During these two weeks, Mr L. was drunk on reality – on sensations and feelings and relations which had been cut off from him, or distorted, for many decades. He loved going out in the hospital garden: he would touch the flowers and leaves with astonished delight, and sometimes kiss them or press them to his lips. He suddenly desired to see the night-city of New York, which (although so close to) he had not seen, or wanted to see, in twenty years: and on his return from these night-drives he was almost breathless with delight, as if New York were a jewel or the New Jerusalem. He read the 'Paradiso' now – during the previous twenty years he had never got beyond 'Inferno' or 'Purgatorio' – with tears of joy on his face: 'I feel saved,' he would say, 'resurrected, re-born. I feel a sense of health amounting to Grace ... I feel like a man in love. I have broken through the barriers which cut me off from love.' The predominant feelings at this time were feelings of freedom, openness and exchange with the world; of a lyrical appreciation of a real world, undistorted by phantasy, and suddenly revealed; of delight and satiety with self and the world – 'I have been hungry and yearning all my life,' said Mr L., 'and now I am full. Appeased. Satisfied. I want nothing more.' He experienced a vanishing of hostility, anxiety, tensions and meanness – and in their place felt a sense of ease, of harmony and safety, of friendship and kinship with everything and everyone which he had never in his life experienced before – 'not even before the Parkinsonism', as he was the first to admit. The diary which he started to keep at this time was full of expressions of amazement and gratitude. '*Exaltavit humiles!*' he wrote on each page: and other exclamations like 'For *this* it was worth it, my life of disease,' 'L-DOPA is a *blessed* drug, it has given me back the possibility of life. It has opened me out where I was clammed tight-shut before,' and 'If everyone felt as good as I do, nobody would think of quarrelling or wars. Nobody would think of domination or possession. They would simply enjoy themselves and each other. They would realize that Heaven was right here down on earth.'

In April, intimations of trouble appeared. Mr L.'s abundance of health and energy – of 'grace' as he called it – became *too* abundant and started to assume an extravagant, maniacal and grandiose form; at the same time a variety of odd movements and other phenomena made their initial appearance. His sense of harmony and ease and effortless control was replaced by a sense of *too-muchness*, of force and pressure, and a pulling-apart – a pathological driving and fragmentation which increased, obviously and visibly, with each passing day. Mr L. passed from his sense of delight with existing reality, to a peremptory sense of mission and fate: he started to feel himself a Messiah, or the Son of God; he now 'saw' that the world was 'polluted' with innumerable Devils, and that he – Leonard L. – had been 'called on' to do battle with them. He wrote in his diary: 'I have Risen. I am still Rising. From the Ashes of Defeat to the Glory of Greatness. Now I must Go Out and Speak to the World.' He started to address groups of patients in the corridors of the hospital; to write a flood of letters to newspapers, congressmen, and the White House itself;[47] and he implored us to set up a sort of evangelical lecture-tour, so that he could exhibit himself all over the States, and proclaim the Gospel of Life according to L-DOPA.

Where, in April, he had had a marvellous sense of ease and satisfaction he now became uneasy and dissatisfied, and increasingly filled with painful, unsatisfiable appetites and desires. His hungers became transmogrified into insatiable passions and greeds. He ascended to heights of longing and phantasy which no reality could have met – least of all the grim and confining reality of a Total Institution, an asylum for the dilapidated and dying,[48] or – as he himself had described it three years earlier – a 'human zoo'. The most intense and the most thwarted of these yearnings were of a sexual nature, allied with desires for power and possession. No longer satisfied with the pastoral and innocent kissing of flowers, he wanted to touch and kiss all the nurses on the ward – and in his attempts to do so was rebuffed, at first with

47. Mr L. never actually sent out any of these letters, and spoke with irony of himself as 'a Parkinsonian Herzog'.

48. The hospital was, in fact, originally called 'The Mount Carmel Home for the Crippled and Dying', and despite having changed its lugubrious name, necessarily retained some of its original character.

smiles and jokes and good humour, and then with increasing asperity and anger. Very rapidly, in May, relationships became strained, and Mr L. passed from a gentle amorousness to an enraged and thwarted erotomania. Early in May he asked me if I could arrange for various nurses and nursing aides to 'service' him at night, and suggested – as an alternative – that a brothel-service be set up to meet the needs and the hungers of DOPA-charged patients.

By mid-May, Mr L. had become thoroughly 'charged up', in his own words, 'charged and super-charged' with a great surplus, a great *pressure*, of libidinous and aggressive feelings, with an avidity and voracity which could take many forms. In his phantasies, in his notebooks, and in his dreams, his image of himself was no longer that of the meek and mild and melancholy one, but of a burly caveman equipped with an invincible club and an invincible phallus; a Dionysiac god packed with virility and power; a wild, wonderful, ravening man-beast who combined kingly, artistic and genital omnipotence. 'With L-DOPA in my blood,' he wrote at this time, 'there's nothing in the world I can't do if I want. L-DOPA is power and irresistible force. L-DOPA is wanton, egotistical power. L-DOPA has given me the power I craved. I have been waiting for L-DOPA for the past thirty years.'[49] Driven at this time by libidinal force, he started to masturbate – fiercely, freely, and with little concealment – for hours each day. At times his voracity took other forms – hunger and thirst, and licking and lapping, biting and chewing, and sucking his tongue – all of which stimulated him and yielded something very similar to sexual pleasure (compare Margaret A., Rolando P., Maria G., *et al.*).

Coinciding with this surge of general excitement, Mr L. showed innumerable 'awakenings' and specific excitements – particular forms of urge and push, repetition, compulsion,

49. Compare the sentiments expressed by Freud about cocaine quoted in the Appendix.

suggestion, and perseveration. He started to talk with great speed, and to repeat words and phrases again and again (palilalia). He continually seized and held different objects with his eyes, and would be unable to relinquish his gaze voluntarily. He showed urges to pant and to clap his hands, and once he had started to do either of these he was unable to stop, but proceeded with continually increasing violence and speed until a sort of clench or freezing set in: these frenzied crescendos – a catatonic equivalent of Parkinsonian hurry and festination – yielded 'a surge of excitement, just like an orgasm'. In the latter half of May, reading became difficult because of uncontrollable hurry and perseveration: once he had started to read he would read faster and faster without regard for the sense or syntax, and unable to stop this festinant reading he would have to shut the book with a snap after each sentence or paragraph, so that he could digest its sense before rushing ahead. Tics appeared at this time, and grew more numerous daily: sudden impulsions and tics of the eyes, grimaces, cluckings, and lightning-quick scratchings. Finding himself distracted and decomposed by this increasing furor and fragmentation, Mr L. made his final effort at control, and decided – at the start of June – on an act of supreme coherence and catharsis – the writing of an autobiography: 'It'll bring me together,' he said; 'it'll cast out the devils. It'll bring everything into the full light of day.'

Using his shrunken, dystrophic index-fingers, Mr L. typed out an autobiography 50,000 words in length, in the first three weeks of June.[50] He typed almost ceaselessly – twelve or

50. Mr L.'s autobiography is a remarkable document, unique of its kind. Its style and content clearly show the conflicts which were raging in Mr L. at this time. For the most part, he shows an extraordinary humour, detachment and passion for accuracy, and provides penetrating and moving descriptions of his early years, the development of his illness and his reactions to this, his fellow patients at the home they all shared, his reactions to L-DOPA, his feeling towards the drug, towards me, and towards others. It is *also* interlarded with

fifteen hours a day, and *when* he typed he indeed 'came together', and found himself free from his tics and distractions, from the pressures which were driving and shivering his being; when he left the typewriter, the frantic, driven, ticcing palilalia would immediately assert its hegemony again.

During this writing, Mr L. felt a returning sense of strength and freedom, and a need of absolute solitude and concentration. He said to his mother at this time : 'Why don't you take off for a week or a month, go to Florida maybe – you could do with a rest. I'm independent now – I won't need you so much. I can do everything I want for myself right now.' His mother was greatly disturbed by these sentiments, and now showed how much *she* was in need of their relationship of symbiosis and dependence. She became greatly agitated, and came to me and to others several times at this period, saying that we had 'taken away' her son, and that she couldn't go on unless he were 'restored' to her : 'I can't bear Len, the way he is at the moment,' she said; 'the way he's so active and full of decision. He has pushed me away. He only thinks of himself. *I* need to be needed – it's the main need I have. Len's been my baby for the last thirty years, and you've taken him away with your darned El-Dopey !'[51]

---

waves and floods of sexual phantasy, jokes, pseudo-reminiscences, etc., which would rise up and engulf him from time to time; some of these are conflated with carnivorous and cannibalistic phantasies, with thoughts of raw meat to satisfy his needs : at this point Mr. L. calls himself 'the Parkinsonian Portnoy'.

51. Mrs L.'s attitude was not uncommon among relatives of our invalid patients. The restoration of activity and independence was by no means always welcomed by some of these relatives, and was sometimes passively or actively opposed. Some of these relatives had built their own lives around the illnesses of the patients, and – unconsciously, at least – did everything they could to reinforce the illness and dependence ensuing. One sees such social and familial reinforcement of illness in neurotic and schizophrenic families, of course, and – as I noted in my last book, *Migraine* – quite commonly also in migrainous families.

In the last week of June, and throughout July, Mr L. returned to his violently frenzied and fragmented state, and now this passed beyond all bounds of control, and brought into action ultimate physiological safeguards which in themselves were highly distressing or disabling.

His sexual and hostile phantasies now assumed hallucinatory form, and he had frequent voluptuous and demoniac visions,[52] and erotic dreams and nightmares each night. His

52. At first, Mr L. ingeniously controlled these hallucinations by confining them to the blank screen of his television set or a picture which hung on the wall opposite his bed. The latter – an old picture of a Western shanty-town – would 'come to life' when Mr L. gazed at it; cowboys on horses would gallop through the streets, and voluptuous whores would emerge from the bars. The screen of the television set was 'reserved' for the production of grinning and leering demoniac faces. Later in July, this 'controlled' hallucinosis (which had some analogies to that of Martha N. and Gertie C.) broke down, and his hallucinations 'escaped' from the picture and screen, and spread irresistibly in his whole mind and being.

ADDENDUM (1974): What I have said about Leonard L.'s hallucinosis requires amplification. Leonard L. had, in fact, been hallucinating for years – long before he ever received L-DOPA (although he was unable or unwilling to admit this to me until 1969). Being particularly fond of 'Western' scenes and films, Leonard L. had, indeed, ordered the old painting of the shanty-town as long ago as 1955 *for the sole and express purpose of hallucinating with it* – and it was his custom to 'animate' it for a hallucinatory matinée after lunch every day. It was only when he was maddened by L-DOPA that this chronic (and comic) and benign hallucinosis escaped from his will and imaginative control, and assumed a frankly psychotic character.

Those who hallucinate are, not unnaturally, usually reticent about their 'visions' and 'voices', etc., for fear that they will be regarded as eccentric or mad; and this was equally true of the large population of post-encephalitic patients resident at Mount Carmel. Moreover these patients also had, of course, very great physical difficulties in communication. It has taken many years for these patients to trust me, to *entrust* me with some of their most intimate experiences and feelings; and thus it is only *now* (in 1974), after we have known each other for almost a decade, that I find myself in a position to make a double observation: first, that at least a third, and

tics, his palilalia, his frenzies increased. His speech became broken by sudden intrusions and cross-associations of thought, and by repeated punning and clanging and rhyming. He started to experience forms of motor and thought 'blocking' very similar to those of Rose R. and Margaret A.: at such times he would suddenly call out, 'Dr Sacks! Dr Sacks! I want . . .', but be unable to complete what he wished to say; the same block was also manifest in his letters to me, which were full of violent, exclamatory starts (usually my name, followed by two or three words – in one such letter, impotently repeated twenty-three times) followed by sudden haltings and blocks. And in his walking and movements such blocks were apparent, which suddenly arrested him in mid-motor stream : he seemed, at such times, to be in collision with an invisible wall.

---

possibly a majority, of the deeply disabled and longest-institutionalized patients are 'chronic hallucinators'; and secondly, that in most cases it would be quite incorrect to use the term 'schizophrenic' of either the patients or their hallucinations. My reasons for saying this are, in essence, as follows : that most of the patients' hallucinations lack the ambivalent, often paranoiac, and in general uncontrollable nature of schizophrenic hallucinations; but that they are, in contrast, very like scenes of normal life, very much like that healthy reality from which these pathetic patients have been cut off for years (by illness, institutionalization, isolation, etc.). The function (and form) of schizophrenic hallucinations, in general, has to do with the *denial of reality*; whereas the function (and form) of the benign hallucinations seen in Mount Carmel has to do with *creating reality*, imagining a full and happy and healthy life of a sort which has been cruelly denied to them through Fate. Thus I regard it as a sign of these patients' health, of their enduring wish to live, and live fully – if only in the realms of imagination and hallucination, which are the only realms where they still enjoy freedom – that they hallucinate all the richness and drama and fullness of life. They hallucinate to *survive* – as do subjects exposed to extreme sensory, motor or social isolation; and for this reason, whenever I learn from a patient that he constructs a rich and benign hallucinatory 'life', I encourage him to the full, as I encourage all creative endeavours which reach out to life.

This period also saw the onset and progress of rapid exhaustions or reversals of response – an up-or-down or 'yoyo' reaction essentially similar to those shown by Hester Y., Margaret A., Maria G., Rolando P., and many of our other most severely affected patients. At such times, Mr L. would pass within minutes (and as his oscillations grew more severe, within seconds) from an intensely aroused and excited state to one of profound exhaustion, associated with severe recrudescence of Parkinsonian and catatonic immobility and rigidity. These switches (of reaction between agitated-manic-ticcy-akathisia and exhausted-depressed-Parkinsonian-akinesia) took place with continually increasing frequency and suddenness – at first related to the times of L-DOPA administration, and controllable to some extent by the times and the dosage: but then 'spontaneously', without any reference to dosage or times. During this period his total daily intake of L-DOPA was reduced from 5 gm. to 0·75 gm. a day, without making the least difference to his pattern of reaction; at this time also we followed the Cotzias schedule of giving him his L-DOPA in small frequent doses – we even tried him on hourly doses of the drug; but this also made no difference to his rapid and violent oscillations of response. All his reactions had become all-or-none. The 'middle-ground' of health, temper, harmony, moderation had almost entirely disappeared at this time, and Mr L. became completely 'decomposed' into pathological immoderations of every sort.

We could only guess at the relative importance of various determinants in this catastrophic reaction – the possibility of L-DOPA accumulating within him; a 'functional' conflagration, whereby one form of excitement led to another; the inevitability of exhaustions or 'crashes' given such stimulation; the lack of real absorbing occupation, or effective catharsis, with the finishing of his book; the deteriorating relationship between him and the nursing staff; or the implicit (if not explicit) demand by his mother for him to be

sick and dependent, and her disapproval or 'veto' of any improvement. It seemed likely that *all* of these factors – as well
as others which we could not formulate – were playing some
part in determining his reactions.

The closing scene of this so-mixed summer was precipitated by institutional disapproval of Mr L.'s ravening libido,
the threats and condemnations which this brought down on
him, and his final, cruel removal to a 'punishment cell' – a
tiny three-bedded room containing two dying and dilapidated terminal dements.[53] Deprived of his own room and all his

53. I thought at this time, and still think, that among the important non-pharmacological determinants of the reactions of these
patients to L-DOPA – and especially the form and severity of their
'side-effects' after a period of enormous improvement – the repressive
and censorious character of the institution they found themselves
in played a considerable part. In particular, the hospital administration frowned upon any manifestations of sexuality among the
inmates and often treated this with an irrational and cruel severity.
Leonard L., Rolando P., Frank G. and many other patients were, I
think, driven at times into depressive or paranoid psychoses by the
combination of a DOPA-induced libidinous arousal and its frustration
or punishment by the conditions and policies of institutional life. If,
as Mr L. suggested, some mode of sexual release had been provided or
permitted, the effects of L-DOPA might – perhaps – have been less
malignant.

A further factor, which doubtless added to Mr L.'s sexual drives and
their guilty moral recoil, was the too-close relation between him and
his mother. His mother – who, in a sense, was herself in love with her
son, as he was with her – became indignant and jealous of Mr L.'s
new thoughts: 'It's ridiculous,' she spluttered. 'A grown man like
him! He was so *nice minded* before – never spoke about sex, never
looked at girls, never seemed to think about the matter at all ... I
have sacrificed my life for Len: I am the one he should constantly
think of; but now all he thinks of is those *girls*!' On two occasions,
Mr L.'s thwarted sexuality became incestuous in direction, which out-
raged (but also titillated) his ambivalent mother. Once she confided
to me that 'Len was trying to *paw* me today; he made the most
horrible suggestions. *He said the worst thing in the world* – Bless
him,' and she blushed and giggled as she said this to me.

belongings, deprived of his identity and status in our post-encephalitic community, degraded to the physical and moral depths of the hospital, Mr L. fell into suicidal depression and infernal psychosis.

During this dreadful period at the close of July, Mr L. became obsessed with notions of torture, death and castration. He felt the room was a network of 'snares'; that there were 'ropes' in his belly which were trying to strangle him; that a gibbet had been set up, outside his room, for his impending and deserved execution for 'sin'. He felt that he was going to burst open, and that the world was coming to an end. He twice injured his penis, and once tried to suffocate himself by burying his head in his pillow.

We stopped his L-DOPA towards the end of July. His psychoses and tics continued for another three days, of their own momentum, and then suddenly came to a stop. Mr L. reverted during August to his original motionless state.

During August he scarcely moved or spoke at all – he had been returned to his original room – but reflected deeply on the preceding few weeks. In September he 'opened up' again to me, tapping his thoughts on his original letter-board. 'The summer was great and extraordinary,' he said (paraphrasing, as he was prone to, a poem of Rilke's[54]), 'but whatever happened then will not happen again. I thought I could make a life and a place for myself. I failed, and now I am content to be as I am; a *little* better perhaps, but no more of – all that.' At his request, then, I restarted Mr L. on L-DOPA in September 1969. He now showed the most extraordinary sensitivity to it – reacting strongly to a total dose of 50 mg. a day, where he had originally required 5,000 mg. a day. His response now was *entirely* pathological; he showed not a trace of therapeutic response, simply tics and tension and

54. Der Sommer war sehr gros.
    Wer jetzt kein Haus hat, baut sich keines mehr.

blocking of thought. 'You see,' he said afterwards, 'I told you so. You will never see anything like April again.'

In the past three years I have, in place of L-DOPA, repeatedly tried the use of amantadine, a drug with effects somewhat similar to, but milder than those of L-DOPA. I have given him amantadine eleven times in all. His reaction to this initially was very favourable, though lacking the intensity of the effects of L-DOPA. For almost ten weeks in the autumn of 1969 Mr L. was able to speak and move with some facility on amantadine without too much in the way of 'side-effects'; but towards the end of the year his reactions to amantadine became more pathological, the therapeutic reaction being displaced by a return to Parkinsonism and 'block', on the one hand, and an accession of tics and restlessness, on the other. With each succeeding use of amantadine the therapeutic effects became less marked and shorter in duration, and the pathological effects more marked. On his eleventh and final trial of amantadine in March 1972, Mr L. showed only pathological reactions to this. He said at this time, 'This is the end of the line. I have *had it* with drugs. There is no more you can do with me.'

Since this final, futile trial of amantadine, Mr L. has recovered his 'cool' and composure. He has, apparently, conquered his hopes and regrets, the violent feeling of promise and threat, which drugs thrust on him for more than three years. He has, finally, assimilated the entire mixed experience, and used his strength and intelligence to accommodate to it. 'At first, Dr Sacks,' he recently said, 'I thought L-DOPA was the most wonderful thing in the world, and I blessed you for giving me the Elixir of Life. Then, when everything went bad, I thought it was the worst thing in the world, a deathly poison, a drug which sent one down to the depths of hell; and I cursed you for giving it to me. I was terribly mixed in my feelings between fear and hope, and hatred and love ... Now I accept the whole situation. It was wonderful, terrible, dramatic and comic. It is finally – *sad*, and that's all there is to it. I'm best left alone – no more drugs. I've learned a great deal in the last three years. I've broken through barriers which I had all my life. And now, I'll stay myself, and you can keep your L-DOPA.'

PERSPECTIVES

PERSPECTIVES

The terrors of suffering, sickness and death, of losing our-selves and losing the world, are the most elemental and in-tense we know; and so too are our dreams of recovery and rebirth, of being wonderfully restored to ourselves and the world.

Our sense that there is *something the matter*, that we are ill or in error, that we have departed from health, that we are possessed by disorder and no longer ourselves – this is basic and intuitive in us; and so too is the sense of *coming to* or awakening, of resipiscence or recovery, being restored to ourselves and the world: the sense of health, of being well, fully alive, in-the-world.

Scarcely less basic are our *perversions* of being. Given cer-tain conditions, we create our own sickness; we imagine and construct innumerable diseases, whole worlds of mor-bidity which can defend or destroy:

> ... As the other world produces *Serpents*, and *Vipers*, malignant and venimous creatures, and *Wormes*, and *Caterpillars*, that en-deavour to devour that world that produces them ... so this world, ourselves, produces all these in us, in producing *diseases*, and *sicknesses*, of all these sorts; venimous and infectious diseases, feeding and consuming diseases, and manifold and entangled diseases, made up of several ones ... O miserable abundance, O beggarly riches!   DONNE

And as we allow diseases, so we can collude with them, and connive at them, greedily embracing sickness and suffering, plotting our own ruin, in a horrible peccancy of body and mind:

> ... We are not onely *passive*, but *active*, in our owne *ruine*; we do not onely stand under a *falling house*, but *pull* it downe upon us; and wee are not onely *executed*, but wee are *executioners*, and *executioners of our selves*.   DONNE

But, by the same token, we can resist and combat our own diseases, employing not only the remedies which physicians and others provide, but resources and strengths of our own which are inborn or acquired. We would never survive without these powers of health, so deep and far-reaching, which are, finally, the deepest and strongest we have. Yet we know so much of the devices of disease, and so little of the powers of health that are in us:

> To well manage our affections, and wild horses of *Plato*, are the highest Circenses; and the noblest Digladiation is in the Theater of ourselves; for therein our inward Antagonists, with ordinary Weapons and down right Blows make at us, but also like Retiary and Laqueary Combatants, with Nets, Frauds and Entanglements fall upon us. Weapons for such combats are not to be forged at *Lipara*; *Vulcan's Art* doth nothing in this Internal Militia ...
>   SIR THOMAS BROWNE

These are the terms in which we experience health and disease, and which we naturally use in speaking of them. They neither require nor admit definition; they are understood at once, but defy explanation; they are at once exact, intuitive, obvious, mysterious, irreducible and indefinable. They are *metaphysical* terms – the terms we use for infinite things. They are common to colloquial, poetic and philosophical discourse. And they are indispensable terms in medical discourse, which unites all of these. 'How are you?', 'How are things?', are metaphysical questions, infinitely simple and infinitely complex.

The whole of this book is concerned with these questions

– 'How are you?', How are things?' – as they apply to certain patients in an extraordinary situation. There are many legitimate answers to this question: 'Fine!', 'So-so', 'Terrible!', 'Bearing up', 'Not myself', etc.; evocative gestures; or simply *showing* how one is, how things stand, without use or need of special gestures or words. All of these are intuitively understood, and *picture* for one the state of the patient. But it is not legitimate to answer this metaphysical question with a list of 'data' or measurements regarding one's vital signs, blood chemistry, urinalysis, etc. A thousand such data don't begin to answer the essential question; they are irrelevant and, additionally, very crude in comparison with the delicacy of one's senses and intuitions:

> The *pulse*, the *urine*, the *sweat*, all have sworn to say nothing, to give no Indication, of any dangerous *sicknesse* ... And yet ... I feele, that insensibly the *Disease* prevailes.   DONNE

The dialogue about how one is can only be couched in human terms, familiar terms, which come easily and naturally to all of us; and it can only be held if there is a direct and human confrontation, an 'I–Thou' relation, between the discoursing worlds of physicians and patients.[1]

1. In *The Revised Confessions* de Quincey tells us how much he suffered from 'the pressure on the heart from the incommunicable'. This pressure, no doubt, is known to all of us; but it may approach the most agonizing level in patients whose sufferings are not only intense, but so *strange* as to seem, at first, beyond the possibilities of communication. Such difficulties in communication, clearly, can arise from the very strangeness, the extraordinary quality, of patients' problems, their experience; but an equal, if not greater, difficulty may be created by physicians themselves who, in effect, decline to listen to their patients, to treat them as equals, and who are prone to adopt – from force of habit, or from a less excusable sense of professional apartness and superiority – an approach and language which effectively *prevent* any real communication between themselves and their patients. Thus patients may be subjected to forms of interrogation and examination which smack of the schoolroom and

The situation is radically different with regard to the subject matter and discourse of logic, mathematics, mechanics, statistics, etc. For here the terms of reference – quantities, locations, durations, classes, functions, etc. – are clear-cut and finite, and thus admit of precise definition, enumeration, estimation and measurement. Moreover, one's attitude in such matters is radically different: one is no longer 'a man in his wholeness wholly attending'; one de-personalizes one's self and the object under survey, making of both an 'It'.[2]

---

the courtroom – questions of the form: 'Do you have *this* . . . do you have *that* . . . ?' which by their categorical nature demand categorical answers (yes and no answers, answers in terms of *this* and *that*). Such an approach forecloses the possibility of learning anything *new*, and prevents the possibility of forming a *picture*, or pictures, of what it is like to be as one is. The fundamental questions – 'How are you?' and 'What is it *like*?' – can only be answered analogically, allusively, in terms of 'as if' and likeness, by images, similitudes, models, metaphors, that is, by *evocations* of one sort and another. There can be no reaching out into the realm of the incommunicable (or the scarcely communicable) unless the physician becomes a fellow traveller, a fellow explorer, continually moving *with* his patients, discovering with them a vivid, exact, and figurative language which will reach out towards the incommunicable. *Together* they must create languages which bridge the gulf between physician and patient, the gulf which separates one man from another.

Such an approach is neither 'subjective' nor 'objective'; it is (in Rosenstock-Huessey's term) '*trajective*'. Neither seeing the patient as an impersonal object nor subjecting him to identifications and projections of himself, the physician must proceed by sympathy or empathy, proceeding in company with the patient, *sharing* his experiences and feelings and thoughts, the inner conceptions which shape his behaviour. He must feel (or imagine) how his patient is feeling, without ever losing the sense of himself; he must inhabit, simultaneously, two frames of reference, and make it possible for the patient to do likewise.

2. I should make it clear that my purpose is to distinguish two modes of clinical approach, and to indicate their complementarity – not to advocate either as against the other. We are faced, as physicians, with two sorts of problem, each requiring its own approach

Here, then, the basic question is: 'What exactly is the case with regard to *this* at this particular time and place?' And

---

and language: one is the problem of *identification*, the other is the problem of *understanding*. Identification, in this sense, is essentially legal in nature – the same term ('case') is used in medicine and law. Faced with a 'case' of something or other, we seek for 'evidence' which will enable us to arrive at a diagnostic decision. This evidence may take various forms – *symptoms* which form the grounds of complaint; *signs* which are regarded as specific to specific disorders; *tests* to confirm or refute our suspicions. When we have gathered the requisite testimony we say, 'This is a case of such-and-such' and 'The requisite treatment is such-and-such': the case has been 'considered' and is now ready to be 'disposed of' or 'closed'. Our sole concern in this judicial process is the treatment of diagnostically relevant criteria, and the search for data which meet these criteria. The business of 'understanding' is nowhere relevant, nor is the question of 'care' for the patient: diagnostic medicine could be entirely carried out by the rote application of rules and techniques, which a computer could undertake as well as a doctor.

Such a mechanical and technological medicine is ethically neutral and epistemologically sound – it advances continually, it has saved countless lives. It only becomes unsound and wrong if it excludes non-mechanical or non-technological approaches, if it displaces clinical dialogue and an existential approach. 'Cases' are abstract; patients are people, people who are suffering, perplexed and fearful. Patients need proper diagnosis and treatment, but they also need understanding and care; they need human relationship and existential encounter, which cannot be provided by any technology.

Thus our theme and plea relates to the *complemantarity* of both approaches – the development of the technical without any forfeit of the human: what Buber has called 'the humanization of technology, before it dehumanizes us'. Such a complementarity is bound to be present if the physician stands in a proper relation to his patients – a relation which is neither sentimental nor mechanical – but one which is based on deep *consideration*, on an inseparable combination of wisdom and care. Thus Leibniz, who amongst so much else was one of the greatest of jurists, regarded legalisms and mechanisms as purely secondary, and defined law and judgement in fundamentally ethical and existential terms – as '*caritas sapientis*'. If we care, and care wisely for our patients, everything else will fall into place.

the answer is couched in terms of when, where, and how much : the world is reduced to pointing and points.[3]

Both types of discourse are complete in themselves; they can neither include nor exclude one another; they are complementary; and both are vital in understanding the world. Thus Leibniz, comparing metaphysical and mechanical approaches, writes :

> I find indeed that many of the effects of nature can be accounted for in a two-fold way, that is to say by a consideration of efficient causes and again independently by a consideration of final causes . . . Both explanations are good, not only for the admiring of the work of a great artificer, but also for the discovery of useful facts in Physics and Medicine. And writers who take these diverse routes should not speak ill of each other . . . The best plan would be to join the two ways of thinking.

Leibniz stresses, however, that metaphysics comes first : that although the workings of the world never contravene mechanical considerations, they only make sense, and become fully intelligible, in the light of metaphysical considerations; that the world's mechanics subserve its design.[4]

If this were clearly understood, no trouble would arise. Folly enters when we try to 'reduce' metaphysical terms and matters to mechanical ones : worlds to systems, particulars to

3. The entire body of the *Philosophical Investigations* is, in a sense, concerned with the distinction between *pointing language* (a language in which 'every word has a meaning. The meaning is correlated with the word. It is the object for which the word stands.') and *evocative language*. Wittgenstein here shows, with extreme penetration and clearness, how a pointing-language (or calculus) is always inadequate to describe the real world, how its use is confined to what is abstract and 'unreal'.

4. These quotations and paraphrases of Leibniz are taken from his *Discourse on Metaphysics* and his *Correspondence with Arnauld*, which, though written in the 1680s, were only published in the 1840s, subsequent to the death of Locke, Hume and Kant.

categories, impressions to analyses, and realities to abstractions. This is the madness of the last three centuries, the madness which so many of us – as individuals – go through, and by which all of us are tempted. It is this Newtonian–Lockean–Cartesian view – variously paraphrased in medicine, biology, politics, industry, etc. – which reduces men to machines, automata, puppets, dolls, blank tablets, formulae, ciphers, systems, and reflexes. It is this, in particular, which has rendered so much of our recent and current medical literature unfruitful, unreadable, inhuman, and unreal.

There is nothing alive which is not individual : our health is *ours*; our diseases are *ours*; our reactions are *ours* – no less than our minds or our faces. Our health, diseases, and reactions cannot be understood *in vitro*, in themselves; they can only be understood with reference to *us*, as expressions of our nature, our living, our being-here (*da-sein*) in the world. Yet modern medicine, increasingly, dismisses our existence, either reducing us to identical replicas reacting to fixed 'stimuli' in equally fixed ways, or seeing our diseases as purely *alien* and bad, without organic relation to the person who is ill. The therapeutic correlate of such notions, of course, is the idea that one must *attack* the disease with all the weapons one has, and that one can launch the attack with total impunity, without a thought for the *person* who is ill. Such notions, which increasingly dominate the entire landscape of medicine, are as mystical and Manichean as they are mechanical and inhuman, and are the more pernicious because they are not explicitly realized, declared, and avowed.[5]

---

5. One must wonder, how could the notion of diseases as *alien* arise? How can one suppose that diseases are not parts of ourselves, and parts of the world, but *outside* Nature, or demonic? For such a supposition is clearly insane. To suppose that diseases, or anything, are alien is the clearest sign of one's own alienation, that one is no longer in touch with oneself and the world.

The notion that disease-causing agents and therapeutic agents are things-in-themselves is often ascribed to Pasteur, and it is therefore salutary to remember Pasteur's death-bed words:

Bernard is right; the pathogen is nothing; the *terrain* is everything.

Diseases have a character of their own, but they also partake of our character; we have a character of our own, but we also partake of the world's character: character is monadic or microcosmic, worlds within worlds within worlds, worlds which express worlds. The disease–the man–the world go together, and cannot be considered separately as things-in-themselves. An adequate concept or characterization of a man (Adam, in Leibniz's example) would embrace all that happened to him, all that affected him, and all that he affected; and its terms would combine contingency with necessity, allowing the perpetual possibility of 'alternative Adams'. Leibniz's ideal is thus a perfectly shaped and detailed history, or disclosure, or biography, an integral combination of science and art.[6]

In our own time, the most perfect examples of such biography (or pathology) are the matchless case-histories of Freud. Freud here shows, with absolute clarity, that the ongoing nature of neurotic illness and its treatment cannot be displayed *except* by biography.

But the history of neurology has nothing, or almost noth-

6. In the case of illness, one's confinement, one's surroundings, one's hopes and one's fears, what one hears, or believes, one's physician, *his* behaviour, are all coalesced in a single picture or drama. Thus Donne, on his sick-bed, writes: 'I observe the Phisician, with the same diligence, as hee the disease; I see he feares, and I feare with him: I overtake him, I overrun him in his feare, and I go the faster, because he makes his pace slow; I feare the more, because he disguises his fear, and I see it with the more sharpnesse, because hee would not have me see it . . . he knows that my fear may disorder the effect, and working of his practice.'

ing, of this sort to offer.[7] It is as if some absolute and categorical distinction had been made between the nature of neurotic and neurological illness, the latter being seen as arrays of 'facts' without design or connection. Everything real and concrete, in a sense, has a history and a life: did not Faraday provide a charming example of this in his 'History of a Candle'? Why should diseases be exceptions? And why especially such extraordinary illnesses as Parkinsonism and post-encephalitic 'syndromes', which have such profound (if generally unregarded) analogies to neurotic illness? If ever an illness and a 'cure' called out for a dramatic and biographic presentation, the story of Parkinsonism and L-DOPA does so. If we seek a 'curt epitome' of the human condition – of long-standing sickness, suffering and sadness; of a sudden, complete, almost preternatural 'awakening'; and, alas! of entanglements which may follow this 'cure' – there is no better one than the story of these patients.

Not that there is any dearth of writing on the subject: a vast flood of papers, articles, reports, reviews, editorials, proceedings of conferences, etc., has poured forth since Dr Cotzias's pioneer paper in February 1967, to say nothing of rhapsodic (and often unscrupulous) advertisements and newspaper articles. But there is, I believe, something quite fundamental which is missing in these. One mulls over whole libraries of papers, couched in the 'objective', styleless style *de rigueur* in neurology; one's head buzzes with 'facts', figures,

7. Among the few exceptions may be mentioned the fascinating and witty 'Confessions of a Tiqueur', at the start of Meige and Feindel's book *Tics*, and the very fine psychoanalytically oriented case-histories of post-encephalitic syndromes given in Jelliffe's two books on the subject (*Post-encephalitic Respiratory Disorders*, Washington, 1927; and *Psychopathology of Forced Movements and the Oculogyric Crises of Lethargic Encephalitis*, Washington, 1932). The finest recent examples of such biographical case-histories have been provided by A. R. Luria (*The Mind of a Mnemonist* and *The Man with a shattered World*, both published by Penguin, 1975).

lists, schedules, inventories, calculations, ratings, quotients, indices, statistics, formulae, graphs, and whatnot; everything 'calculated, cast-up, balanced, and proved' in a manner which would have delighted the heart of Thomas Gradgrind.[8] And nowhere, *nowhere*, does one find any colour, reality, or warmth; nowhere any residue of the living experience; nowhere any impression or picture of what it *feels* like to have Parkinsonism, to receive L-DOPA, and to be totally transformed. If ever there were a subject which needed a non-mechanical treatment, it is this one; but one looks in vain for life in these papers; they are the ugliest exemplars of assembly-line medicine: everything human, everything living, pounded, pulverized, atomized, quantized, and otherwise 'processed' out of existence.

And yet – it is the most enchanting of subjects, as dramatic, and tragic, and comic as any. My own feelings, when I first saw the effects of L-DOPA, were of amazement and wonder, and almost of awe. Each passing day increased my amazement, disclosing new phenomena, novelties, strangenesses, whole worlds of being whose possibility I had never dreamt of – I felt like a slum-child suddenly transplanted to Africa or Peru.

This sense of worlds upon worlds, of a landscape continually extending, reaching beyond my sight or imagination, is one which has always been with me, since I first encountered my post-encephalitic patients in 1966, and first gave them L-DOPA in 1969. It is a very mixed landscape, partly familiar, partly uncanny, with sunlit uplands, bottomless chasms, volcanoes, geysers, meadows, marshes; something like Yellowstone – archaic, prehuman, almost prehistoric,

8. 'Thomas Gradgrind, Sir – peremptorily Thomas – Thomas Gradgrind. With a rule and a pair of scales, and the multiplication tables always in his pocket, sir, ready to weigh and measure any parcel of human nature, and tell you exactly what it comes to. It is a mere question of figures, a case of simple arithmetic.'

with a sense of vast forces simmering all round one. Freud once spoke of neurosis as akin to a prehistoric, Jurassic landscape, and this image is still truer of post-encephalitic disease, which seems to conduct one to the dark heart of being.[9]

9. The use of this Conradian phrase (though Conrad was not in my conscious thoughts as I wrote!) epitomizes a certain *doubleness* of attitude, a complexity of feeling which I cannot wholly resolve. A number of those who read the original edition of this book, and who saw the film made about it, spoke of various scenes and phenomena as being 'shocking', 'extraordinary', and even 'horrible'; one reviewer went so far as to say that the film made him 'lose his faith in God'. My own 'faith in God', or feeling about the world, is not as simple or as brittle as that of this obviously sincere and good-hearted man; nevertheless, I have to confess that my own experiences with these patients in *Awakenings* also gave me an unprecedented sense of shock, and was instrumental in introducing into my world-picture a complexity and depth which it had lacked before (or which, at least, I had never consciously allowed or avowed).

I was forced to hear words and use terms which I had never previously allowed into scientific descriptions. Thus I note of Hester Y. that her sudden awakening filled me, and all those around her, with 'awe', and that we found her awakening 'just like a miracle'. I quote the words of Ida T.: 'wonderful, wonderful! ... that dopey's a *Mitzphah*!' and of Maria G.'s parents: 'A miracle from Heaven ... a completely new person'. On the other hand, I note the 'dark' side of patients' awakenings; that Frances D. (who called L-DOPA 'Hell-DOPA') found herself face to face with 'very deep and ancient parts of herself, monstrous creatures from her unconscious, and from unimaginable physiological depths below the unconscious ... prehistoric and pre-human landscapes ...'; and that even in a patient as prosaic and good-humoured as Lillian W. there was a sense of the anarchic, the absurd, the grotesque, of crises and symptoms so surrealistic and strange as to seem lacking not only in moral nature, but in any intelligible nature at all.

All of this shocked me, in a fundamental way, shocked my pre-existing ideas of the world. *Credo ut intellegam*: my *Credo* had always been one of Simplicity and Order, Light and Reason, of Nature as ultimate Harmony and Calm. But now I was abruptly faced with a fierceness, a wildness, a strangeness in Nature, something which seemed *Pandemoniac*, the very reverse of order and calm. I felt like a sailor who has been confidently sailing on a calm, friendly sea,

Wittgenstein once remarked that a book – like the world – could convey its subject-matter by *examples*, anything further being redundant. My prime intention, in this book, has been to provide examples.

Hitherto we have travelled, in imagination, *with* our patients, tracing with them the course of their lives, their illness, and their reactions to L-DOPA. Now, we can remove ourselves from this itinerary, from history and happening,

---

who all of a sudden is assailed by an unbelievably violent, fantastic storm; or like the heroine-victim of St *Mawr*, who, thinking to establish a sweet and neat New England garden in New Mexico, finds herself assaulted, engulfed, by a huge wild jungle, by the monstrous fertile forces of primitive Nature.

I was forced to wonder if my previous world-views had not been too pallid, too superficial, and altogether too 'rational' – mere skimmings or skatings on the surface of reality; if I had not been denying the fierce complexity of Nature, profoundly important determinants of being – forces below the surface of the conscious, forces below the surface of the world, powers beyond powers, depths beneath depths, extending into the infinite depths of our world-home, the cosmos. On the surface there was Apollonian light and calm, everything 'rational and reconciled'; beneath – I knew not what chthonic or Dionysiac depths. As my first sight of Yellowstone revealed to me monstrous, plutonic powers and depths, neither visible nor imaginable under 'ordinary' circumstances, so the extraordinary phenomena presented by my patients hinted at unseen, unsuspected, and almost *wanton* human depths, innumerable 'Ids' below the lowest level of which Freud spoke – or perhaps one vast 'Id', an ancient savage core of power like the primordial energy of the cosmos itself. This deepest 'Id' of all – neither 'good' nor 'evil', moral nor immoral, rational nor irrational, orderly nor unruly (unless all of these at once, complected together); this endlessly resourceful, creative Force seemed to be the very spirit of Nature itself, the urge *to be* (and to persist and grow in self-being), that ever-living, ever-struggling, self-realizing *conatus* of which Spinoza and Leibniz spoke in identical terms.

Thus, when I speak of being led to 'the dark heart of Being', I imply nothing base, Manichean, or arcane, nothing diabolic or morally dark. I imply altitude, depth, the abyss, the heights – a vision of the numinous centre of things, the radiant spirit of the phenomenal world.

and gaze more fully at certain *aspects* of the landscape, at patterns-of-reaction which have special importance.

We have no need to look farther afield – above or below or behind or beyond anything which we have seen so far. We have no need to chase after 'causes', or theories and explanations – anything which lies *outside* our observations:

Everything factual is, in a sense, theory ... There is no sense in looking for something behind phenomena: they *are* theory.

GOETHE

We have no need to go beyond the evidence of our senses. But what we need is an approach, a language, which is adequate for the subject. The terms of existing neurology, for example, cannot begin to indicate what is happening with the patient; we are concerned not simply with a handful of 'symptoms', but with a *person*, and his changing relation to the world. Moreover, the language we need must be both particular and general, combining reference to the patient and *his* nature, and to the world and *its* nature. Such terms – at once personal and universal, concrete and metaphorical, simple and deep – are the terms of *metaphysics*, or colloquial speech. These terms, of course, are those of '*health*' and '*disease*', the simplest and deepest terms we know. Our task – in the context of patients' reactions to L-DOPA – is to explore the meaning of these terms, to avoid superficial definitions and dichotomies, and to *feel* (beyond the range of formulations) the intimate, essential nature of each.

The quantitative welfare statistics of existing studies of L-DOPA are really a paradigm of the Benthamite felicific calculus ('the greatest good of the greatest number'), or of F. Y. Edgeworth's 'Hedonical Calculus'. The brevity and use of such an actuarial approach can be conceded at once, whereas its limitations (and cruelties) are covert and implicit, and need exposure to the full light of day. The utilitarian approach is not couched in terms of particulars and universals, and its terms necessarily hide both from sight; it gives us no insight whatever into the general design of behaviour, or into the ways in which this is exemplified in particular patients; it positively stands in the way of such insight.

If we are to learn anything *new* from our study, we must pay attention to the precise forms and relationships of all phenomena seen, to 'health' and 'disease' in terms of design. We need infinite terms for infinite states (worlds), and must go to Leibniz, not Bentham, for appropriate concepts. The Leibnizian 'optimum' – health – is not a numerical quotient, but an allusion to the greatest fullness of relationship possible in a total world-manifold, the organization with the greatest richness and reality. Diseases, in this sense, depart from the optimum, for their organization or design is impoverished and rigid (although they have frightening strengths of their own). Health is infinite and expansive in mode, and reaches out to be filled with the fullness of the world; whereas disease is finite and reductive in mode, and endeavours to reduce the world to itself.

Health and disease are alive and dynamic, with powers and propensities and 'wills' of their own. Their modes of being are inherently antithetical: they confront one another in perpetual hostility – our 'Internal Militia', in Sir Thomas Browne's words. Yet the outcome of their struggle cannot be pre-determined or pre-judged, any more than the outcome of a chess-game or tournament. The rules are fixed but the strategy is not, and one can learn to outplay one's antagonist, Sickness. In default of health, we manage, by *care*, and control, and cunning, and skill and luck.

Health, disease, care – these are the most elemental concepts we have, the only ones adequate to bear the discussion. When we give L-DOPA to patients, we see first an emergence from sickness – an AWAKENING; then a relapse, and a multiplication of problems and troubles – TRIBULATION;

finally, perhaps, the patient reaches a sort of 'understanding' or balance with his problems – this we can call AC-COMMODATION. It is in terms of this sequence – Awakening ... Tribulation ... Accommodation – that we can best discuss the consequences of L-DOPA.[10]

AWAKENING

Virtually all patients with true Parkinsonism show some sort of 'awakening' when given L-DOPA.[11] This is true of

10. Many other metaphorical triads might be used, e.g.:

Being-Well	Being-Ill	Bearing-up
Satisfaction (Benefaction)	Dissatisfaction (Malefaction)	Assuefaction
Peace	War	Reconciliation
Union	Disunion	Reunion
Unspoiltness	Spoilage (Degeneration)	Recovery (Regeneration)
Grace	Dis-grace (Lapse, Fall)	Courage
Rootedness (Autochthony)	Uprootedness	Re-rootedness
At-homeness	Departure	Return

Such allegorical sequences recapitulate, in a way, the original course of these patients' lives and illnesses, before the advent of L-DOPA; they recapitulate in a more general way the course of all our lives, and of history and culture; they constitute a paradigm of being human and being alive in the world.

11. A few patients may fail to show awakening on L-DOPA and instead be thrust into deeper illness; moreover, the response may be quite different at different times in a single patient. Thus, among post-encephalitic patients at Mount Carmel not described in this book, one initially became comatose with the administration of L-DOPA, but when given it a year later showed a dramatic awakening. Another (Seymour L.), when first given L-DOPA in April 1969, showed a dramatic but very short-lived awakening, which was

all but three (Robert O., Frank G., Rachel I.) of the patients described in this book, and of all but a score of the two hundred Parkinsonian patients to whom I have given L-DOPA. In general – though this is not always the case – awakening

---

compromised within a month by respiratory crises, side-to-side lunging movements of the neck and trunk, hallucinations, tics, etc., necessitating discontinuance of the drug; when given a *minute* dose of L-DOPA (100 mg. daily) twenty months later, he showed a disastrous reaction, being immediately precipitated into a state of greatly exacerbated Parkinsonism and catalepsy, followed by coma; but when placed on L-DOPA for the *third* time, in October 1972, he not only did well, but has maintained this excellent reaction up to the time of writing (October 1974). It is *perhaps* germane to say that Seymour L. is a man of most unusual intelligence, courage and goodness-of-heart, and that he went through a protracted period of the most intensive soul-searching and self-examination after his disastrous and near-fatal reaction to L-DOPA at the end of 1970. I have seen similar sequences with other patients, for example Gertie C., who was put on L-DOPA again early in the summer of 1974, after a gap of almost four years, and has since maintained a stable, happy, and tranquil reaction and a renewed ability for speech. I cannot judge whether such unexpectedly auspicious responses to renewed administration of L-DOPA have some simple physiological explanation, or whether they have occurred in consequence of a great inner act of psychophysiological '*accommodation*' (as described in the section on this). I am inclined to suspect the latter, because in *general*, unhappily, the chances of doing well on L-DOPA diminish with every successive trial.

Patients with 'pseudo-Parkinsonism' (e.g. Parkinsonian-like pictures associated with disease of the cortex – a not uncommon situation in elderly patients) show virtually no awakening at all. I drew attention to this in 1969 (see *Lancet*, 13 September 1969, pp. 591–2) and suggested at this time that trial with L-DOPA might thus be useful in distinguishing such patients from true Parkinsonians.

The aetiology of the Parkinsonism, in itself, is not of significance in modifying reactions to L-DOPA: thus toxic Parkinsonism, associated with manganese or carbon monoxide poisoning, may respond well to L-DOPA. Among my own patients who have done well when given L-DOPA have been three who suffered from syphilitic Parkinsonism (Wilson's 'syphilitic mesencephalitis') associated with tabes.

is most profound and most rapid in patients with the severest disease, and may be virtually instantaneous in patients with 'imploded' (or 'Black Hole') types of Parkinsonism-catatonia (e.g. Hester Y.). In patients with ordinary Parkinson's disease, awakening may be extended over a matter of days, although it usually reaches its zenith within two weeks or so. In post-encephalitic patients, as our case-histories have shown, awakening tends to be much prompter and more dramatic; moreover, post-encephalitic patients, in general, are much more sensitive to L-DOPA, and may be awakened by a fifth or less of the doses required for 'ordinary' patients.

An 'ordinary' patient may be in excellent (behavioural) health apart from his Parkinsonism, and this itself may be mild, and of relatively short duration; for such a patient, therefore, getting well or awakening chiefly consists in a reduction or apparent abolition of his Parkinsonism; there *are* other aspects to awakening, even in such patients, but these are much more readily studied in profoundly and chronically disabled post-encephalitic patients, who suffer from a great number of disabilities in addition to Parkinsonism. These patients, we have seen, may show profound reductions not only of their Parkinsonism, but of innumerable *other* problems – torsion-spasms, athetosis, chorea, tics, catatonia, depression, apathy, torpor etc., etc. – from which they concurrently suffered. Such patients recover, not from one malady, but from a multitude of illnesses, and in extremely short order. All manner of disorders, which are not usually taken to have a dopamine-substrate or to be amenable to L-DOPA, may nevertheless vanish as the Parkinsonism vanishes. Such patients, in short, may experience a virtually *total* return to health, a recovery which is over and above anything one

---

The term 'awakening', (or 'behavioural arousal') was used as early as 1960, with regard to the effects of L-DOPA on animals, and was used by Cotzias *et al.* in their pioneer paper.

could predict from our knowledge of the location and functions of L-DOPA, etc., or from our currently accepted physiological picture of the brain. That such virtually simultaneous-instantaneous awakenings occur is not only of profound therapeutic interest, but of momentous physiological and epistemological interest.

Certain feelings are invariably experienced during a profound awakening, and are described by patients in figurative terms very similar to those which an 'outside' observer would invoke. The sudden relief of Parkinsonism, catatonia, tensions, torsions, etc., is experienced as a deflation or detumescence, a sudden relief of an internal pressure; patients often compare it to passing flatus, eructation, or emptying of the bladder. And this is exactly how it looks to an external observer: the stiffness or spasm or swelling disappears, and suddenly the patient is 'relaxed', and at ease. Patients who comment on the 'pressure' or 'force' of their Parkinsonism, etc., are clearly not speaking in physical terms, but in ontological or metaphysical terms which correspond to their experience. The terms of 'pressure' or 'force' indicate something about the *organization* of illness, and give a first inkling of the nature of ontological or 'inner' space in these patients; and in all of us.

This return-to-oneself, resipiscence, 'rebirth', is an infinitely dramatic and moving event, especially in a patient with a rich and full self, who has been *dispossessed* by disease for years or decades (e.g. Hester Y.). Furthermore, it shows us, with wonderful clarity, the dynamic relation of sickness to health, of a 'false self' to the real self, of a disease-world to an optimum-world. The automatic return of real being and health, *pari passu* with the drainage of disease, shows that disease is not a thing-in-itself, but parasitic on health and life and reality: an ontological ghoul, living on and consuming the grounds of the real self ('draining the *da-sein*', in

Binswanger's term). It shows the dynamic and implacable nature of our 'internal militia'; how opposed forms of being fight to possess us, to dispossess each other, and to perpetuate themselves.[12]

That a return to health or resipiscence is *possible*, in these patients with half a century of the profoundest illness, must fill one with a sense of amazement – that the potential for health and self can *survive*, after so much of the life and structure of the person has been lost, and after so long and exclusive an immersion in sickness. This also is of major importance, not only therapeutically, but theoretically as well.[13]

12. This reciprocity between health (real-being, *da-sein*) and sickness (false-being, non-being) is quite apparent even in the absence of L-DOPA. One sees, in practice, again and again, how Parkinsonism may suddenly burst into apparency – from a previously inapparent, latent or virtual condition – if a person becomes ill (in some other way), profoundly exhausted, shocked, depressed, etc., how it takes over and flourishes with the ebbing of health; one sees, equally clearly, how it may then 'go away' again – retreat into inapparency, latency, virtuality – with the return of strength and abounding health. Thus, two years ago, I had occasion to see an old lady who, the day before falling and breaking her hip, had been 'full of life', and had shown not the least sign of Parkinsonism (or none that was recognized); the following day, when I saw her, she was in some pain, but – more significantly – had suffered, and showed, an existential collapse, a sense that she was 'finished' and that death was near, a draining away of her vitality and *da-sein*; *now*, in addition to looking half-dead, she was deeply Parkinsonian; three days later, she 'was herself' once again – she felt full of life and no longer showed the least trace of Parkinsonism. She has continued in excellent health since this time, and has not again shown any manifest Parkinsonism. I have no doubts, however, that it is *there* (in potential, in propensity, latent, dormant, *in posse*), and will again come to the forefront if her health, her real-being, is injured or lost.

13. The comparison of such awakenings to so-called '*lucid intervals*' will at once occur to many readers. At such times – despite the presence of massive functional or structural disturbances to the brain – the patient is suddenly and completely *restored to himself*. One

If we are to understand the *quality* of awakening, and of the awakened state – health – we must depart from the physiological and neurological terms which are generally used, and heed the terms which patients themselves tend to use. Currently used neurological and neuro-physiological terms

observes this, again and again, at the height of toxic, febrile, or other deliria: sometimes the person may be recalled to himself by the calling of his name; then, for a moment or a few minutes, he is himself, before he is carried off by delirium again. In patients with advanced senile dementias, or pre-senile dementias (e.g. Alzheimer's disease), where there is abundant evidence of all types regarding the massive loss of brain structure and function, one may also – very suddenly and movingly – see vivid, momentary recalls of the original, lost person.

Again, there is described, and I have seen, the sudden 'sobering' effect of illness, tragedy, bereavement, etc., on profoundly deteriorated, 'burnt-out', hebephrenic schizophrenics; such patients – who may have been 'decomposed' into a swarm of mannerisms, impulsions, automatisms and mocking 'selflets' for decades – may *come together* in a moment faced with an overwhelming reality.

But one need not look for such far-out examples. All of us have experienced sudden composures, at times of profound distraction and disorganization; sudden sobriety, when intoxicated; and – especially as we grow older – sudden total recalls of our past or our childhood, recalls so complete as to be a re-being. All of these indicate that one's self, one's style, one's *persona* exists as such, in its infinitely complex and particular being; that it is not a question of this system or that, but of a total organization which must be described as a self. Style, in short, is the deepest thing in one's being. An extraordinary example of this is provided by a number of letters which I once saw, written by Henry James when he was in a terminal, extremely febrile, pneumonia delirium: these letters show clear evidences of delirium, but their *style* is unmistakably and uniquely that of Henry James, and indeed, of 'late' Henry James.

Many neuropsychologists, pre-eminently Lashley, have spent their lives 'in search of the Engram': the work of Lashley, in particular, has conclusively shown how individual skills and memories may survive massive and varied extirpations of the brain. Such experimental observations, like careful and thoughtful clinical observations (most notably those of Luria, as set out in *The Man with a Shattered*

have reference to alterations of energy-level and energy-distribution in the brain; we must also use energetic and economic concepts, but in a radically different way from the way in which they are generally used.

We have already spoken (pp. 50–51.) of the two schools

World), indicate that one's *persona* is in no way 'localizable' in the classical sense, that it cannot be equated with any given 'centre', 'system', 'nexus', etc., but only with the intricate totality of the whole organism, in its ever-changing, continuously modulated, afferent-efferent relation with the world. They show, instead, that one's ontological organization, one's entire being – for all its multiplicity, all its shimmering, ever-shifting succession of patterns (Hume's 'bundle of perceptions', Proust's 'collection of moments') – is nevertheless a coherent and continuing entity, with a historical, stylistic and imaginative continuity, with the unity of a life-long symphony or poem; that it is not a thing-in-itself, but a special being-in-relation, a being-there in the world, a minute but active and self-aware microcosm of the world. We see that our beings are at once unique yet communal, inherent in us, specific to us, but also in perpetual co-relation with the world : that our selves are entelechies or monads in nature.

The reader will perhaps concede that a person who is sufficiently 'together' as a person may indeed retain his 'togetherness' in the face of overwhelming structural brain damage; but what – he will say – what of the integrity of the self in severe neurotic and schizophrenic disintegrations? Have I myself not spoken freely of 'dissociation', 'disintegration', 'decomposition', etc.? Have I not spoken of 'splitting' and 'selflets'? Clearly I must qualify these terms, if I am to maintain that everyone has a definite, entire, and (in a sense) inviolable self ... I feel readier to attempt this on the basis of recent clinical experience, in particular the experience of working with a number of very deeply disturbed and 'disintegrated' schizophrenics, as I have done in the two years which have passed since the original writing of this book. My initial approach to these patients (this was a theoretical and heuristic, not a personal, approach) was partly Kraepelinian and partly Freudian; that is to say, I looked for 'symptoms', on the one hand, and 'processes', on the other; and, needless to say, I found an abundance of both. But I *also* found (as I find with my friends!) that these patients could not be 'reduced' to their 'component parts', either in classical or Freudian terms; I found that I

in classical neurology – the holists and topists, or, in their
own vernacular – the 'lumpers' and 'splitters'. Holists refer
to the 'total energy' of the brain as if this were something
uniform, undifferentiated, and quantifiable. They speak, for
example, of arousal and activation, of increased activity in

---

could not approach them, either heuristically or practically, if I did
so in a purely *empirical* way. No matter how scattered or regressed
the patient, I found that other sorts of concepts were essential to
understanding (and to treatment). This radical revision of thought
and attitude was far from easy; it entailed an epistemological and
emotional crisis very similar to that described by Hume when he
found that his empirical approach to human nature had arrived
nowhere, and had to be given up entirely to make a re-approach possible; at this point (very beautifully described in the closing pages of
Book I of his *Treatise*) Hume realized that the concept of 'Personal
Identity' *could not be arrived at, but could only be started from* –
that 'personal identity' (in contemporary terms) was an existential 'given' in existential 'space', and not a concatenation of 'atomic
facts' in 'logical space'. Thus Hume switched in mid-course from
an empirical to an existential philosophy, and was thereafter concerned to trace how this 'given' identity, endowed with passions,
imagination and moral intelligence, develops by *acting in*, and *being
acted on by* the world. Similarly, I had to switch in mid-stream, and
could only begin to understand (and reach an understanding *with*)
my schizophrenic patients by reaching for that moral, aesthetic
and imaginative *core* which (I believed) lay 'beneath' their seemingly incoherent rantings and ravings. (Thus I note of Robert O.: 'The
former Mr O., one couldn't help feeling, was still present somewhere,
watching and controlling, somewhere *behind* the broken-up ravings'
p. 122.)

If a patient only allows fantastic, hieroglyphic or surrealistic
communication, then *this* is the form which one's communication
must take. But dialogue is dialogue, whatever form it takes, and
sooner or later – at least, in my experience – the defences, the distractions, the delusions die down, and one comes face-to-face with
the patient himself, with that central Identity which was hidden
before, with that 'Thou' one can engage in a genuine dialogue.
(Thus I note of Frances D., recovering from a period of deep psychic
disturbance: 'The denials, the projections, the identifications, the
transferences, the postures and the impostures ... fell away like a

an activating-system – an increase which can be defined and (in principle) measured by counting the total number of impulses which pass up this system. In more idiomatic terms, it is said that patients are 'turned on' or 'switched on' by L-DOPA. The limitation, and finally, the unreality, of such terms is that they are purely quantitative, and that they speak of magnitudes without reference to qualities. In reality, one *cannot* have magnitudes destitute of quality. Although patients do speak of feeling more energy, more 'pep', more 'go', etc., they clearly distinguish the qualities of pathology and health : in the words of one patient awakened by L-DOPA – 'Before I was *galvanized*, but now I am *vivified*.'

Topists, by contrast, envisage a mosaic of different 'centres' or 'systems', each imbued with a different kind of energy; they see energy as parcelled or partitioned in innumerable packages, all of which are 'correlated' in some mysterious way. Thus, patients on L-DOPA may be given a 'vigilance-rating', a 'motility-rating', an 'emotivity-rating', etc., and correlation-coefficients established between these. Such notions are completely alien to the experience of the patient, or to that of a sympathetic observer who *feels with* his patients. For *nobody* is conscious of their 'emotivity', for example, as distinct from their 'vigilance' : one is conscious

---

carapace, revealing "the old Miss D." – the real self – underneath' – p. 84).

Thus, in answer to questions about the existence and integrity of the Self in severe mental disease, I believe that though one can be 'beside oneself' or 'lose oneself' for years on end, the Self itself is still present, always present, intact, entire – however withdrawn or buried it may be. I think that all psychotic distortions and splinterings of the Self are relatively superficial, even though they may dominate the clinical picture. I think the ravages of physical and mental disease are both superficial; that there is something unfathomably deep beyond their reach; that this is the best and strongest and realest thing we have; and that once upon a time this was called the Soul.

only of feeling alive, attentive, aware – and of the total, infinite character of one's attention and awareness. To break
up this unity into isolated components is to commit an epistemological solecism of the first order, as well as to be blind
to the feelings of one's patients.

Awakening consists of a change in awareness, of one's
total relation to one's self and the world. All post-encephalitic patients (all *patients*), in their individual degrees and
ways, suffer from defects and distortions of attention: they
feel, on the one hand, cut-off or withdrawn from the world,
on the other hand immersed, or *engrossed*, in their illness.
This pathological in-turning of attention on itself is particularly marked in cataleptic forms of illness, and is beautifully
illustrated by a cateleptic patient who once said to me: 'My
posture continually yields to itself. My posture continually
enforces itself. My posture is continually suggesting itself.
I am totally absorbed in an absorption of posture.'

Awakening, basically, is a reversal of this: the patient
ceases to feel the presence of illness and the absence of the
world, and comes to feel the absence of his illness and the
full presence of the world.[14] He becomes (in D. H. Lawrence's
words) 'a man in his wholeness wholly attending'.

14. Instinctively and intuitively all patients use certain metaphors
again and again with regard to the transformations wrought by L-
DOPA; one sometimes feels that such metaphors are an inherent part
of our experience and heritage, like Borges's 'eternal metaphors' or
Kant's *synthetic a priori*, or (though I dislike the mysticism which
accrues to the notions) Platonic or Jungian 'archetypes'. Thus, there
are the universal images of rising and falling, which come naturally
and automatically to every patient: one *ascends* to health and happiness and grace, and one *descends* to depths of sickness and misery.
But a dangerous confusion can also arise: there are enticing ascensions and 'fraudulent heights' of mania, greed, and pathological
excitement; and although these are quite different from the solid
elevation of health, yet they may be confused with and 'compensate'
for it. Another universal metaphor is that of *light* and *darkness*: one
emerges from the darkness and dimness of disease, into the clear light

Thus the awakened patient *turns* to the world, no longer
occupied and preoccupied by his sickness. He turns an eager
and ardent attention on the world, a loving and joyous and
innocent attention, the more so because he has been so long
cut-off, or 'asleep'. The world becomes wonderfully vivid
again. He finds grounds of interest and amazement and
amusement all round him – as if he were a child again, or
released from gaol. He falls in love with reality itself.

Reunited with the world and himself, the entire being and
bearing of the patient now changes. Where, previously, he
felt ill at ease, uncomfortable, unnatural and strained, he
now feels at ease, and at-one with the world. All aspects of
his being – his movements, his perceptions, his thoughts, and
his feelings – testify simultaneously to the fact of awakening. The stream of being, no longer clogged or congealed,
flows with an effortless, unforced ease : there is no longer the
sense of '*ça ne marche pas*', or stoppage inside.[15] There is a

---

of health, and perhaps the radiance of grace. And here, again, a confusion may arise, for sickness has brilliance and false lights of its
own. Both images, for example, are brought together in D. H. Lawrence's lines :

> I have mounted up on the wings of the morning.
> And I have dredged down to the zenith's reversal.

– a couplet which could epitomize the rise and fall of patients on L-
DOPA.

15. This partly mechanical, partly infernal, sense of inner stoppage, or of a senseless, maddening going-which-goes-nowhere, so
typical of Parkinsonism and neurosis, is nowhere better expressed
than in Lawrence's last poems and letters.

> Men that sit in machines
> among spinning wheels, in an opotheosis of wheels,
> sit in the grey mist of movement which moves not,
> and going which goes not,
> and being which is not.

> ... going, yet never wandering, fixed yet in motion,
> the kind of hell that is real, grey and awful
> the kind of hell grey Dante never saw ...

great sense of spaciousness, of freedom of being. The instabilities and knife-edges of disease disappear, and are replaced
by poise, resilience, and ease.

These feelings, variously coloured by individual disposition and taste, are experienced, with greater or less intensity,
by every patient who becomes fully awakened from the use
of L-DOPA. They show us the full quality – the zenith of
real being (so rarely experienced by most 'healthy' people);
they show us what we have known – and almost forgotten;
what all of us once had – and have subsequently lost.

This sense of a return to something primal, to the deepest
and simplest thing in the world, was conveyed to me, most
vividly, by my patient Leonard L. 'It's a very sweet feeling,'
he said (during his own so-brief awakening), 'very sweet
and easy and peaceful. I am grateful to each moment for
being itself . . . I feel so contented, like I'm at home at last
after a long hard journey. Just as warm and peaceful as a cat
by the fire.' And this was exactly how he *looked* at that
moment–

> . . . Like a cat asleep on a chair, at peace, in peace,
> and at one with the master of the house, with the mistress,
> at home, at home in the house of the living,
> sleeping on the hearth, and yawning before the fire.
>
> Sleeping on the hearth of the living world
> yawning at home before the fire of life
> feeling the presence of the living God
> like a great reassurance
> a deep calm in the heart
> a presence

This is the hell of nullity, of senselessness, of unreality, distinguished
by Erigena from the hell of anguish, pain, pettiness and active torment. Parkinsonism perfectly epitomizes the anatomy of such hells
because it consists of nothing else – it has neither complications nor
compensations to soften or enrich its bleak topography.

as of the master sitting at the board
in his own and greater being,
in the house of life.

D. H. LAWRENCE

TRIBULATION

Thanne schal be greet tribulacionn.

WYCLIF BIBLE

For Fortune lays the Plot of our Adversities in the foundation of
our Felicities, blessing us in the first quadrate, to blast us more
sharply in the last.

SIR THOMAS BROWNE

For a certain time, in almost every patient who is given L-
DOPA, there is a beautiful, unclouded return to health; but
sooner or later, in one way or another, almost every patient
is plunged into problems and troubles. Some patients have
quite mild troubles, after months or years of good response;
others are uplifted for a matter of days – no more than a
moment compared to a life-span – before being cast back
into the depths of affliction.

No simple statement can be made as to which patients get
into most trouble first, nor can any firm prediction be made
as to how and when trouble will present itself. But it is reasonable to say that patients who were in the greatest trouble
originally – whether their troubles were neurological, emotional, socio-economic, or whatever – *tend* (other things being equal) to get into the greatest trouble on L-DOPA.[16]

16. So general a statement requires addition and qualification. By
and large, patients with ordinary Parkinson's disease – who constitute the vast majority of our present Parkinsonian population –
can expect the longest periods of unclouded response, and the mild-
est 'side-effects' when these finally come; whereas patients with
post-encephalitic Parkinsonism appear much more prone to early and

There has been a widespread, indeed universal, tendency to lump all these troubles into the category of 'side-effects', a term which is at once dismissive and reassuring. Sometimes the term is used for convenience, without carrying any particular implications;[17] more commonly, following the precedent of Cotzias, and a widely accepted medical practice, the term is used to denote some essential distinction from effects which are desired or expected – a distinction which allows them to be *excised*, if one wishes. Nothing is pleasanter than such an assumption, and nothing so requires dispassionate inquiry. This is very well realized by clear-minded patients, often better than by the physicians who treat them.[18]

---

drastic adverse responses. But there are exceptions, and important ones, to any such 'rule': *no* Parkinsonian patient, however favourable his 'starting-situation', can be *guaranteed* a long period of favourable response; conversely, one sees profoundly disabled post-encephalitic patients – like Magda B., and others whose histories are not given in this book – who astonish themselves and everyone by doing famously on L-DOPA, and *continuing* to do so. The incalculable nature of individual responses (which is hidden by the statistical presentations usually used) indicates how numerous and complex must be the determinants of response, and how many of them must be *latent* (*in posse*), strengths and weaknesses unexpected because unseen. There is, however, one group of patients who are almost invariably tipped into disaster by the use of L-DOPA: these are patients with supervening dementia; they are the most vulnerable of all to L-DOPA, and not only to L-DOPA but to stresses of all kinds. The story of Rachel I. exemplifies the special dangers which attend the giving of L-DOPA to such patients. I shall not dilate further on this particular problem here, but will refer interested readers to two papers of mine: 'Effects of L-DOPA in Patients with Dementia' (*Lancet*, 6 June 1970), and 'Effects of L-DOPA in Parkinsonian Patients with Dementia' (*Neurology*, 20, pp. 516–19).

17. Thus one of my own publications, a letter in the *Lancet* (9 May 1970, p. 1006), was editorially entitled 'Side-effects of L-DOPA in Post-encephalitic Parkinsonism', a title I had not chosen myself, and which was implicitly at odds with the observations it contained.

18. One such patient, now in Mount Carmel, when admitted to a large neurological hospital in New York, for the ninth time, for the

The term 'side-effects' is objectionable, and to my mind untenable, on three sets of grounds: practical, physiological, philosophical. First, the vast majority of what are now called 'side-effects' had long ago been observed as characteristic responses of 'normal' animals given L-DOPA; in this situation, where there were no therapeutic assumptions, intentions or insistences, there was no thought of introducing such categorical distinctions. Secondly, the use of such a term hides the actual structure and interrelation of 'side-effects', and therefore prevents any study of this. The enormous number and complexity of 'side-effects' from L-DOPA, though an affliction to patients, is uniquely instructive if we wish to learn more of the nature of disease, and of being; but the possibility of such learning is foreclosed if we take the term 'side-effects' to be the end of the matter. Thirdly, to speak of 'side-effects' here (or in the context of technology, economics, or anything whatever) is to divide the world into arbitrary bits, and deny the reality of an organized *plenum*.

The therapeutic corollary of all this is that we may commit ourselves (and our patients) to chimerical hopes and searches for 'abolishing side-effects', while excluding from our attention the very real ways in which they *can* be modified, or be made more bearable. Nobody has ever commented more pungently on the futility of chopping down 'side-effects', as opposed to the necessity of looking at the 'whole complexion and constitution' of what is actually happening, than our metaphysical poet as he lay on his sick-bed:

Neither is our *labour* at an end, when wee have cut downe some *weed*, as soone as it sprung up, corrected some *violent* and dan-

---

'treatment of side-effects' – in her case, a violent head-thrusting from side to side – said to her physician: 'These are *my* head-movements. They are no more a "side-effect" than my head is a "side-effect". You won't cut them out unless you cut off my head!'

gerous *accident* of a *disease*, which would have destroied *speedily*;
nor when wee have pulled up that *weed*, from the very root,
recovered *entirely* and *soundly*, from that *particular disease*; but
the whole *ground* is of an *ill nature*, the whole soile *ill disposed*;
there are inclinations, there is a propensenesse to *diseases* in the
body, out of which without any other *disorder*, *diseases* will grow,
and so wee are put to a continuall labour upon this *farme*, to a
continuall studie of the whole *complexion* and *constitution* of our
body.

DONNE

All patients, then, move into trouble on L-DOPA; not into
'side-effects', but into *radical trouble*: they develop, once
more, their 'propensenesse to diseases', which can sprout and
flower in innumerable forms. Why should this be so, we are
compelled to wonder? Is it something to do with L-DOPA
per se? Is it a reflection of the individual reactivity of each
patient – of a universal reactivity all organisms show, when
exposed to continued stimulation or stress? Does it depend
on the expectations and motives of patients, and of physicians and others who are significant at this time? Are the
overall life-style and life-circumstances relevant? All of these
questions are real and important; all must be asked, and test-
ed if possible; all of them overlap and dovetail to form the
total *plenum* of patients' being-in-the-world.

We see, in Donne, a great variety of words relating to the
nature of disease: disposition, inclination, propensity, complexion, constitution, etc., a richness of language which both
distinguishes and unites two aspects of disease – its *structure*
and *strategy*. Freud reminds us repeatedly that we must
clearly distinguish the *liability to illness* from the *need for
illness*: it is one thing, for example, to be migraine-prone, and
another to want an attack as an excuse for breaking an unpleasant appointment. Schopenhauer's thesis is that the
world presents itself to us under two aspects – as Will and
Idea – and that these two aspects are always distinct and

always conjoined; that they totally embrace, or *inform*, one another. To speak in terms of either alone is to lay oneself open to a destructive duality, to the impossibility of constructing a meaningful world: this is exemplified in the epistemological inadequacy of such statements as 'He did badly on L-DOPA out of sheer spite,' or 'He did badly on L-DOPA because he had too much (too little) dopamine in the brain.' The spite may indeed have been there, and the alteration of dopamine may indeed have been there, both significant, both crucial, both aspects of the way he was doing. But neither consideration alone can afford us an adequate picture, or the possibility of an adequate picture, of the total situation. Perhaps the patient's spite was the 'final cause', and his dopamine the 'efficient cause'; both considerations, both ways of thinking, as Leibniz reminds us, are useful, and both *need to be joined*. But how shall we unite the 'final cause' with the 'efficient cause', the will with the matter, the motive with the molecule, when they seem so remote, and disparate, from each other? Here again – as always – we are rescued from the wastes of mechanism and vitalism by common sense, common language, metaphysics: by terms which unite in their two-facedness the concepts of structure and intention – words like *plan* and *design*, and by the innumerable exemplifications of such words which colloquial speech presents to us, and which we – as scientists – so often feel impelled to reject and ignore.

For a brief time, then, the patient on L-DOPA enjoys a perfection of being, an ease of movement and feeling and thought, a harmony of relation within and without. Then his happy state – his world – starts to crack, slip, break down, and crumble; he lapses from his happy state, and moves towards perversion and decay.[19] We are forced to use words

19. Awakening is characterized by perfect satisfaction, a perfect filling of the organism's needs. At such a time the patient says (as did Leonard L., in effect): 'I have what I need, I need no more. I have

of this nature, however unexpected they may seem in this context, if we are to gain any dynamic understanding of the development of those dissolutions and departures and perversions which constitute the essence of downfall, of disease.

---

enough, and all is well'; *he* says this, and (we may imagine) all his starved cells are saying this as well. Being-well is 'enoughness' – satisfaction, contentment, fulfilment, assuagement. To the question, 'How much?' of a drug should be given, there is only one correct answer, and that is 'Enough!' But, alas! this happy state, this state of 'enoughness', never endures.

> 'There lives within the very frame of love
> A kind of wick or snuff that will abate it,
> And nothing is at a like goodness still,
> For goodness, growing to a plurisy,
> Dies in his own too-muchness.'

After a time 'enoughness' is lost, and thereafter there is *no longer* any correct dose to give: 'enoughness' is replaced by 'not-enoughness' and 'too-muchness', and it is no longer possible to 'balance' the patient. Nothing is sadder than this insidious loss of balance, the steady attrition of therapeutic latitude, of health; nevertheless it occurs – and seemingly inevitably, in every patient who is given L-DOPA. One's wish, the temptation, is to deny it occurs, and to promise the patient that the 'right' dose, the 'right' response, has only been temporarily or fortuitously lost, and can be found once again by ingenious manipulations and 'titrations' of dosage. To do so is to lie, or at least to delude – to raise expectations which cannot be met.

The problem of 'titration' – giving so much of a substance to obtain so much of a response – which is so easy and straightforward in chemistry (where one has simple stoichiometric equivalence) sooner or later becomes *the* problem with the continued administration of L-DOPA (or with the administration of any drug designed to alter behaviour). Let us review the sequence of responses we have seen in all our patients – the sequence of responses which occurs in *any* patient maintained on L-DOPA. To begin with, we see a simple, solid, beneficial response – the patient *gets better*, after he has been given so much of the drug; and it seems, for a while, that his new-found improvement can be maintained on a fixed 'maintenance-dose' of L-DOPA: at *this* stage, therefore, the notion of 'titration', of a simple

What we need so much – and not only in medicine – is an anatomy of wretchedness, an epistemology of disease, which will follow Burton, Schopenhauer, Freud, etc., and extend their considerations to all other (monadic) 'levels': one must see, for example, that Galen's *circulus vitiosus*, the vicious circle, is a universal of pathology at all possible levels; and that this is equally true of exorbitance and extravagance, and of all self-augmenting deviations from the ease,

---

stoichiometric balancing or commensuration between dose and response, seems to have been achieved, and to be perfectly feasible. But *then*, invariably, 'complications' occur, and these have the following general pattern: First, patients become more and more 'sensitive' to the effects of L-DOPA, sometimes to a quite extraordinary degree (as with Leonard L., who initially required 5,000 mg. a day, but later responded to a hundredth of this dose). Secondly, we see qualitative alterations in response to L-DOPA, so that reactions which were originally simple and straightforward now become increasingly complex, variable, unstable and paradoxical – they may become, indeed, *impossible to predict* (at which point infinitesimal alterations of dosage may precipitate responses *incalculable* in magnitude or kind). At such a time we can no longer converge on any correct or appropriate dose of L-DOPA (we see this very clearly in the case of Frances D.,) – there *is* no longer any such thing as a correct dose, as 'enough'. We are now in a veritable double-bind – there is no longer any evidently right thing to do, and whatever we do is the wrong thing to do. At this stage, then, there is no mind-point of response any longer; the patient is no longer titrable with L-DOPA; there is no longer any equivalence between dose and response; there has ceased to be any commensurability between stimulus and response.

There may be, as I have suggested, a number of possible reasons for this; but there is one basic idea which cannot be stressed enough: as long as L-DOPA serves as a *complement* to patients, meeting and filling their hunger, their needs, no problem arises; but when, thereafter, it serves as a *stimulant*, combatting Parkinsonism rather than making up a deficiency, an inherently unstable *opposition* develops, an irresoluble tug-of-war between incommensurable forces – something essentially akin to a neurotic conflict. These considerations are put in more general (cybernetic) terms in the footnote to p. 319.

the harmony, the unforcedness of health. So Donne, in his relapse into sickness, continually asks himself, What went wrong? And why? Might it have been avoided? etc., and by inexorable stages is driven to the most universal concept of disease and 'propensenesse' to this.

The first symptom of returning disease, of going wrong, is *the sense* that something is going wrong. This so-obvious point cannot be emphasized too strongly. The patient does not experience a precisely formulated and neatly tabulated list of symptoms, but an intuitive, unmistakable sense that 'there is something the matter'. It is not reasonable to expect him to be able to define exactly what is the matter, for it is the indefinable sense of 'wrongness' that indicates to him, and to us, the *general* nature of his malaise: the sense of wrongness which he experiences is, so to speak, his first glimpse of a *wrong world*.[20] This sense of wrongness carries with it a precursory quality, of a perfectly precise kind: whatever is experienced conveys or intimates what will or may be experienced in the future, the expansion and evolution of an already-present character.[21] Thus, Donne, experiencing the first 'grudging' of his illness, writes:

20. Of interest, in this connection, is a case of epilepsy described by Gowers. The affected patient invariably suffered from an abrupt and authentic sense of *wrongness* ('whatever was taking place before the patient would suddenly appear to be *wrong* – i.e. morally wrong . . .') immediately before convulsion and unconsciousness.

21. An interesting and perhaps essential formal model of this quality is to be found in Cantor's concepts of infinite sets and transfinite cardinals. The laws of ordinary, inductive mathematics do not apply to these, for the 'least part' of such transfinites are equal to the whole, and convey their infinite (i.e. world-like) quality. All of us have perhaps thought of this reflexive quality with regard to an infinite series of maps: the map which contains a map of the map, which contains a map of the map of the map, etc. Indeed, this image has been specifically mentioned to me by a number of patients who find themselves embedded in interminable reflexive states of precisely this type.

In the same instant that I feele the first attempt of the disease, I feele the victory.

Unease and discord – in the most general of senses – are the sign and source of returning disease. The forms and transforms are infinitely varied, and never the same in any two patients. Individuality is inherent in disease, as in everything; diseases are 'perverse' individual creations – worlds, base worlds, simpler and starker than the worlds of health.

Common to all worlds of disease is the sense of pressure, coercion and force; the loss of real spaciousness and freedom and ease; the loss of poise, of infinite readiness, and the contractions, contortions and postures of illness: the development of pathological rigidity and insistence.

In patients with ordinary Parkinson's disease, the first 'side-effects' of L-DOPA are most easily seen in movement and action: in a certain haste, alacrity, and precipitancy of movement, in the exaggerated force and extent of movements ('synkinesis') and in the development of various 'involuntary' movements (choreatic, athetotic, dystonic, etc.). In post-encephalitic patients, for various reasons, excesses of 'temperament' are particularly prominent, and these perhaps indicate more clearly the general form of disease. One sees this particularly clearly in such patients as Rolando P., Margaret A., Leonard L., etc., but one also sees it in patients with common Parkinson's disease, like Aaron E.

Paradoxically, deceptively, such exaggerations first appear as excesses of health, as exorbitant, extravagant, inordinate well-being; patients such as Leonard L. slip by degrees, almost insensibly, from supreme well-being to pathological euphorias and ominous ectasies. They 'take off', they exorb, beyond reasonable limits, and in so doing sow the seeds of their subsequent breakdowns. Indeed, exorbitance is *already* a first sign of breakdown: it indicates the presence of an unmeetable need. Defect, dissatisfaction, underlie exorbitance: a 'not-enoughness' somewhere leads to greed and 'too-muchness', to a voracity and avidity which *cannot* be met.[22]

If we ask, Where is the defect, the dissatisfaction, the avidity?, we must recognize that it may be anywhere, in the *plenum* of being: that it may be in their molecules, their motives, or their relations with the world. Unsatisfied need, insatiable greed, defines the eventual position of *all* patients on L-DOPA. This leads us to an inexorable economic conclusion – that there is a lacuna somewhere, an unassuageable gap, to be found in the situation of every single patient. Such a gap may be of any type – a chemical or structural hiatus in the midbrain itself; a wound or lacuna in emotional being; an isolation approaching Limbo in relation to the world: one way or another, there is a gulf which cannot be filled *and stay filled*; not, at least, through the agency of L-DOPA alone. A chasm develops between supply and demand, between need and capacity; an inner division of being takes place, so that there is a simultaneous suffering from surfeit and starvation – 'one halfe lackes meat, and the other stomacke' – in the metaphor which Donne applies to his sickness.

22. If we review the evidence before us, we are led to an astonishing, yet obvious comparison. A sense of 'not enough!', of dissatisfaction; a craving for 'more!', which fails to satisfy; an avidity for 'still more!', which *still* fails to satisfy, and which feeds or increases the craving for more; an irresistible tendency which defeats its own end, continually goaded by frustration, continually tempted towards futile exorbitance, into a tantalizing spiral of self-thwarting desire ... surely the pattern is all too familiar! We are compelled to recognize a precise formal analogy (and homology) between pathological propensity and sin, and must rank both together as ontological peccancy, instead of separating them, as we usually do, by a completely arbitrary, dualistic dichotomy: the 'level' is of no consequence – the basic plan is the same. The concept of the identity (isology) of sickness and sin is central to all metaphysics. It is a notion we can neither dismiss nor dispense with.

We see from their responses to the continued and continual administration of L-DOPA – if we did not see it before – that these patients have needs over and above their need for L-DOPA (or brain-dopamine); and that beyond a certain point or period no mere *substance* – however 'miraculous' – can compensate, indemnify, or cover up these other needs. These patients not only lack meat, but stomach as well: what will happen if we stuff a man who lacks some of his stomach? These considerations are passed over in the current insistence that patients can be 'titrated' with L-DOPA indefinitely, in a perfect commensuration of supply and demand. They can be 'titrated' with L-DOPA *at first*, as eroded ground can be watered, or a depressed area given money; but sooner or later, complications occur; and they occur because there is complex trouble in the first place – not merely a parching or depletion of one substance, but a defect or disorder of *organization* itself, invariably in the brain, and elsewhere as well.

This danger, this dilemma, was quite clearly recognized by Kinnier Wilson, forty years ago (see p. 54): he says, in effect, that there is just so much we can do, by restoring to pathological cells their missing 'pabulum', but that beyond this there is futility and danger if we try to 'whip up' the patient's impoverished and decaying cells. Whether we try to stuff cells beyond their capacity, or whether the cells themselves show an incontinent 'avidity', and 'try' to assimilate or function beyond their capacity, the end-result will be the same. Moreover, a static metaphor – like stuffing a man who lacks half his stomach – is not adequate to describe what actually occurs; the image of 'whipping up' decayed and flagging cells, and of their accelerated breakdown under this stress, is much more germane to the eventual consequences of L-DOPA. For what we see, in every patient maintained on L-DOPA, is that his tolerance for the drug becomes less and less, while his need for the drug becomes greater and greater: in short, that he gets caught in the irresoluble vicious circle of 'addiction'.[23]

Let us now plot the steps by which this occurs, the successive positions of the patient as he plays the losing game he cannot stop.[24] He becomes over-stimulated, over-reactive,

23. Such dangers and dilemmas are in no sense peculiar to the use of L-DOPA. They tend to occur, one way or another, with the prolonged use of all cerebral stimulants and depressants, with all drugs which have supposedly specific effects on behavioural disorders. Perhaps the closest analogy is the use of stimulants (amphetamines) to combat the intense sleep and drowsiness of narcoleptic patients – who, in the severest cases, may tend to sleep twenty-four hours a day, to sleep away the whole of their lives; such sleepers may be brilliantly awakened by the use of amphetamines, and be able to resume normal life for weeks or months; but, sooner or later – as with patients on L-DOPA – they tend to show both a waning and a spreading of effect, the advent of psychoses and other 'side-effects' of amphetamines, along with a recurrence of their original sleep. Similar considerations apply to the use of amphetamines, cocaine, or other stimulants to combat 'neurasthenia' and neurotic depressions (see Appendix). Especially similar patterns of response occur with the prolonged use of tranquillizers to combat emotional and motor excitements. Thus the phenothiazide or butyrophenone tranquillizers are often superbly effective in the *short-term* treatment of neuroses and psychoses, and may restore the patient to a merciful calm, but *thereafter* there comes an ever-increasing likeliness of drug-induced Parkinsonism, dyskinesia, and other 'side-effects', along with a recurrence of the original neurosis. Such effects are especially germane with regard to the extraordinary effects of haloperidol (so-called anti-DOPA) on Gilles de la Tourette or multiple-tic syndrome (a disorder associated with an excess of brain-dopamine). Almost all such patients at first show a 'miraculous' reduction or abolition of their tics; but many of them, sooner or later, run into a series of 'tribulations' – Parkinsonism, apathy, and similar 'side-effects' – along with a recurrence of their original tics; the most fortunate, the toughest – like patients on L-DOPA – finally achieve a more or less acceptable 'accommodation' or *modus vivendi*.

24. The process of sickening, going-down, deteriorating, etc., has always been visualized as a circular process, with a peculiarly terrible force and shape of its own. Morbid process and propensity were

over-excited – exorbitant; but underlying all this is an increasing need or deficit; he is, so to speak, striving to gain by illegitimate means what he is no longer attaining by legitimate means. Or, to return to our economic metaphor: he is no longer 'earning his keep'; his real assets and reserves are continually dwindling; he is subsisting on a loan, on borrowed time and money, and this – while it preserves appearances – further depletes his own reserves and earning-power,

---

classically identified with sin and peccability – hence Galen's vicious circle: the fundamental image of Dante's 'Inferno'.

If we are to picture, more fully, the inherent dynamism of health and disease, and the reciprocal (*parasitic*) relation between them, we must employ an elaboration of this image, viz. a *double* spiral, double helix, or twin-vortex. We must also indicate that the curvature, angle, or gradient of these spirals is neither constant nor linear, but increases in a hyperbolic way.

This spiral-of-deterioration – so similar in structure to inflationary spirals – starts with an *insufficiency* (a not-enoughness) of supply or amenity, which is felt as a dissatisfaction or increase of need; this is projected as increased demand, which cannot be met (without strain) by depleted resources. The demand is increased, or inflamed, so to speak, placing an ever-heavier strain on ever-more-eroded resources. This leads to an ever-widening gap or incommensurability between supply and demand, an ever-decreasing chance of 'catching-up' or equilibrating: the possibility of meeting needs, of real resolution, is continually attenuated to an ever less less-ness; the never-ending spiral proceeds to infinity (infinitesimality).

Pari passu with this trajectory into dwindling amenity is a mirror-trajectory into pathological propensity. Needs and demands which cannot be met by reality turn towards substitute or compensatory amenities, for which they display an ever-increasing avidity. The satisfaction yielded by substitute activities is essentially *hollow*, and therefore unreal (or pseudo-real), and this continually inflates pathological appetites (*greeds*), which become ever more insatiable and exorbitant in quality. The nature of this pathological propensity is essentially extortionate, and, if unchecked, must lead to the death of real being ('The wages of sin is death').

A model of this kind seems to me invaluable, if not indispensable, in understanding the *economics* of pathology or disease.

and brings nearer the day of reckoning, of repayment; he is experiencing a transitory 'boom', but sooner or later the 'crash' must come.[25]

Our patients, then, ascend higher and higher into the heights of exorbitance, becoming more active, excited, impatient, increasingly restless, choreic, akathisic, more driven by tics and urges and itches, continually more hectic, fervid and ardent, flaming into manias, passions and greeds, into climactic voracities, surges, and frenzies ... until the crash comes at last.[26]

25. This pattern – of a single supreme moment, which once attained can never be attained again – is all too familiar with regard to alcohol, opium, stimulants, and other 'addictive' drugs. De Quincey writes (*Confessions*, Everyman edition, p. 185): '... the movement is always along a kind of arch; the Drinker rises through continual ascents to a summit or *apex*, from which he descends through corresponding steps of declension. There is a crowning point in the movement upwards, which once attained cannot be renewed.'

26. I have emphasized, in this and preceding descriptions, what I take to be a generic *tendency* ('exorbitance') common to *all* excitations in this phase of reaction. This mode of description departs from that of classical neurology, which describes excitations as localizations, in either holistic or topistic terms. If one speaks in these terms, one will speak of the following items in response to L-DOPA: an increase in the magnitude of each excitation, a spread of excitation to other areas of the brain, and a continuous proliferation of 'new' excitations (*de novo*), until the brain is lit up with innumerable excitations. Pavlov – who is both holist and topistic in approach – ascribes each widening distribution of excitations partly to the centrifugal spread of charge in a homogeneous brain-conductor ('irradiation'), and partly to the sequential stimulation of anatomically or functionally contiguous systems ('chain-reaction').

Allied to the images of *illumination* (Sherrington's 'myriad of twinkling lights' and Pavlov's 'bright halo with wavering borders' – both images of awakening and consciousness) are those of *conflagration*: flares being lit in the cerebral city, until it finally goes up in flames; a fire being lit in the cold house of being, which first warms, then consumes, the whole of the house. Notions of proliferation call forth images of *growth*: the 'side-effects' of L-DOPA growing into a gigan-

The form and tempo of 'crashing' are immensely variable in Parkinsonian patients; and in many of the stabler, more fortunate patients, there is more the feeling of gentle subsidence and detumescence, than of a sudden violent crash. But whatever the form and tempo it takes, there is descent from the dangerous heights of pathology – a descent which is at once protective, yet also destructive.[27] Patients do not descend to the ground, as a punctured balloon would sink to the ground. They sink or crash below the ground, into the subterranean depths of exhaustion and depression, or the equivalents of these in Parkinsonian patients.

In patients with ordinary Parkinson's disease (Aaron E., for example), these crashes may not occur for a year or more, and may be relatively mild when they do occur. Their 'akinetic episodes' (as the crashes are usually called) tend, at first, to be short and slight, and to come on two or three hours after each dose of L-DOPA. Gradually they become more severe and longer, increasingly abrupt in onset and offset, usually losing their relation to times of giving L-DOPA.

The qualities of these states are varied and complex, more

---

tic homunculus or behavioural monstrosity, or forming a more-than-Amazonian jungle – L-DOPA as a 'Boomfood' or cerebral manure. A fictional illustration of drug-induced exorbitance is given in H. G. Wells's The Food of the Gods.

27. Generically similar reactions have been described by Pavlov, in experimental animals submitted to 'supra-maximal' stress. Such animals, after a time, show diminutions or reversals of response, entering into 'paradoxical' and 'ultra-paradoxical' phases. Pavlov speaks, in such cases, of 'transmarginal inhibition consequent upon supra-maximal excitation', and regards this inhibition as protective in type. Goldstein, working with patients, describes essentially similar phenomena, and regards them as basic biological reactions; Goldstein speaks here of an 'excitation-course' rising to a peak, with reversal of responses, or 'equalization', after this peak. One sees too, at the level of single neuronal units, how response to continued massive stimulation is always bi-phasic, the unit adapting to, or resisting, further stress.

so than is usually described in the literature: among these qualities are lassitude, fatigue, somnolence, torpor, depression, neurotic tension and – specifically – a recrudescence of Parkinsonism itself. Such states vary from mildly unpleasant and disabling to intensely distressing and disabling; in Aaron E. for example, they were far more disabling and unpleasant than his original (pre-DOPA) state, the more so because they occurred with such suddenness, and so unpredictably.

In post-encephalitic patients, these crashes tend to be far more severe, and may occur within seconds, and scores of times daily (as in Hester Y., for example). But their complexity and severity are highly instructive, and show us more clearly what goes on at such times. One sees from the reactions of such patients that one is not dealing with any mere exhaustion of response – an assumption which is rather generally made, and taken as the basis of hopefully therapeutic 'titration' of drug-dosage.[28] There is, no doubt, an element of exhaustion in these variations of response; but their instantaneity, profundity, and complexity show us that other transformations – of a fundamentally different nature – are *also* occurring. Thus, in Leonard L., Rolando P., Hester Y., etc., we see virtually instantaneous changes from violently explosive, 'expanded' states to intensely contracted, 'imploded' states – or, in the astronomical image suggested by Leonard L., from 'super-nova' states to 'Black Holes', and

28. Thus, in the summer of 1970, Cotzias *et al.* published a table with recommended alterations of drug-dosage for different clinical states. If akinetic episodes occurred, the dosage of L-DOPA was to be increased by 10%; if they *still* occurred, by another 10%. Such recommendations, to my mind, can be dangerously misleading in the management of patients; moreover, they lack any sound theoretical basis. It is only fair to add that Cotzias, and many other neurologists, are now readier to relinquish such fixed rotas and tables and rules-of-thumb, and to play each patient 'by ear', with a full appreciation of the *individual* nature of all responses, and their real complexity.

back again. The two states we see – which at various times have been called 'up' states and 'down' states – show a precise formal analogy of structure; they represent different phases, or transforms, of each other; they depict for us, as for our patients, the opposite 'poles' of an ontological continuum.[29]

The 'down' states, then, do not represent simple and – so to speak – 'normal' exhaustions, with the protective and recuperative capacities of such exhaustions; nor can they be adequately represented as 'protective inhibitions' (in Pavlov's term) or protective 'equalizations' (in Goldstein's term). They are much less benign, for they consist of total *recoils* or rebounds or reversals of response, which fling patients, in an almost uncontrollable trajectory, from pole to pole of their being or 'space'.[30] The opposite of each exorbit-

29. These deeply pathological states seem to lead us towards exceedingly strange yet possible images of 'inner space' in such patients; and such images, it must be stressed, occur spontaneously to imaginative patients. Thus the 'shape' of behaviour, when reduced to exorbitances, becomes that of an *hour-glass*, with a 'waist' fined down to almost-zero proportions; or, putting the matter less concretely, of an infinite yet closed ontological space, everywhere hyperbolic, and negatively curved: a space, moreover, which allows *no exit*, for it runs into itself like a Möbius strip. And *this* image, too, may be expressed by some patients: thus Leonard L., when most torturingly enclosed, compared himself to a fly which was trapped in a Klein bottle. Such images – of an essentially relativistic 'ontological space' – require a detailed and formal elaboration, if they are to be anything more than intriguing and suggestive.

30. Pavlov – speaking of similar switch-backs in experimental animals, and in manic-depressive patients – talks of 'waves of excitation followed by troughs of inhibition'. Many patients, similarly, speak of waves running through them, or of being tossed up and down like a boat in heavy seas. These undulant images seem entirely appropriate, if one departs from the notion of simple, sinusoidal waves, and instead visualizes torrential excitements which *surge hyperbolically*, getting steeper and steeper, as they get higher and higher, and thus have the potential of infinite height. Such waves – fortu-

ance is a counter-exorbitance, and patients may be bounced between these as in a frictionless space: their extremities and excursions tend to *increase*, in a frightening paradigm of positive feed-back or 'anti-control'; and 'between-states' (control-states) tend to *decrease* towards zero. Thus, once such ontological oscillations or reverberations have started, the possibilities of 'normality' become smaller and smaller, and 'in-between' states are less and less seen. Almost all of my patients, who have found themselves in such situations, use the image of a *tight-rope* to express how they feel: and this, indeed, is almost literally true, for they have become ontological funambulists above a pit of disease; or, in an allied metaphor, they seek a vanishing still-point amid total exorbitance – thus Leonard L.'s tortured wish: 'If only I could find the eye of my hurricane !'

With the continuation of such states – which may be highly persistent despite withdrawal of L-DOPA (see Rachel I., for example) – further splits or decompositions may occur, exorbitances splitting into facets or aspects, sharply differentiated 'equivalents' of being; Hester Y., for example, showed this 'crystalline' splitting and was able to describe it particularly clearly. This further schism leads to an ontological delirium, with behaviour refracted into innumerable facets, and instantaneous jumps between these facets or aspects.[31]

---

nately – do not occur in terrestrial seas; they reflect forces and spaces of an extraordinary type; they only occur in a non-linear space, which we must endeavour to imagine as best we can.

31. Consideration of these sparkling effervescent deliria, and of the kinematic vision and 'standstills' with which they may be associated (see Hester Y.), leads us to an aspect of 'inner space' even stranger and more difficult to imagine than the curved spaces we have looked at; kinematic phenomena show us a dimensionless 'space' where there is a succession without extension, moments without time, and change without transit: in short, the world of quantum mechanics.

These considerations, to my mind, depict the *general* form or design of reactions to L-DOPA. They have not departed from the general ground of physiological energetics or economics. They have outlined, in the sparest detail, various energetic-economic positions, or phases, of brain-state, and their interrelations, something which would be susceptible, in principle, to a precise mathematical exposition.

The administration of L-DOPA is a *general* treatment, which one hopes to match with brain-reactions or phases. One would suspect on theoretical grounds, as one finds in practice, that it becomes increasingly less possible to match dose-level and brain-phase. For dose-level has only a single dimension or parameter: we can increase or decrease the dose – nothing else (altered spacing of doses can be subsumed under this); whereas brain-reaction and behaviour flower into many dimensions, which cease to become describable or determinable in linear terms. To insist or suppose that responses can always be 'titrated' by dose-level is to pretend that the brain is a sort of barometer, to make a reduction of its real complexity. 'Biological organization cannot be reduced to physico-chemical organization,' Needham reminds us, 'because nothing can ever be reduced to anything.' And one finds, in practice, that once patients have entered complex states of perturbation and turbulence, their reactions to L-DOPA become singularly difficult to predict – if not, at times, inherently unpredictable. Once akinetic episodes have started to occur, for example, their severity may sometimes be modified by increasing L-DOPA, sometimes by decreasing L-DOPA, and sometimes by neither – all depending. Depending on two or ten or fifty variables, themselves interdependent, and complexly linked. Jevons used to compare complex economic situations to *weather*, and we must use the same image here: the brain-weather or ontological weather of these patients becomes singularly complex, full of inordinate sensitivities and sudden changes, no longer susceptible to an item-by-item analysis, but requiring to be seen as a whole, as a *map*.

To imagine that such a meteorological situation can be 'played' by the application of fixed formulae and rules of the most simplistic type is to play blind-man's-buff in the world of reality;[32] to be an alchemist or an astrologer – a purveyor of 'secrets'; to be 'a mathematical chimaera bombinating in a biological vacuum' (to borrow Huxley's paraphrase of the original Rabelais). The therapeutic game cannot be played this way, whatever our wishes; but – to the extent that it can be played at all – it can be played 'by ear', by an intuitive appreciation of what is actually going on. One must drop all presuppositions and dogmas and rules – for these only lead to stalemate or disaster; one must cease to regard all patients as replicas, and honour each one with individual attention, attention to how *he* is doing, to *his* individual reactions and propensities; and, in this way, with the patient as one's equal, one's co-explorer, not one's puppet, one may find therapeutic ways which are better than other ways, tactics which can be modified as occasion requires. Given a 'policy-space' no longer simple or convergent, an intuitive 'feel' is the only safe guide: and in this the patient may well surpass his physician.

I must emphasize once more – to avoid needless misunderstanding or distress – that the patients considered in this book do not constitute, nor are meant to constitute, a 'fair sample' of the Parkinsonian population-at-large; the fact that many of our patients have run into exceedingly severe,

32. It is, of course, not fortuitous that those who are most apt to speak of L-DOPA as 'a miracle drug' (see pp. 47–52) are also most prone to publish complicated tables and formulae and rules for proper dispensing of the Magical Stuff. Such mystical and mechanistic attitudes can not only endanger patients, but are deeply unscientific in that they go with an improper attitude to Nature – the arrogant feeling that Nature exists to be commanded and *ruled*, instead of the humble feeling that we exist to honour and woo her.

complex, and intractable problems is an index of *their* situation, which is far worse, in almost every way, than the situation of their more fortunate Parkinsonian brethren outside institutions. Their reactions to L-DOPA, in almost every way, are hyperbolic and extreme: they experience the most intense Awakenings, and they go on to the most intense Tribulations; quantitatively, their reactions far outstrip in magnitude those likely to be seen in the vast majority of Parkinsonian patients; but the quality of their reactions is the same, and casts light on the reactivity and nature of *all* Parkinsonian patients, and of *all* human beings.

We find, in their reactions to L-DOPA, that there is another universal quality which cannot be understood in the energetic and economic terms we have hitherto used. It is necessary, but never sufficient, to speak of their reactions as 'ups', 'downs', 'exorbitances', 'exhaustions', 'recoils', 'decompositions', 'schisms', etc.; for their reactions are equally imbued with a *personal* quality, which is expressed in dramatic or histrionic terms; the person shows forth in all his reactions, in a continual disclosure or epiphany of himself; he is always enacting himself in the theatre of his self.[33] Entire memory-theatres are set in motion; long-past scenes are recalled, re-enacted, with an immediacy which effaces the passage of time; scenes past and scenes possible are called into being – presentiments and presentations of what might once have been, of what could still yet be, given an imaginable difference at any one time. L-DOPA, in this way, can

33. The concepts of mechanics, and the concepts of theatre, are radically different, yet need to be joined: they are joined legitimately in the notions of *actors* and *acting*, and illegitimately in the notions of *puppets* and *reflexive reaction*. The first of these is a living, biological notion; the second a mystical, Golemical notion – a degraded and degrading travesty of life. The physiology of the last three centuries has been skewered on just such Cartesian notions – the puppet, the doll, the Golem, etc.; the same fantasy is imaginatively explored in Faust's *homunculus*, and Frankenstein's *monster*.

serve as a sort of strange and personal time-machine, bringing to each patient time past and time possible, *his* past and
his possible, into the palpable 'Now'. Worlds past and
worlds possible pass like apparitions before him, intensely
real – yet not real, as ghosts tend to be. The actual, the possible, the virtual, commingle in that uncanny but beautiful
coming-together, that multiplicity of being we can only call
transport (one sees this, most clearly, in the visionary Martha N.). Rose R. awoke to *her* 1926, and not to anyone else's
1926; Frances D. was recalled to *her* long-past respiratory
idiosyncrasies, which were not like anyone else's idiosyncrasies; Miriam H., in her crises, experienced a (hallucinatory)
recall of an 'incident' in *her* past, not an incident in anyone
else's past; Magda B. experienced hallucinations of *her* husband, his presence, his absence, his infidelities to *her*, not of
anyone else's husband. How absurd to call such phenomena
'side-effects'! Or to imagine that they can be understood
without reference to the experience and personality, the total
make-up, of each patient.[34] We cannot understand the nature

34. The anamnestic powers of L-DOPA seem to be among its
most remarkable effects, those which (in the original, Platonic sense)
indicate most clearly the nature of 'Awakening'. The *quality* of reminiscence induced by L-DOPA is absolutely characteristic and highly
instructive. It does not consist of a vague reminiscent streaming, or
the regurgitation of 'facts' deliberately learnt. It consists of the
sudden, spontaneous, and 'involuntary' recall of *significant moments
from the personal past*, recalled with such sharpness, concreteness,
immediacy, and force as to constitute, quite literally, a re-living or
re-being. The character of this living memory, in which self and
world, image and affect, are totally and inseparably fused, is utterly
different from that of mechanical or 'rote' memory (the literal regi-
stration of 'information' or 'data', in the sense such terms are used
with regard to computers). These sudden revocations of personal
memories have nothing of the 'dead' quality of re-run documentaries,
but are experienced as intensely moving re-livings of one's past,
vital recollections (akin to those of the analysand or artist) by which
one recollects one's 'lost' identity, one's continuity with the forgotten

of such reactions without reference to the nature of each
patient; nor the nature of each patient without reference to
the nature of the world : thus we are led to see (what everybody once knew) that the constitution of Nature, and all
natures, is essentially dramatic ('All the World's a stage
...') and presents itself epiphanically on all possible occasions:

> Though the World be Histrionical ... yet be thou what thou
> singly art, and personate only thy self ... Things cannot get out
> of their natures, or be or be not in despite of their constitutions

– as our metaphysical physician, Sir Thomas Browne, reminded us so clearly three centuries ago. One has, it is true, a
number of natures, which in their totality constitute one's
whole possible nature – a point raised by Leibniz in his famous example of 'alternative Adams'. This too is brought
out with great clarity in responses to L-DOPA: thus Martha
N., when given L-DOPA on five different occasions, showed
different patterns of response on each occasion; all of these

---

past. The quality of these recaptured moments shows us the quality
of experience itself, and reminds us (as Proust is continually at pains
to show) that our memories, our selves, our very existences, consist
entirely of *a collection of moments*:

'A great weakness, no doubt, for a person to consist entirely in a
collection of moments; a great strength also; it is dependent upon
memory, and our memory of a moment is not informed of everything that has happened since; this moment which it has registered
endures still, lives still, and with it the person whose form is
outlined in it' (Proust, A *la recherche du temps perdu*).

What is true of personal history is true of all history – 'History
is a pattern of timeless moments' (Eliot). These timeless moments are
not clock-moments, chronological cross-sections of an arbitrary,
abstract, 'absolute' Time; they are *events*, moments of summation,
revelation, epiphany – *kairoi*, not *chronos* –

> ... a lifetime burning in every moment
> And not the lifetime of one man only.

                                                           ELIOT

responses had dramatic unities[35] of their own – they represented a spray or bouquet of 'alternative Marthas', although one was pre-eminent, most full and most real, and
this – as she knew – was the *real* Martha-self. In the case of
Maria G. – who was deeply schizophrenic – the situation on
L-DOPA was more complex and tragic; for Maria G.'s *real*

35. The constitution of *dramatic* (or 'organic') unities is radically
different from that of *logical* (or mechanical) unities, although it at no
point contravenes the latter. The concepts used in logical operations
are the basic mathematical ones so comprehensively described by
Whitehead and Russell; whereas those employed in dramatic presentations are the 'biological' ones of imitation, suggestion, sympathy,
attunement, affinity, community, compossibility, etc. – all of these,
as Leibniz stresses, being 'social' relations.

Thus one observes of dogs that they 'like company' or 'need
company', and one feels (if one has a dog) that this sociability is
something essential and primary, which *cannot* be reduced to a
question of 'reflexes', 'drives', 'stimuli', 'instincts', etc. Yet this
is precisely what Descartes did – hence Sherrington's comment that
Descartes writes as if he had never had, or been friendly with, a dog;
and Cartesian physiology has, ever since, been a dog-less, friendless,
lifeless science concerned with 'preparations' rather than beings. In
a Leibnizian physiology, by contrast, the presiding concept is social
and dramatic. The organism is not seen as a mechanical concatenation
or network, shackled together by extrinsic, mechanical forces and
bonds; but as an amity, a comity, a company, a congress, every 'element' (or monad) a complete social being, with a vivid 'awareness'
of the presence of all others, all fitting together in a perfection of ease,
in a total, intrinsic, dramatic omneity, in (pre-established) harmony,
compossibility, courtesy and beauty.

Disease, thus considered, is not a mere impairment of supply or
commodity, but a radical breakdown of amenity and courtesy, a mutilation of social being, awareness, and discourse – a radical alienation
from the full grounds of being. This, in Leibnizian terms, is one
half of disease; the other half is implied in Leibniz's question (in
Principles of Nature and of Grace): 'Why should there be something
rather than nothing? The *something* which develops in place of full
being, which fills, so to speak, the existential *vacuum* of disease, is a
substitutive or compensatory organization of a crude-rigid-narrow
and 'self-centred' sort.

self only showed itself for a few days, before being decomposed or replaced by swarming 'selflets' – miniature, pathological impersonations of herself.[36]

Thus we are led to a deeper and fuller concept of 'awakening', embracing not only the first awakening on L-DOPA but all possible awakenings which thereafter ensue. The 'side-effects' of L-DOPA must be seen as a summoning of possible natures, a calling-forth of entire latent repertoires of being. We see an actualization or extrusion of natures which were dormant, which were 'sleeping' *in posse*, and which perhaps might have been best left *in posse*. The problem of 'side-effects' is not only a physical but a metaphysical problem: a question of how much we can summon one world, without summoning others, and of the strengths and resources which go with different worlds. That infinite equation, which represents the total being of each patient from moment to moment, cannot be reduced to a question of systems, or to a commensuration of 'stimulus' and 'response': we are compelled to speak of whole natures, of worlds, and (in Leibniz's term) of the 'compossibility' between them.

Thus, we are brought back once more to our torturing

36. The tendency to exorbitance and the tendency to schism are clearly quite separate (though they play on each other); they represent the two fundamental tendencies to be seen in disease. One observes such splits of behaviour (or, in Pavlov's term, 'ruptures of higher nervous activity') in all organisms pushed beyond a certain limit of stress and strain; the limit itself varies very widely and so does the *level* at which splitting occurs. Martha N., for example, tended to a high-level 'molar' splitting (hysterical dissociation), even before she received L-DOPA; Maria G. tended to 'molecular' splitting (schizophrenic disintegration), which was clearly present, though constrained, before the administration of L-DOPA; Hester Y. had an immensely stable 'ego' or personality, but went to pieces at a *lower* level (tics) when given L-DOPA. It seems to me unlikely that anyone could tolerate excitement or pressures of the order of those seen in Hester Y., and *not* show splitting at one level or another.

'Why?' Why did so many of our patients, after doing so well at first, spoil, 'go bad', move into all sorts of trouble? Clearly, they had in them the *possibilities* of great health: the most deeply ill patients were able to become deeply well for a time. Thereafter, apparently, they 'lost' this possibility, and in no case were able to retrieve it again; such, at least, is the case in all the Parkinsonian patients I have seen. But the notion of 'losing' a possibility in such a way is difficult to comprehend, on both theoretical and practical grounds: why, for example, should a patient who retained the possibility of 'awakening', through fifty years of the severest illness, 'lose' it, in a few days, after receiving L-DOPA? One must allow, instead, that their possibilities of continued well-being were actively precluded or prevented because they became *incompossible* with other worlds, with the totality of their relationships, without and within. In short, that their physiological or social situations were incompossible with continuing health, and therefore disallowed or displaced the first state of well-being, thrusting them into illness again.

The descent into illness, once started, may proceed by itself, moving incontinently further by innumerable vicious circles, positive feed-backs, chain-reactions – a first strain causing other strains, a first breakdown other breakdowns, perversion summoning perversion, with the dynamism and ingenuity which is the essence of disease:

> Diseases themselves hold Consultations, and conspire how they may multiply, and join with one another, and exalt one anothers force . . .   DONNE

In this spiral of deterioration, the need for illness joins hands with the liability to illness, that conjoint perversion which is pathological *propensity*. The first of these, necessarily, must be a major factor in the lives of some of our most deeply disabled and deeply regressed patients, whose illness has been

the main part of their lives. In such patients, the sudden removal of illness will leave a *hole*, so to speak, a sudden existential vacuum, which needs to be filled and filled quickly
with real life and activity, before pathological activity is
sucked back again to fill it. The perverse need for illness –
both in patients themselves, and sometimes in those who are
close to them – must be a major determinant in causing
relapse, the most insidious enemy of the will-to-get-better:

BURNLEY: 'How does poor Smart do, Sir; is he likely to re-
    cover?'
JOHNSON: 'It seems as if his mind has ceased to struggle with
    the disease; for he grows fat upon it.'

                                                          BOSWELL

Whenever ... advantage through illness is at all pronounced,
and no substitute for it can be found in reality, you need not look
forward very hopefully to influencing (it) through your therapy.

                                                            FREUD

It is certain that the compensations of disease, and the desti-
tutions of 'external' reality, can only be a *part* of the matter; but they are a part which we are well-placed to study,
and sometimes to modify.

Such considerations can hardly be avoided, for instance,
with regard to Lucy K., Leonard L. and Rose R. Lucy K. had
spent the greater part of her life in a state of symbiotic and
parasitic dependence on her mother; her mother was the
most needed person in her life, and at once the most loved
and most hated, and Lucy's illness and dependence, conversely, were the most important parts of her mother's life.
Lucy K. had scarcely awoken on L-DOPA before she turned
to me and demanded marriage, rescue, and removal from her
mother; when I indicated that this was impossible, she fell
back within hours into the depths of her sickness. Leonard
L. had a similar if somewhat milder pathological relation
with *his* mother, and she, as we have seen, herself broke

down when he got better; Leonard saw, all too clearly, that his mother's well-being was incompossible with his own well-being; and shortly after this he too relapsed. Perhaps the saddest case is that of Rose R., who 'came to' joyously to the world of 1926 – and found that '1926' no longer existed; the world of 1969, into which she awoke, was incompossible with the world of 1926, and so she went back to '1926'. In these three cases, the overall situation was pathological beyond remedy: the needs of these patients were incompossible with reality. In other patients – most clearly exemplified by Miron V. – a much happier situation eventually resulted, the 'side-effects' of L-DOPA being greatly reduced by the establishment of good feelings and relations, of central securities which had lapsed in their lives.

Thus, finally, we come to the only conclusion we can: that patients on L-DOPA will always do as well as their total circumstances will allow; that altering their chemical circumstances may be a prerequisite to any other alteration; but that it is not, in itself, enough. The limitations of L-DOPA are as clear as its benefits, and if we hope to reduce the one and increase the other we must go *beyond* L-DOPA, beyond all purely chemical considerations, and deal with the *person* and his being-in-the-world.

ACCOMMODATION

> Or to take arms against a sea of troubles
> And by opposing end them?

It is characteristic of many neurologists (and patients) that they mistake intransigence for strength, and plant themselves like Canutes before advancing seas of trouble, *defying* their advance by the strength of their will. Or, like Podsnaps, they *deny* the sea of troubles which is rising all round them:

'I don't want to know about it; I don't choose to discuss it;
I don't admit it!' Neither defiance nor denial is of the least
use here: one takes arms by learning how to negotiate or
navigate a sea of troubles, by becoming a mariner in the seas
of one's self. 'Tribulation' dealt with trouble and storm;
'Accommodation' is concerned with weathering the storm.

The troubles experienced are not ordinary troubles, and
the weapons which are needed are not ordinary weapons:

Weapons for such combats are not to be forged at *Lipara*;
Vulcan's Art does nothing in this internal militia . . .

                                                                BROWNE

The weapons of use in the tribulations of L-DOPA are those
we all use in conducting our lives: deep strengths and reserves, whose very existence is unsuspected; common sense,
forethought, caution, and care; special vigilance and wiles
to combat special dangers; the establishment of right relations of all sorts; and, of course, the final acceptance of what
must be accepted. A good part of the tribulations of patients
(and their physicians) comes from unreal attempts to transcend the possible, to deny its limits, and to seek the impossible: accommodation is more laborious and less exalted, and
consists, in effect, of a painstaking exploration of the full
range of the real and the possible.[37]

37. Accommodation lacks the *glamour* of Awakening. It lacks its
sudden, spontaneous, 'miraculous' quality. It does not come of 'itself'
– easily and effortlessly. It is *earned, worked for* – with infinite effort
and courage and trouble. It does not reflect some local change in the
basal ganglia, and can in no sense be regarded as localized process:
it is an achievement of character, of Negotiation, in its widest possible sense. What is achieved in this way, with work and difficulty,
is secure and enduring – unlike the facile 'flash' of Awakening, which
goes, as it comes, too easily, too quickly . . . The qualities of the first
DOPA-Awakening are essentially those of innocence and joy – like
an anomalous return to earliest childhood: the Awakened, in this
sense, irrespective of their age, come to resemble the 'once-born' of
whom William James speaks. Tribulation is an ordeal, a dark night

All the operations involved in coming to terms with one-self and the world, in face of continual changes in both, are subsumed in Claude Bernard's fundamental concept of 'homeostasis'. This is essentially a Leibnizian concept, as Bernard himself was the first to point out: homeostasis means achieving the optimum which is possible in (or compossible with) particular circumstances – in short, 'making the best of things'. We have to recognize homeostatic endeavours at all levels of being, from molecular and cellular to social and cultural, all in intimate relation to each other.

The deepest and most general forms of homeostasis proceed 'automatically', below the level of conscious control. Such activities occur in all organisms submitted to stress, and involve depths and complexities about which we know all too little. Our deepest and most mysterious strengths are called forth from these levels.

Some of the patients described in this book – Rose R., Rolando P., Leonard L., etc. – were never able to achieve a 'satisfactory' accommodation, and were forced either to cease taking L-DOPA altogether or to accept a very miserable *modus vivendi*. Other patients described in this book – and perhaps the majority of 'ordinary' Parkinsonian patients placed on L-DOPA – did, eventually, achieve a more satisfactory coming-to-terms. Common to all such patients is a gradual diminution of the effects of L-DOPA, leading at length to a sort of plateau. The achievement of this plateau involves both a gain and a loss: a fairly stable and satisfactory level of functioning, *minus* the drama of full 'awaken-

---

of the soul, which challenges to the utmost those who must face it. A number are broken and fail to survive; others endure and are *forged* by their suffering. These survivors – the Accommodated – have (in James's words) 'drunk too deeply of the cup of bitterness ever to forget its taste, and their redemption is into a universe two storeys deep'. These, then, are the 'twice-born', who after bitter division, physiological and social, finally achieve a real reunion, a reconciliation of the deepest and stablest kind.

ing' or 'side-effects'. Such patients are no longer very well or very ill; their Awakenings and Tribulations are both in the past; they have emerged into relatively even water, into a state which is nevertheless much 'better' than their pre-DOPA state. Our first history (Frances D.) exemplifies this passage.

I know of no simple way, no set of criteria, which allows one to predict whether a satisfactory coming to terms of this sort will occur. Certainly the severity of the original Parkinsonism or post-encephalitic illness is not itself a good index: thus I have seen patients with quite mild Parkinson's disease experience intractable 'side-effects' from which they never emerged, and at the other extreme one sees patients like Magda B., who do well and stay well despite the devastating severity of the original disease.

This indicated that *other* parts of the brain (or the organism) must determine or co-determine the powers and potential of deep homeostasis. It is clear, for example, that functional integrity of the cerebral cortex is such a prerequisite, for accommodation tends to be undermined if the cortex is impaired.[38]

But even these basic processes cannot, I think, account for the range and extent of accommodation. One must allow the possibility of an almost limitless repertoire of functional reorganizations and accommodations of all types, from cellular, chemical, and hormonal levels to the organization of the self – the 'will to get well'. One sees again and again, not merely in the context of L-DOPA and Parkinsonism, but in cancer, tuberculosis, neurosis – *all* diseases – remarkable, unexpected and 'inexplicable' resolutions, at times when it seems that everything is lost. One must allow – with surprise, with delight – that such things happen, and that they

38. As in Rachel I. Pavlov's 'protective inhibition' and Goldstein's 'equalization ... towards the mean' were described with special reference to cortical processes.

can happen to patients on L-DOPA as well. Why they should happen, and what indeed is happening, are questions which it is not yet in our power to answer; for health goes deeper than any disease.

When we rise to the level of accommodations which are accessible (in part) to consciousness, and (in part) to deliberate control, we find what we have found at every stage in our discussion: that the 'private' sphere, the sphere of individual actions and feelings, is everywhere commingled with the 'public' sphere, with the human and non-human environment. We cannot really separate individual endeavours from social endeavours, as these assist (or impede) the patient's being-in-the-world; the patient's therapeutic endeavours depend on the world's compliance, and other therapeutic endeavours depend on the patient's compliance. There must be a working together to realize the possible.

Physicians often speak of 'preventive', 'precautionary', or 'supportive' measures, as if these were different in kind from 'radical' measures. This distinction disappears the more we look into it: the therapeutic measures which we will touch on now are no less radical than taking L-DOPA, and they are an essential complement to taking L-DOPA. As the central concept of disease is dis-ease, the central concept of therapy is ease: everything which promotes the ease of the patient reduces his pathological potentials, and assists the fullest coming to terms which is possible.

All patients who continue to receive L-DOPA show a reduction of tolerance, becoming particularly in need of ease, and particularly intolerant of strain or un-ease. The need for rest becomes especially important, whether in the form of night-sleep, 'naps', 'taking it easy', or 'relaxation'. One invariably sees, with patients on L-DOPA, a resurgence of 'side-effects' if their rest or sleep is less than their needs. One observes this even in out-patients with Parkinson's disease, who at best show not a trace of trouble (like George W.).

What is 'adequate rest' can only be found by each individual patient, and may be considerably in excess of 'normal' needs; I have under my care a number of patients who enjoy excellent health if they sleep twelve hours a day, and intractable 'side-effects' if they sleep any less.[39]

The intolerance of strain is equally marked, whether the strain is imposed by fever or by pain, disability, frustration, anxiety or anger. One repeatedly sees, with patients who seem 'almost normal' on L-DOPA, this peculiar intolerance to all forms of stress.[40] But life involves *action* besides 'relaxa-

39. The special need for additional sleep, rest, or recuperation, in these frail, struggling, convalescing-accommodating patients must, I think, be interpreted in metaphysical as well as physical terms. One recaptures during sleep (or 'relaxation' in general) an elemental sort of strength, a reunion with the world and the grounds-of-one's being. This is explicit in Heidegger's and Binswanger's existential notions of 'Care'. It is poetically intimated by Sir Thomas Browne: '... whilst we sleep within the bosome of our causes, we enjoy a being and life in three distinct worlds ...'; and in Lawrence's beautiful images of reunion and renewal:

> And if tonight my soul may find her peace
> in sleep, and sink in good oblivion,
> and in the morning wake like a new-opened flower
> then I have been dipped again in God, and new-created.

It is analysed by Freud, in terms of libido-theory (A *General Introduction to Psychoanalysis*, 1926, pp. 424–6): 'Sleep is a condition in which all investments of objects, the libidinal as well as the egoistic, are abandoned and withdrawn into the ego. Does this not shed a new light upon the recuperation afforded by sleep? ... In the sleeper the primal state of the libido-distribution is again reproduced, that of absolute narcissism, in which libido and ego-interests dwell together still, united and indistinguishable in the self-sufficient self.' And it is experienced by us all. Physiologists have never been able to explain the need for sleep, seen in all living beings, in purely physical terms.

40. This was strikingly exemplified on one occasion when I saw Aaron E. He had returned home at this time, and was ostensibly quite normal, but came back to see me for periodic check-ups. On one of these return-visits I was dismayed to see a rather violent chorea,

tion'; one can be at ease in an easy-chair only for so long, before the impulse to move assumes imperative force; and if one cannot move when one needs to, unease is extreme. Impediment to movement is a main symptom in all of these patients, and the distress thus caused is liable to call forth a variety of other symptoms. In order to break this vicious spiral of distress and disorder, various devices are needed to make movement easy. The use of such devices is an indispensable adjunct to the use of L-DOPA, and allows accommodations of critical importance.

Only a few such devices and accommodations can be mentioned. One is the use of 'auto-command' and 'pacing', employed with such success by Frances D. and others.[41] A variant of this is the use of external command and suggestion, where auto-command is impossible – a matter of critical importance with all Parkinsonians. The therapeutic power of music is very remarkable, and may allow an ease of movement otherwise impossible. The design of furniture, and interior design, is equally important in allowing free movement. Mechanical difficulties must be smoothed away, for they may constitute a critical danger to patients on L-DOPA.[42] In these and similar ways, the extent to which a

---

grimacing, and tics, which he had never shown previously. When I inquired if there was anything making him uneasy, he replied that he had taken a taxi to hospital, and that the taxi-meter was continually ticking away: 'It keeps ticking away,' he said, 'and it keeps *me* ticcing too!' On hearing this, I immediately dismissed the taxi, and promised Mr E. we would get another one and pay all expenses. Within thirty seconds of my arranging all this, Mr E.'s chorea, grimacing and ticcing had vanished.

41. The use of visual command, in this way, is beautifully illustrated in Purdon Martin's *The Basal Ganglia and Posture*.

42. Thus, at the Highlands Hospital, where it is well realized that a curve rather than an angle can make all the difference to a Parkinsonian patient, the main promenade is in the form of an oval. This environmental accommodation greatly facilitates patients' walking. On the other hand, it may facilitate it so much that they *cannot*

mutual accommodation can be reached between the symptom-prone patient and his environment determines (or co-determines) the consequences of L-DOPA.[43]

---

stop walking. In Mount Carmel, by contrast, where everything tends to be sharp and angled rather than curved and smoothed, Parkinsonian patients can easily walk up and down the regular stairs (see p. 62 and accompanying footnote), but tend to get jammed in the irregular, crowded, and zig-zag corridors whenever they have to make a *shift* of direction. Thus sharpnesses and smoothnesses, steps and curves, each have their own advantages and disadvantages. A consequence of the contradictory nature of Parkinsonian symptoms is that Parkinsonian patients need a contradictory *milieu*; but this would involve them in all sorts of logical and ontological paradoxes, like those Alice encountered in the Looking-Glass World.

43. We have seen that Parkinsonian and post-encephalitic patients, especially when over-stimulated or 'galvanized' by L-DOPA, tend to *exorbitances* of various kinds – incontinences, intemperances, departures from measure and moderation. Thus the essence of 'mutual accommodation' is *the re-achievement of measure and moderation,* by existential and ecological (as opposed to pharmacological) means. How can we adapt to each other, in the best possible way, the patient's exorbitance (his *milieu interne*) with his human and non-human environment (his *milieu externe*)? There seem to me three possible forms of such homeostasis, all (in their different ways) interesting, valuable and limited.

The first, seemingly the simplest, turns out to be the most tricky, the least tenable, in theory and practice. This first method would be to *counter* exorbitance, directly : to 'measure' the amount of immoderation, and cancel it out with exactly the same measure of moderation. Thus we would be seeking a *control by feedback*, cybernetic devices of one sort or another (these could be internal or external, and could be based on illusion or reality – for we have indicated that Parkinsonism is internally generated, and is based, *inter alia*, on metrical illusions of various kinds). Such controls would be feasible if we were dealing with fairly simple (e.g. linear and constant) disturbances of magnitude : examples of such simple disturbances would be *tachykinesia* and *tachyphemia*, as opposed to *festination* (which is far more complex). Thus we have seen that Hester Y., when excited, displayed an abnormal celerity of movement (so much so that she resembled a film speeded up), and that Miriam H., analogously, would show an abnormal celerity of speech (speaking at 500 words

In these and a thousand and one other ways some Parkinsonian patients, and patients on L-DOPA, become astute and expert navigators, steering themselves through seas of

a minute, without missing a syllable). It is important to emphasize that these celerities were most marked when these patients were *alone*, or felt themselves alone: thus Hester would rush and dart when alone in a room, but move at a more 'normal' pace if she were moderated by *other things* or *other people* (which, to anticipate, constitute the second and third kinds of moderation to be discussed); similarly Miriam would only speed up in her speech when she 'forgot' the presence of others, when she was, as it were, enveloped in monology. At such times, they *felt* they were moving and talking 'normally', i.e. they suffered a sort of *tachyscopic illusion* which blinded them to their own tachykinesia and tachyphemia. Could not such a tendency and such an illusion be countered by the introduction of a commensurate resistance or retardation in the medium of their movements, or a commensurate illusion of 'bradyscopy'? Such measures *do* work, in a limited way: thus Hester's tendency to walk too fast was moderated if she had to walk *uphill* (as it was aggravated if she had to walk *downhill*); it was also moderated if she *thought* she was walking uphill (when, in reality, she was walking on the level). Indeed she once asked me if it might not be possible to make a special pair of glasses for her which would distort appearances so that all the level corridors would seem to her to be going uphill. (I was unsure whether this would be ontologically possible, let alone optically possible.) In a case of festination, where movements simultaneously become faster and smaller, due to the envelopment of the patient in a hyperbolically contracting space–time, the business of constructing a sort of 'rectifying glass' (which would rectify their magnified or minified space–time) would, of course, be far more difficult; perhaps, indeed, it would be *theoretically* impossible. And as for the situation where a patient is suffering from a contradictory coupling of festination and cunctation (which is quite common, as in precipitation–procrastination in neurotic patients) – what could one do here? The patient is *already* suffering from precisely corresponding and conflicting impulses ('Hurry !', 'Hold !', 'Faster !', 'Slower !'), which urge him continually to move too fast/too slow, to do too much/too little, to act too soon/too late (along with the illusion that everything around him is moving too fast and/or too slow, and that everything is happening too soon and/or too late). Could such an ontological delirium or 'double-bind' be controlled or moderated

trouble which would cause less expert patients to founder on the spot. The extent to which such ruses and wiles can be learned and employed depends, among other things, on the

using its own terms? The answer, quite clearly, is 'No!' Problems created by a perverse and paradoxical logic cannot be solved by the use of such a logic. If compulsion is countered by counter-compulsion, then the counter-compulsion may in turn require countering by a counter-counter-compulsion; and similarly with illusions, counter-illusions, etc. We are led into a chimera, an infinite regress, a veritable _Through the Looking Glass_ maze of mirrors. Parkinsonism is irresoluble in Parkinsonian terms, as irrationality is irresoluble in irrational terms. We see, therefore, why a seemingly simple, cybernetic approach becomes infinitely complex, if not impossible, with Parkinsonian patients.

It will have been borne in upon the reader that the ever-mounting difficulties encountered in (and _generated by_) such cybernetic procedures are precisely analogous to those encountered in (and generated by) the use of L-DOPA – _once the patient has entered exorbitance._ Once the patient has lost the 'happy mean', we cannot _directly_ restore it to him (or him to it): we make correction upon correction upon correction upon correction, and _still_ we find he is uncorrected: he is absolutely incorrigible and incommensurable. Whether we try chemical titration (with the use of L-DOPA), or existential–ecological titration (with the methods we have sketched, or by adaptations of Skinnerian or Pavlovian methods), we are alike doomed to failure. Once the patient has entered exorbitance (or immeasurability, incommensurability, insatiability, etc. – whatever term we care to use), _he cannot be 'titrated', he cannot be 'balanced'_, whatever procedures we try to use. He cannot even _theoretically_ be balanced, because the 'happy mean' is not a mathematical mean – it is not (as Aristotle makes it) the geometrical _mid-point_ between two hyperbolic extremes: such a vanishingly small, indeed dimensionless 'point' has none of the qualities (spaciousness, latitude, etc.) of health.

We cannot _directly_ straighten a Parkinsonian warp – as we cannot straighten a crooked stick. If we are to achieve moderation or rectitude, we must do it _indirectly_ – by calling the Parkinsonian out of his warped and exorbitant mode-of-being into a correct and moderate mode-of-being. In short, we must give him _a measure, a structure, by_ which he can rectify his activity, for this is what he needs – measured and organized activity. We have already indicated (in the footnote to p. 62) the two sorts of measure which he can use, the two

inventiveness and resourcefulness of individual patients, on their attitude and the attitude of those around them, and on the opportunities for studying one's being-in-the-

sorts of measure which *all of us* use; and in the following footnote we will give various concrete examples of these. Here we will speak in more general terms, but terms which are practicable, and germane to the business of living the fullest, freest, best-organized life which is possible for any Parkinsonian, given the resources and limits of his internal and external situation.

We have repeatedly referred to the usefulness of steps, lines, ticks, clocks, routines, pacings, etc. – scales, measures, series, patterns, disposed in a fixed and regular and conventional space–time. All of these can provide (in Luria's terminology) 'syntagms' or 'algorithms' for the structuring and coordination of experience and behaviour; they provide (again in Luria's terms) 'logico-grammatical' or 'quasi-spatial' paradigms or schemes.

All of us (by 'us' I mean *human* animals, as opposed to non-human animals, who are so admirably guided by their own, biological, 'clocks' and 'scales') require and use artificial, abstract, conventional measures – *standards* – of this sort, standards for consensus and communication. The Parkinsonian, who is 'far out', whose behaviour has become so different from, so incommensurable with, ordinary conduct, stands in special need of such formalities and conventions; but he also stands in special peril from them. (One sees a dangerous hypertrophy of the mechanical, the standardized, the conventional in 'total institutions' of various sorts – monasteries, convents, hospitals, asylums, barracks, battleships, Leviathans, super-states, etc., which have in effect reduced their inmates to robots or puppets.) A subtle and sensible balance is needed, a propriety of relation, so that the Parkinsonian patient can have the mechanical and the systematic *at his service, without himself becoming enslaved to them.*

Complementary to such fixed, abstract, metrical, logical and *non-living* devices and measures, complementary to such systems and syntagms, is the real world, infinite in variety, aspect and depth, infinitely concrete, infinitely metaphorical, infinitely formal yet infinitely expressive, infinitely ordered yet infinitely free. The real world, whether in Nature or Art or social relationship, is – finally – the only thing which can give the Parkinsonian (which can give any of us) that fullness, ease and spontaneity of action which constitutes happiness, health, freedom and life.

Thus, in summary, we can compare three modes-of-being, which

world.[44] In general, post-encephalitic patients seem to be far wilier and cannier in this regard than 'ordinary' Parkinsonians; they have usually had (even before the advent of L-DOPA) decades of experience in the stormy seas of themselves;

---

are fundamentally different and incompossible with each other (although they can coexist, *immiscibly*, to varying extents). One is *being Parkinsonian* (which, in Aristotelian terms, is being 'incontinent' and 'intemperate'); the second is *being controlled* ('contained'); the third we might call being *re-tempered* (restored to the latitude, the temper, of health).

44. One such patient (the head-nodding patient previously referred to: p. 286, n. 18) had managed to maintain an independent life outside institutions for years, in face of almost incredible difficulties – difficulties which would instantly have broken a less determined or resourceful person. This patient – Miss Z. – had long since found that she could scarcely start, or stop, or change her direction of motion; that once she had been set in motion, she had no control. It was therefore necessary for her to plan all her motions in advance, with great precision. Thus, moving from her arm-chair to her divan-bed (a few feet to one side) could never be done *directly* – Miss Z. would immediately be 'frozen' in transit, and perhaps stay frozen for half an hour or more. She therefore had to embark on one of two courses of action: in either case, she would rise to her feet, arrange her angle of direction exactly, and shout 'Now!', whereupon she would break into an incontinent run, which could be neither stopped nor changed in direction. If the double doors between her living-room and the kitchen were open, she would rush through them, across the kitchen, round the back of the stove, across the other side of the kitchen, through the double doors – in a great figure-of-eight – until she hit her destination, her bed. If, however, the double doors were closed and secured, she would calculate her angle like a billiard-player, and then launch herself with great force against the doors, rebounding at the right angle to hit her bed. Miss Z.'s apartment (and, to some extent, her mind) resembled the control-room for the Apollo launchings, at Houston, Texas: all paths and trajectories pre-computed and compared, contingency plans and 'fail-safes' prepared in advance. A good deal of Miss Z.'s life, in short, was dependent on conscious taking-care and elaborate calculation – but this was the only way she could maintain her existence. Needless to say, many forms of taking-care and calculation, of somewhat less

they have painfully acquired their wiles and their insight:
unsung, post-encephalitic Odysseuses, dispatched (by Fate) on
Odysseys of themselves.

'Deep' accommodation, rest, care, ingenuity – all of these

---

elaborate kind, can become purely automatic and second nature to
patients, and no longer demand any conscious attention. This
entire subject is penetratingly discussed in the last chapter of A.
R. Luria's *The Nature of Human Conflict*. Luria speaks here, and in
allied contexts, of the necessity of devising 'algorithms of behaviour'
– behavioural prostheses, calculated but invaluable *substitutes* for
the ease, naturalness, and intuitive sureness which have been undermined by disease. Such 'algorithms' are, of course, artifices and,
above all, *artificial metrics*; but they may represent almost the only
way in which patients with profound disorders of force and metrica-
tion can achieve *some* control of their own incontinent tendencies.
They are analogous to the use of a metronome by musicians who have
a defective or distorted sense of timing and rhythm.

Radically different – the true ideal – would be the restoration of a
'natural' rhythm and movement – the 'kinetic melody' (in Luria's
term) natural and normal to each particular patient: something
which would not be a mere scheme or diagram or algorithm of behaviour, but a restoration of genuine spaciousness and freedom. We
have seen, again and again, that patients' own kinetic melodies *can*
be given back to them, albeit briefly, by the use of an appropriate flow
of *music*: one is reminded here of Novalis's aphorism – 'Every sickness is a musical problem, and every cure a musical solution.' Other
'natural' motions of Nature and Art are equally potent if experienced
visually or tactually. Thus, I have known patients almost totally
immobilized by Parkinsonism, dystonias, contortions, etc., capable
of riding a horse with ease – with ease and grace and intuitive control, forming with the horse a mutually influencing and natural
unity; indeed the mere *sight* of riding, running, walking, swimming,
of any natural movement whatever – as a purely visual experience
on a television screen – can call forth by sympathy, or suggestion,
an equal naturalness of movement in Parkinsonian patients. The art
of 'handling' Parkinsonian patients, learned by sensitive nurses and
friends – assisting them by the merest intimation or touch, or by a
wordless, touchless moving-together, in an intuitive kinetic sympathy of attunement – this is a genuine art, which can be exercised
by a man or a horse or a dog, but which can *never* be simulated by

are essential for the patient on L-DOPA. But more important than all of them, and perhaps a prerequisite for all of them, is the establishment of proper relations with the world, and – in particular – with other human beings, or *one* other human being, for it is human relations which carry the possibilities of proper being-in-the-world. Feeling the fullness of the presence of the world depends on feeling the fullness of another *person*, as a person; reality is given to us by the reality of people; reality is taken from us by the unreality of un-people; our sense of reality, of trust, of security, is critically dependent on a human relation. A *single* good relation is a life-line in trouble, a pole-star and compass in the ocean of trouble : and we see, again and again, in the histories of these

---

any mechanical feedback; for it is only an ever-changing, melodic, and *living* play of forces which can recall living beings into their own living being. Such a subtle, ever-changing play of forces may also be achieved through the use of certain 'natural' devices, which *intermediate*, so to speak, between afflicted patients and the forces of Nature. Thus while severely affected Parkinsonians are particularly dangerous at the controls of motorcars and motorboats (which tend to *amplify* all their pathological tendencies), they may be able to handle a sailing boat with ease and skill, with an intuitive accuracy and 'feel'. Here, in effect, man–boat–wind–wave come together in a natural, dynamic, union or unison; the man feels at one, at home, with the forces of Nature; his own natural melody is evoked by, attuned to, the harmony of Nature; he ceases to be a *patient* – passive and pulsive – and is transformed to an *agent* – active and free. Such observations (which might be multiplied a hundredfold) show us that the greatest of all remedies for Parkinsonism – as for all sicknesses, aberrations, and departures from Nature – is Nature herself : *Vis Medicatrix Naturae* – that deep and mysterious healing force to which we can turn when all else fails :

> 'Healing',
> Papa would tell me,
> 'is not a science,
> but the intuitive art
> of wooing Nature.'
>
> W. H. AUDEN (*The Art of Healing*)

patients, how a single relation can extricate them from trouble. Kinship is healing; we are physicians to each other – 'A faithful friend is the physic of life' (Browne). The world is the hospital where healing takes place.

The essential thing is feeling *at home* in the world, knowing in the depths of one's being that one has a real place in the home of the world. The essential function of such hospitals as Mount Carmel – which house several millions of the world's population – is that they should provide *hospitality*, the feeling of home, for patients who have lost their original homes. To the extent that Mount Carmel acts as a *home*, it is deeply therapeutic to all of its patients; but to the extent that it acts as an *institution*, it deprives them of their sense of reality and home, and forces them into the false homes and compensations of regression and sickness. And this is equally true of L-DOPA, with the unreal 'miraculous' expectations which attend it, with its false promise of a false home in the bosom of a drug. Tribulations of every kind were at a maximum for our patients in the autumn of 1969 – a time when the hospital changed its character, when human relations of all sorts became strained or undermined (including my own relation with our patients), and when neurotic hopes and fears reached exorbitant heights. At this period, patients who had attained accommodations previously, who *had* felt reasonably at home with themselves and the world, were deprived of their accommodations, and profoundly unsettled: unsettled socially, physiologically, at all possible levels.

Many of these patients have now *re*-settled, *re*-accommodated, *re*-attained good relations, and with this are doing much better on L-DOPA. One sees this, with great clarity, in the case of Miron V., as he was restored to his work, his place in the world; and one sees it, most movingly, with regard to Magda B., Hester Y., and Ida T., who were restored to their children, and the love of their families.[45] One sees it in *all* patients, insofar as they are able to love themselves and the world.

One sees that beautiful and ultimate metaphysical truth, which has been stated by poets and physicians and metaphysicians in all ages – by Leibniz and Donne and Dante and Freud : that Eros is the oldest and strongest of the gods; that Love is the *alpha* and *omega* of being; and that the work of healing, of rendering whole, is, first and last, the business of Love.

45. The most dramatic, if shortest-lived, example of such accommodation is given by Leonard L., who was delivered from his severe 'side-effects' and tribulations on L-DOPA during the twenty days in which he wrote his Autobiography, and at no other time; these were days of complete metaphysical sobriety, of proper relation to himself and the world.

EPILOGUE

And so we come to the end of our tale. I have been with these patients for almost seven years, a considerable part of their lives and mine. These seven years have seemed like a single long day: a long night of illness, a morning awakening, a high noon of trouble, and now a long evening of repose. They have also composed a strange sort of Odyssey, through the deepest and darkest oceans of being; and if our patients have not reached an ultimate haven, some of them have fought through to a staunch, rock-girt Ithaca, an island or home against the perils around them.

It is given to these patients, through no wish or fault of their own, to explore the depths, the ultimate possibilities of human being and suffering. Their unsought crucifixions are not without consequence, if they afford help or illumination to others, if they lead us to a deeper understanding of the nature of affliction and care and cure. This sense of genuine and generous, if involuntary, martyrdom is not unknown to the patients themselves – thus Leonard L., speaking for them all, wrote at the end of his Autobiography: 'I am a living candle. I am consumed that you may learn. New things will be seen in the light of my suffering.'

What we *do* see, first and last, is the utter inadequacy of mechanical medicine, the utter inadequacy of a mechanical world-view. These patients are living disproofs of mechanical thinking, as they are living exemplars of biological thinking. Expressed in their sickness, their health, their reactions, is the living imagination of Nature itself, the imagination we must match in our picturing of Nature. They show us that

Nature is everywhere real and alive and that our thinking about Nature must be real and alive. They remind us that we are over-developed in mechanical competence, but lacking in biological intelligence, intuition, awareness; and that it is this, above all, that we need to regain, not only in medicine, but in *all* science.[1]

In the years I have known them – and, most of all, in their years on L-DOPA – those patients have been through a range and depth of experience that is not granted to, or desired by, the majority of people. Many of them, by superficial criteria, appear now to have come full-circle, and to be back where they were, in their starting-position; but this, in actuality, is by no means the case.

They may still (or again) be deeply Parkinsonian, in some instances, but they are no longer the people they were. They have acquired a depth, a fullness, a richness, an awareness of themselves and of the nature of things, of a sort which is rare, and only to be achieved through experience and suf-

---

1. James Joseph Sylvester, poet and mathematician, student of Leibniz and Goethe, speaking of an analogous awakening in Mathematics ('. . . if the day only responds to the promise of its dawn . . .'), depicts in unforgettable terms the real, spacious, and *alive* quality of mathematical thinking:

'Mathematics is not a book confined within a cover and bound between brazen clasps, whose contents it needs only patience to ransack; it is not a mine, whose treasures may take long to reduce into possession, but which fill only a limited number of veins and lodes; it is not a soil, whose fertility can be exhausted by the yield of successive harvests; it is not a continent or an ocean, whose area can be mapped out and its contour defined: it is limitless as that space which it finds too narrow for its aspirations; its possibilities are as infinite as the worlds which are forever crowding in and multiplying upon the astronomer's gaze: it is as incapable of being restricted within assigned boundaries or being reduced to definitions of permanent validity, as the consciousness, the life, which seems to slumber in each monad, in every atom of matter, in each leaf and bud and cell, and is forever ready to burst forth into new forms of vegetable and animal existence' (*Address on Commemoration Day at Johns Hopkins*, 1877).

fering. I have tried, insofar as it is possible for another person, a physician, to enter into or share their experiences and feelings, and, alongside with them, to be deepened by these; and if they are no longer the people they were, I am no longer the person I was.[2] We are older and more battered, but calmer and deeper.

The flash-like drug-awakening of Summer 1969 came and went; its like was not to be seen again. But something else has followed in the wake of that flash – a slower, deeper, imaginative awakening, which has gradually developed and lapped them around in a feeling, a light, a sense, a strength, which is not *pharmacological*, chimerical, false or fantastic: they have – to paraphrase Browne – come to rest once again in the bosom of their causes. They have come to re-feel the grounds of their being, to re-root themselves in the ground of reality, to return to the first-ground, the earth-ground, the home-ground, from which, in their sickness, they had so long departed. In them, and with them, this is the home-coming I have felt. Their experiences have guided me, and will guide some of my readers, on that endless journey which leads to home:

... He found, on his arrival at Waldzell, a pleasure at home-coming such as he had never experienced before. He felt ... that during his absence it had become even more lovely and interesting – or perhaps he was now seeing it in a new perspective, having returned with the heightened powers of perception ... 'It seems to me,' he confided to his friend Tegularius ... 'that I have spent all my years here asleep ... It is now as though I have awakened, and can see everything sharply and clearly, bearing the stamp of reality.'

HERMANN HESSE, *Magister Ludi*

> And the end of all our exploring
> Will be to arrive where we started
> And know the place for the first time ...

ELIOT

2. '*Respondeo etsi mutabor*' – Rosenstock-Huessy.

APPENDIX

FREUD AND COCAINE

The astonishing story of Freud's dalliance with cocaine is brilliantly related in Ernest Jones's biography (see volume 1, pp. 86–108: 'The Cocaine Episode'). The following quotations and paraphrases are taken from this.

Freud, in the mid-1880s, in the midst of arduous labours of every kind, poor, scarcely known, and hungry for fame, 'was constantly occupied with the endeavour to make a name for himself by discovering something important in either clinical or pathological medicine'. One of the endeavours which beguiled him was the notion of giving the world a wonderful drug. The 'side interest' which so enthralled him sprang from the notion that depression, lassitude and neurotic suffering were due to a deficiency in the brain – a 'neurasthenia', and that this deficiency could be made good by the administration of cocaine. Cocaine, indeed, could scarcely be thought of as a drug at all – it merely restored one to normality: thus Freud wrote of the ' exhilaration and lasting euphoria, which in no way differs from the normal euphoria of the healthy person ... In other words, you are simply normal, and it is soon hard to believe that you are under the influence of any drug.' Not the least desirable of its effects was to restore the sense of energy and virility: thus, in a letter to his fiancée, Freud wrote: 'Woe to you, my Princess, when I come ... you shall see who is the stronger, a gentle little girl who doesn't eat enough or a big wild man who has cocaine in his body. In my last severe depression I took coca again and a small dose lifted me to the heights in a wonderful fashion. I am just now busy collecting the literature for a song of praise to this magical substance.'

This 'song of praise' aroused enormous interest, and was couched in a style which never recurred in his writings: in Jones's words, '... with a personal warmth as if he were in love with the content itself. He used expressions uncommon in a scientific paper, such as "the most gorgeous excitement" ... he heatedly rebuffed the "slander" that had been published about this precious drug.'

Freud's active interest in cocaine lasted from 1884 to 1887, and passed through three phases: extravagant enthusiasm; anxiety and doubt, concealed by his dogmatic rebuffs of all 'slanders'; and, finally, a relinquishing and repudiation of his notions, followed by a long-lasting sense of reproach.

WILLIAM JAMES AND NITROUS OXIDE

William James was deeply interested throughout his life in the 'mystagogic' powers of alcohol and drugs. The following personal account is taken from *The Varieties of Religious Experience*, pp. 304–8.

'The next step into mystical states carries us into a realm that public opinion and ethical philosophy have long since branded as pathological, though private practice and certain lyric strains of poetry seem still to bear witness to its ideality. I refer to the consciousness produced by intoxicants, especially by alcohol. The sway of alcohol over mankind is unquestionably due to its power to stimulate the mystical faculties of human nature, usually crushed to earth by the cold facts and dry criticisms of the sober hour. Sobriety diminishes, discriminates, and says no; drunkenness expands, unites, and says yes. It is in fact the great votary of the *Yes* function in man. It brings its votary from the chill periphery of things to the radiant core. It makes him for the moment one with truth. Not through mere perversity do men run after it. To the poor and the unlettered it stands in the place of symphony concerts and of literature; and it is part of the deeper mystery of life that whiffs and gleams of something that we immediately recognize as excellent should be vouchsafed to so many of us only in the fleeting earlier phases of what is in its totality so degrading a poisoning ...

'Nitrous oxide and ether, especially nitrous oxide, when sufficiently diluted with air, stimulate the mystical consciousness to an extraordinary degree. Depth beyond depth of truth seems revealed to the inhaler. This truth fades out, however, or escapes, at the moment of coming to ... Some years ago I myself made some observations on this aspect of nitrous oxide intoxication. One conclusion was forced upon my mind at that time, and my impression of its truth has ever since remained unshaken. It is that our normal waking consciousness, rational consciousness, as we call it, is but one special type of consciousness, whilst all about it, parted from it by the filmiest of screens, there lie potential forms of consciousness entirely different ... No account of the universe in its totality can be final which leaves these other forms of consciousness quite disregarded ... they forbid a premature closing of our accounts with reality. Looking back on my own experiences, they all converge towards a kind of insight to which I cannot help ascribing some metaphysical significance. The keynote of it is invariably a reconciliation. It is as if the opposites of the world, whose contradictoriness and conflict make all our difficulties and troubles, were melted into unity ... To me (this sense) ... only comes in the artificial mystic state of mind.'

HAVELOCK ELLIS AND MESCAL

The following is taken from 'Mescal: a Study of a Divine Plant', a paper written by Havelock Ellis for *Popular Science Monthly*, May 1902, pp. 52–77.

'Under mescal, as far as I have been able to observe, [the exuberant motor manifestations of hashish] seldom appear. Mescal may at one stage produce a sense of well-being, vigour and intellectual lucidity, but there is no actual motor exhilaration, or loss of self-control ... Every sense is affected ... Mescal seems to introduce us into the world in which Wordsworth lived or sought to live. The "trailing clouds of glory", the tendency to invest the very simplest things with an atmosphere of beauty, a "light that never was on sea or land", the new vision of even "the simplest flower that blows", all the special traits of Wordsworth's peculiar poetic vision correspond as exactly as possible to the actual and effortless experiences of the subject of mescal.'

Havelock Ellis notes that no sooner were the effects of the 'divine plant' described, than attempts were made to use mescal therapeutically, especially (as with cocaine) in the treatment of *neurasthenia*. The shortcomings of such therapeutic endeavours Havelock Ellis ascribes to energetic and economic considerations, above all others: 'Mescal', he writes, '... rapidly over-stimulates and exhausts the nervous and cerebral apparatus, more especially on the sensory side ... The day has gone by when it could be supposed that a stimulant put anything into a system. It acts not by putting energy into the system but by taking it out ... So that by the use of [mescal and] other stimulants ... we not only draw on our capital, we actually dissipate and waste it.'

GLOSSARY

A book such as this necessarily uses a number of unfamiliar words referring to its special subject-matter. In general, I have tried to indicate the meanings of these, by context, as they occur. The following short glossary is designed as a reader's companion, to help him visualize the peculiar disorders of movement, posture, will, appetite, sleep, etc. which constitute a major part of the subject-matter of this book. Such terms are analogous to the much more familiar words with which we discuss emotional and neurotic disorders. The following words merge and overlap in meaning, as do the disorders they denote.

ABOULIA. Lack of will or initiative. Especially favoured, at one time, in descriptions of neurotic 'paralyses of the will', true aboulia is perhaps only seen with organic disease or damage to the brain – as in *encephalitis lethargica*, following extensive leucotomy, etc. It is often, but not necessarily, associated with profound apathy. The opposite of aboulia is *hyperboulia* – excess of will, wilfulness, urgency, appetency; similarly the opposite of apathy (or apathism) is *erethism* – morbid excitement, itching, thrusting, urging, pushing. Similar antithetical pairs are *anergy–hyperergy* (lack of energy, excess of energy), and *adynamia–hyperdynamia* (lack of force, excessive force).

AGRYPNIA. Total inability to sleep, absolute resistance to sedation – the acme of insomnia. This disorder, fatal if it lasts much longer than a week, is also only seen in diseases and intoxications – especially *encephalitis lethargica* and ergot-poisoning.

AKATHISIA. Inability to keep still; intense urge to move; restlessness or fidgets in their most extreme degree.

AKINESIA. Total lack of movement, or inability to make voluntary movements, for any reason whatever – seen in its most profound degree in post-encephalitic illness. One speaks, similarly, of *aphonia* (inability to make sounds), *amimia, aphrenia* (stoppage of thought), etc.

ALGOLAGNIA.   Lust for inflicting or suffering pain.

AMETRIA, AMORPHIA.   Deficiencies, respectively, in judgement of *scale* and judgement of *form* (as *dysmetrias* and *dysmorphias* are systematic misjudgements of these). The causes and varieties of such aberrant or misjudged movement are multiform (their occurrence and treatment in post-encephalitic patients is discussed on p. 62 footnote).

AMIMIA.   Literally a loss of *mimesis*, of mimetic, histrionic and expressive capacities. The term is often used of the fixed and rather inexpressive face, voice and posture of many Parkinsonian patients. It should be stressed that this 'amimia' is secondary, not primary: Parkinsonians may have a full repertoire of *internal* expressions and gestures which have been denied full external expression due to the constraint (or enfeeblement) of akinesia. Sometimes, radiantly and unexpectedly, vivid expressions *do* 'break through' (see inset). Parkinsonians over-driven by L-DOPA (like patients with Gilles de la Tourette syndrome) may become *hyper-mimetic* – full of histrionic excesses, grimaces and gesticulations, very suggestible, and prone to involuntary imitations, tics, mannerisms, etc.

ANABLEPSY. Forced upward gaze – the opposite of *catablepsy*: disorders especially seen in the *oculogyric crises* of sleeping-sickness, but also in hysteria, hypnosis, ecstasy, etc.

APHAGIA.   Inability to swallow.

APHONIA.   See *akinesia*.

APHRENIA.   See *akinesia*.

APRAXIA, AGNOSIA.   Difficulties in action or perception due to inadequate understanding. Such difficulties are often associated with damage to the cerebral cortex, and may occur with brain tumours, strokes, senility, etc. They do *not* occur in Parkinsonism, where the difficulties are in *undertaking*, not in *understanding*.

ATHETOSIS.   'Mobile spasm', in Gowers's term; 'involuntary' writhing-movements of the face, tongue and extremities – a form of *dystonia*.

AUTOMATISM.   Forced obedience to external stimuli or commands, as opposed to *command-negativism*: seen most dramatically in catatonia, but also in Parkinsonism and obsessive or hysterical neurotic disorders (see also *echolalia*, *palilalia*, etc.).

BLEPHAROSPASM. Spasm of the eyelids, which may be continuous (*blepharotonus*) or fluttering (*blepharoclonus*).

BLOCK. Resistance (at any level) to thought or movement. Seen most strikingly in catatonia, often associated with command-negativism; but also in Parkinsonian 'freezing', and in neurotic impediments of thought, feeling, speech and action. 'Involuntary' at lower levels, but associated with a sense of 'stickiness' or reluctance at higher levels.

BRADYKINESIA. Slowness of voluntary movement, extremely characteristic of Parkinsonism; one speaks, similarly, of *bradyphemia*, *bradyphrenia*, etc. Similar slowings are common in depression.

BRUXISM. Grinding of the teeth, allied to *trismus* (forced clenching). Common not only in post-encephalitic illness, but in states of neurotic tension, and in response to amphetamines.

BULIMIA. Literally 'ox-hunger'. A violent and insatiable appetite. Bulimia – like all exorbitances – easily switches to its opposite – violent refusal to eat, loathing of food, *anorexia*, voracity-in-reverse.

CATALEPSY. The tireless, timeless, effortless maintenance of postures – including perceptual postures and thought-postures (fascination, enthralment, etc.). As characteristic of hysteria and hypnosis as of catatonia; but also seen, at a lower level, in Parkinsonism.

CATATONIA. So-named about a century ago, but described and depicted since the dawn of recorded history: comprising, in its most familiar forms, catalepsy and the holding of statuesque postures, command-automatism or negativism, extreme suggestibility (either positive or negative), etc. Less familiar is *catatonic frenzy* ('amok'), to which catatonic immobility may suddenly turn. Although common in schizophrenia (especially schizophrenic panic), catatonia is also common in non-schizophrenic post-encephalitic patients, and may also be induced by hypnosis or drugs. Accompanied by an arrest, a deepening, and an intensification of attention, catatonia is perhaps more familiar as ecstasy, trance, rapture and extreme 'concentration'. Catatonia may be regarded as 'intermediate' in level between Parkinsonism and neurotic disorder.

CHOREA. An involuntary, desultory, flickering movement (or motor scintillation), which tends to dance from one muscle-group to another: a movement more primitive than tics, but more highly organized than jactitations and myoclonic jerks.

COMA. A state of deep unconsciousness, with loss of awareness and all higher activities: a state only seen with severe brain-damage or intoxication. It is opposed to *stupor* (in which there is preservation of crude protective responses, and sometimes mental activity of a disorganized, delirious type); and to states of abnormal lethargy (*torpor*), from which patients can be fully, if briefly, aroused.

COPROLALIA. Exclamatory swearing and use of hostile and obscene epithets, in a compulsive and convulsive manner, interlarded with *sotto voce* muttering and cursing. Especially associated with ticcing, and other over-active and impulsive states.

CUNCTATION. Dawdling, delaying, resisting, hindering – the opposite of *festination* (haste).

Cunctation–festination form the corresponding opposites of Parkinsonian behaviour, as procrastination–precipitation form the opposite poles of neurotic behaviour.

It is in similar terms ('obstructive'–'explosive') that William James analyses 'the pathological will' (see p. 24, n. 6).

DYSTONIA, DYSKINESIA. Generic terms for abnormalities of muscle-tone and movement, and thus including such disorders as Parkinsonism, *athetosis*, *torticollis*, etc.

ECHOLALIA. The forced repetition of someone's words again and again; *palilalia*, similarly, is the repetition of one's own words, phrases or sentences; *echopraxia* and *palipraxia* are forced repetitions of movements or actions. Such symptoms are common in catatonia and are analogous to *catalepsy* (which is a forced repetition or echoing of postures).

EMPROSTHOTONOS. Forced flexion of the head on the chest, as opposed to forced throwing-back of the head (*opisthotonos*).

ERETHISM. Pathological excitement of an itching, goading, urging type – especially used of onanistic and venereal excitements.

EXOTROPIA. Divergent squint (or *stabismus*) of the eyes.

FESTINATION. Forced hurrying of walking, talking, speech or thought – perhaps the most characteristic feature of Parkinsonism. Festinating steps tend to become smaller and smaller, until finally the patient is 'frozen' – stepping internally, but with no space to step in:

> '... movement which moves not
> and going which goes not ...'

GEGENHALTEN. Sometimes called *paratonia*. A forced resistance or reluctance to passive movement, akin to, yet distinct from Parkinsonian, negativistic and neurotic resistances. Its antonym (I suppose) would be 'mithalten' (going-with, compliance), though I am not sure that I have ever heard the term used.

HYPERKINESIA. Increased force, impetus, speed, violence, and spread of movement; usually associated with excess of 'background' movement (*synkinesia*); and often with impulsiveness, impetuosity, irritability, insomnia, etc. Hyperkinesias are the opposite of *akinesias*, whether the latter be Parkinsonian, catatonic or neurotic in nature. Akinesia and hyperkinesia are interconvertible – '*kinesia paradoxa*' often quite suddenly and explosively so: such sudden switches are seen not only in manic-depression, but in hysteria, Parkinsonism, and especially catatonia.

HYPERTONIA. Excessive muscular tone – due to spasticity, Parkinsonism, nervous tension, local irritation, etc. That of Parkinsonism tends to affect opposing muscles symmetrically, producing a plastic or 'lead-pipe' rigidity. A striking effect of L-DOPA (even in non-Parkinsonians) is to render muscular tone less than normal – *hypotonic* – sometimes so much so that normal postures cannot be maintained. Thus the muscles and postures of Parkinsonians tend to be *hard*, whereas those of choreics and anti-Parkinsonians tend to be *soft* (so called '*chorea mollis*').

HYPOKINESIA. Reduced force, impetus, or spread of movement – a diminution of movement short of complete *akinesia*.

MYOCLONUS. Sudden violent jerks of a primitive and lowly organized type, involving anything from fractions of muscle-groups (*myokymia*, myofibrillary twitchings) to the entire body-musculature (lighting-spasms, '*blitzkrampf*'). Such movements may be experienced by all of us, e.g. as we are falling asleep.

NARCOLEPSY. One of the many sleep-disorders particularly common in post-encephalitic patients. Narcolepsy is sudden, irresistible sleep, sometimes only a few seconds in length, and usually filled with vivid dreams; often associated with this are *cataplexy* (sudden loss of all muscle-tone, often brought on by excitement or laughter), *sleep-paralysis* (inability to move for several seconds or minutes after waking), *sleep-talking, sleep-walking,* nightmares, night-terrors, and excessive restlessness and movement during sleep (see also *sleep disorders*).

OCULOGYRIC CRISES. Attacks of forced deviation of gaze, often associated with a surge of Parkinsonism, catatonia, tics, obsessiveness, suggestibility, etc., etc.

OPHTHALMOPLEGIA. Paralysis of gaze.

OPISTHOTONOS. See *emprosthotonos*.

OREXIA. Incontinent gluttony, voracity, greed. Its privative (*ánorexia*) may be used to denote either simple loss of appetite, or positive refusal to eat, voracity-in-reverse. (All negative or privative words here – *akinesia, aboulia,* etc. – may also be used to denote a simple lack, a contrariety, or both).

PALILALIA, PALIPRAXIS. See echolalia.

PERSEVERATION. A tendency to indefinite continuation, or repetition, of nervous processes – self-stimulating, self-reinforcing, self-maintaining, scarcely controllable: a basic pathological state, the antithesis of '*block*' (see *catalepsy, echolalia, rigidity,* etc., which are instances of such inertia).

PULSION. Push, thrust – of an uncontrollable type. Thus one speaks of Parkinsonian propulsions, retropulsions, lateropulsions, etc. Variously qualified as *impulsions, compulsions, repulsions,* etc., the term and concept necessarily pervade descriptions of experience and behaviour at *every* level.

RIGIDITY. A primary symptom in Parkinsonism, but also manifest at higher levels, as *gegenhalten* (paratonic rigidity), catatonic rigidity, hysterical rigidity, and neurotic rigidities and obstinacies. The transfixion of a limb (or the entire body, or all being) by the dynamic opposition of opposing innervations, producing a state of *clench,* or *spasm.* If the opposing impulses alternate, instead of coinciding, we see *tremor, flutter, hesitancy, vacillation*, etc. – also basic phenomena in Parkinsonism and neurosis.

SATYRIASIS. Excessive sexual appetency, urgency or hunger: the venereal equivalent of *bulimia*.

SEBARRHOEA. Increased secretion of sebum, causing greasiness of the skin.

SIALORRHOEA. Increased salivation.

SLEEP. Unusual forms and transforms of sleep were particularly common in the early days of the sleeping-sickness, and have become familiar again as 'paradoxical' effects of L-DOPA. Such sleeps tend to be imperative, often sudden, profound, and usually resistant to interruption: they are of two basic types – swoon-like sleeps, wells of perseveration, into which patients may sink deeper and deeper (analogous to *catalepsy*), or inhibitions and obstructions of consciousness (analogous to *block*). If suddenly awoken from such pathological sleeps, patients may instantly fly into a rage or frenzy – a phenomenon analogous to 'kinesia paradoxa', or to the notorious explosiveness of depressed or catatonic patients (see also *narcolepsy*).

TACHYKINESIA. Excessive speed of movement – often associated with excessive force and abruptness; very characteristic of Parkinsonism (especially when activated by L-DOPA), of frenzies, manias, and tic-disorders; one speaks, similarly, of tachyphemia, tachyphrenia, etc.

TIC. A sudden, complex, compulsive movement – more highly organized and constant in form than myoclonic jerks, jactitations, chorea, etc. A tendency to tic – seen in its most florid form in tic-disease (Gilles de la Tourette disease) – is *also* common in neurotic and especially schizophrenic disorders, and in (active or activated) Parkinsonism. Tics of immobility, or tonic tics, resemble catalepsy, and indicate the functional similarity of such tics with catatonia. Higher-level tics tend to proliferate, to induce *counter-tics*, and to be built up into idiosyncratic mannerisms, affectations, impostures, etc.

TONUS–CLONUS. General terms denoting, respectively, co-incidence or alternation of opposing responses: such terms are used not only with reference to Parkinsonism, catatonia, etc., but with reference to epilepsies, at the highest levels, and spinal cord disorders, at the lowest levels.

TORTICOLLIS.   Maintained asymmetric spasm of neck-muscles, forcing the head to one side – a dystonic symptom which may be 'organic' (e.g. Parkinsonian) or 'functional' (e.g. hysterical) in nature. One speaks, similarly, of *tortipelvis*. The general term *torsion-spasm* denotes contorting spasms affecting the trunk and neck (compare *athetosis*). Similar writhing movements and contortions may, of course, affect being-as-a-whole : thus one may speak of a *moral athetosis*, and torturing states of *emotional torsion*.

MORE ABOUT PENGUINS
AND PELICANS

Penguinews, which appears every month, contains details of all the new books issued by Penguins as they are published. From time to time it is supplemented by *Penguins in Print*, which is a complete list of all titles available. (There are some five thousand of these.)

A specimen copy of *Penguinews* will be sent to you free on request. For a year's issues (including the complete lists) please send 50p if you live in the British Isles, or 75p if you live elsewhere. Just write to Dept EP, Penguin Books Ltd, Harmondsworth, Middlesex, enclosing a cheque or postal order, and your name will be added to the mailing list.

In the U.S.A.: For a complete list of books available from Penguin in the United States write to Dept CS, Penguin Books Inc., 7110 Ambassador Road, Baltimore, Maryland 21207.

In Canada: For a complete list of books available from Penguin in Canada write to Penguin Books Canada Ltd, 41 Steelcase Road West, Markham, Ontario.

PSYCHOTHERAPY AND EXISTENTIALISM

Selected Papers on Logotherapy

VIKTOR E. FRANKL

In *Psychotherapy and Existentialism* Dr Frankl presents his major papers, which have earned him universal acclaim.

Confronted with the horrors of the Nazi concentration camps, Dr Frankl formulated logotherapy (psychotherapy which recognizes man's search for meaning) as a response to his own need for a sustaining meaning to life. From these personal experiences he has developed a theory of man – stressing man's freedom to transcend suffering – which provides an antidote to nihilism and is a positive force against the increased sense of inner void or 'existential vacuum' that characterizes the main neuroses of our time.

Dr Frankl's important work has formed the basis of the Third Viennese School of Psychotherapy and is the most significant contribution to psychoanalysis since the pioneering work of Freud and Adler.

'Today Frankl is one of the most famous of all psychiatrists. The incredible attempts to dehumanize man at the concentration camps of Auschwitz and Dachau led Frankl to commence the humanization of psychiatry' – Professor Gerald F. Kreyche, DePaul University, Chicago

Not for sale in the U.S.A. or Canada

THE DOCTOR AND THE SOUL

From Psychotherapy to Logotherapy

VIKTOR E. FRANKL

Why do I go on living? Is there any meaning to life? Can a doctor help a patient 'to shape his suffering into inner achievement'?

In this important book Dr Viktor Frankl, the internationally acclaimed Viennese psychiatrist, discusses these questions and defines his revolutionary theory of logotherapy (psychotherapy which recognizes man's search for meaning) and the concept of the 'will-to-meaning'. Drawing on his experiences in Nazi concentration camps, Dr Frankl maintains, contrary to Freud, that the most important need of the individual is to find a *meaning* in life and that the frustration of this need results in neurosis, suffering and despair. Thus the role of the modern doctor is an increasingly important one – as he will be called upon to assist his patients to find a meaning in life.

'The views which Dr Frankl put forward both here and in his other writings represent the most important contributions in the field of psychotherapy since the days of Freud, Adler and Jung. And his style is far more readable' – Sir Cyril Burt

Not for sale in the U.S.A. or Canada

THE MAN WITH A SHATTERED WORLD

A. R. LURIA

'This book', writes Professor Luria, 'is about a person who fought with the tenacity of the damned to recover the use of his shattered brain.'

A young soldier, having sustained a severe brain injury, suffers impairment of vision, loss of memory and the ability to speak, read and write. As though he were a child, he has to relearn to identify, to recall and understand, to speak, then to read and write. Professor Luria, a distinguished neuropsychologist, worked with Zasetsky for over twenty years as co-explorer of his condition, and together they built up a new life for Zasetsky. Quoting extensively from the patient's diary the author presents a distilled, readable analysis of his conclusions, offering a valuable contribution to research in this field.

This volume is a tribute to the skill and patience of a doctor, and a testimony to the incredible spirit of his patient who fought with such courage and endurance to return to normal life.

Not for sale in the U.S.A. or Canada

ASYLUMS

*Essays on the Social Situation of
Mental Patients and Other Inmates*

ERVING GOFFMAN

What really goes on in a mental hospital? Are asylums genuine havens of rest from the pressures of society, or can they create even more crippling tensions in those already disturbed? How do mental patients adjust to their new life? And are their adjustments so very different from the reactions of members of other 'total institutions' such as army camps, monasteries, prisons and boarding schools?

In these four controversial essays Erving Goffman explores various types of closed community, all of which seek to mould their inmates to some socially approved purpose. He writes as an observer, not an official; and, like the British 'anti-psychiatrists', he is more concerned to interpret the experience of the patients than to justify the system which contains them. His first essay is a general portrait of life in a total institution; the other three consider special aspects of this existence: the sense of betrayal and loss of identity which afflicts the new patient; the flourishing underlife of prisons and hospitals by which inmates retain some self-respect; and the role of the staff in presenting to the inmate their view of his situation.

Not for sale in the U.S.A.

THE CHILD, THE FAMILY, AND
THE OUTSIDE WORLD

D. W. WINNICOTT

Long clinical experience gave Dr Winnicott a unique
standing in child psychiatry and few experts did
more to present the world of children and parents
to the general public.

Beginning at the natural bond between mother and
child – the bond we call love, which is the key to
personality – Dr Winnicott deals in turn in this
volume with the phases of mother/infant, parent/child,
and child/school. From the problems – which are not
really problems – of feeding, weaning, and innate
morality in babies, he ranges to the very real difficulties
of only children, of stealing and lying, and of first
experiments in independence. Shyness, sex education in
schools, and the roots of aggression are among the
many other topics the author covers in a book which,
for its manner of imparting knowledge simply and
sympathetically, must be indispensable for intelligent
parents.

'His style is lucid, his manner friendly, and his years of
experience provide much wise insight into child
behaviour and parental attitudes' –
British Journal of Psychology

Not for sale in the U.S.A.

PLAYING AND REALITY

D. W. WINNICOTT

Dreaming – as opposed to day-dreaming –, playing, creativity, cultural experience and the often hidden rivalry between a male and a female element in the individual are among the apparently random topics discussed by Dr Winnicott in this study. There is a connection, however, and it is shown to lie in what are termed 'transitional objects' and phenomena – the rags, dolls and teddy-bears which provide a child's first 'not-me' experience.

The author suggests that the transient and too often neglected phase between subjective infancy (in which even the mother's breast is assumed to be an extension of self) and the more objective perceptions of childhood may be the source of a variety of later attitudes.

With its case-histories (including a peculiarly effective impression of an analytical session), its comments on the motivation of artists and its tentative and attractive manner of thinking aloud, Dr Winnicott's last book makes a fitting epilogue to his famous books on childhood. It exposes the roots of that *joie de vivre* he frequently awakened in others – adults as well as children.

Not for sale in the U.S.A.